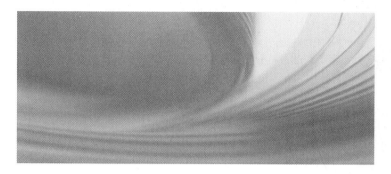

Reading, Understanding, and Applying

Nursing Research

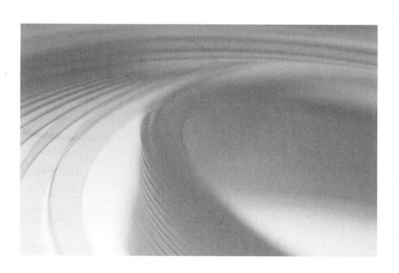

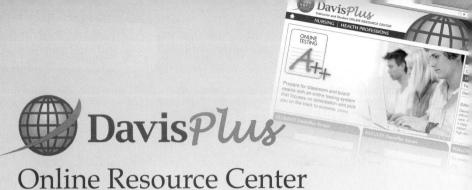
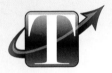
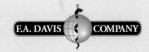

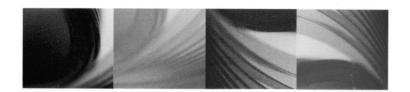

Reading, Understanding, and Applying
Nursing Research

FOURTH EDITION

JAMES A. FAIN, PhD, RN, BC-ADM, FAAN

Dean and Professor

University of Massachusetts Dartmouth
College of Nursing
North Dartmouth, Massachusetts

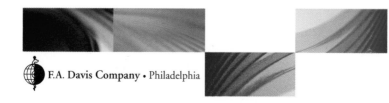

F.A. Davis Company • Philadelphia

F. A. Davis Company
1915 Arch Street
Philadelphia, PA 19103
www.fadavis.com

Printed in the United States of America

Last digit indicates print number: 10 9 8 7 6 5 4 3

Publisher, Nursing: Joanne Patzek DaCunha, RN, MSN
Director of Content Development: Darlene D. Pedersen
Project Editor: Echo Gerhart
Electronic Project Editor: Tyler Baber
Design and Illustration Manager: Carolyn O'Brien

ISBN 978-0-8036-4463-2

To Linda and our children, Lauren, Jillian, and Timothy

PREFACE

Research plays an integral part in determining the roles and responsibilities of nurses. Involvement in research can range from conducting an independent research study to critically appraising the research literature. Enhancing knowledge of research and practicing research skills can help nurses increase their appreciation of how research influences the quality of patient care.

This fourth edition of *Reading, Understanding, and Applying Nursing Research* has been updated while retaining all important features of previous editions. With students now being more sophisticated in the use of technology and inclined to use it, the fourth edition allows students to access learning activities, review questions and more to help increase recognition and understanding of the research process online at DavisPlus.com. The book continues to be directed toward undergraduate students, RNs returning to school, and practicing nurses. This edition continues to emphasize how to read research reports, evaluate them critically, and apply findings to practice by providing more examples of nursing research throughout the book. Steps of the research process are illustrated with excerpts from studies that have been published in nursing literature.

The fourth edition continues to organize content into three parts. Part 1, Nature of Research and the Research Process, presents the importance of nursing research. In addition, several documents present suggested research activities for nurses. The idea that data obtained through sound research methods provide the necessary foundation for best practices (evidence-based nursing) is likewise introduced in Part 1. Part 2, Planning a Research Study, discusses specific aspects of the research process, providing students with information they need to understand inductive and deductive reasoning, along with the formation of research questions and hypotheses from a conceptual model or theoretical framework. Part 3, Utilization of Nursing Research, introduces suggested strategies for evaluating and critiquing research reports along with guidelines for utilization of research findings.

Specific objectives of this edition are to provide students with (1) an understanding of the steps of the research process, (2) a sound ethical knowledge base, (3) the skill to critically evaluate a problem and purpose statement, (4) the knowledge of what specific statistical procedures can be used to answer various research questions and/or hypotheses, (5) the knowledge of randomized clinical trials as a methodological "gold standard" and why use of other types of design is so often necessary in nursing research, and (6) a sense of confidence in their ability to read research reports. In addition, an *Instructor's Guide* is provided, which includes a chapter corresponding to each chapter in the book, with answers to review, multiple-choice, and critical-thinking questions. Finally, an additional test bank of multiple-choice questions and answers is provided.

As with previous editions, student learning objectives are presented at the beginning of every chapter, along with a glossary of terms, and a summary of key ideas is presented at the end of every chapter. A popular feature in previous editions focused on the presentation of excerpts from published research reports. Updated examples of published research from actual journal articles are included in each chapter to help students improve their skills in reading and understanding research reports.

The quality of patient care depends largely on the quality of nursing research. The ability to understand components of the research process and to integrate scientific knowledge with practice to make informed judgments and valid clinical decisions is critical. *Reading, Understanding, and Applying Nursing Research* provides the skills necessary to help students understand what researchers are trying to communicate in published research reports. As consumers of nursing research, the emphasis is on assisting students to understand and evaluate the research reports being discussed. *Reading, Understanding, and Applying Nursing Research* provides a clear and practical presentation of these skills.

—JAMES A. FAIN

REVIEWERS

JANET G. ALEXANDER, EdD, MSN, RN, CNE
Professor & Director, Accelerated Second-Degree BSN Program
Samford University, Ida V. Moffett School of Nursing
Birmingham, Alabama

MAUREEN C. CREEGAN, BSN, MA, EdM, EdD, RN
Professor of Nursing
Dominican College
Orangeburg, New York

MARY ISAACSON, PhD, RN
Assistant Professor of Nursing
Augustana College
Sioux Falls, South Dakota

VALERIE LUNSFORD, RN, BSN, MSN, PhD
Professor
Goldfarb School of Nursing at Barnes Jewish College
Saint Louis, Missouri

LYNX CARLTON McCLELLAN, RN, DSN
Clinical Associate Professor
University of Alabama in Huntsville
Huntsville, Alabama

CHRIS M. WOOD, OP, RN, PhD, GNP
Associate Professor
Goshen College Department of Nursing
Goshen, Indiana

ACKNOWLEDGMENTS

Sincere thanks are extended to the many individuals who contributed to the development of this textbook. Specifically, I wish to acknowledge those individuals who have been most closely involved in the production of the textbook. Thanks to the publisher, F. A. Davis Company, and Joanne P. DaCunha, RN, MSN (acquisitions editor), whose support and patience from the beginning were essential. A special thanks to Sarah M. Granlund, freelance developemental editor assigned to the textbook, for her careful reading of the entire manuscript and helpful comments and suggestions for improving the exposition.

Finally, I would like to thank my wife, Linda, and children, Lauren, Jillian, and Timothy, along with the many students over the years who have contributed directly and indirectly through their interest and support.

—JAMES A. FAIN

CONTENTS

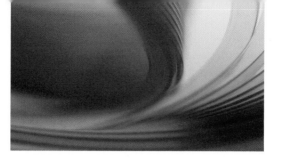

PART 1

Nature of Research and the Research Process

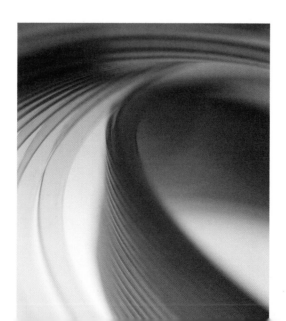

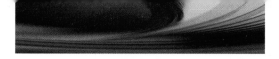

1

INTRODUCTION TO NURSING RESEARCH

James A. Fain, PhD, Rn, Bc-Adm, Faan

LEARNING OBJECTIVES:

By the end of this chapter, you will be able to:
1. Describe the importance of nursing research for nurses.
2. Explain how the scientific method is applied in nursing research.
3. Describe the nurse's role as a consumer of research.
4. Identify strategies for executing research responsibilities.

GLOSSARY OF KEY TERMS

Empirical data. Documented evidence (data) gathered through direct observation rather than a researcher's subjective belief.

Nursing research. A systematic process of investigating problems to gain knowledge about improving care that nurses provide.

Nursing science. The body of knowledge that is unique to the discipline of nursing.

Objectivity. Ability to distance the research process as much as possible from the scientist's personal beliefs, values, and attitudes.

Qualitative research. An approach for generating knowledge using methods of inquiry that emphasize subjectivity and the meaning of an experience for the individual.

Quantitative research. An approach for generating knowledge based on determining how much of a given behavior, characteristic, or phenomenon is present.

Replication. The ability of researchers to repeat a study using the same variables and methods or slight variations of them.

Research consumer. Readers of nursing research whose objective is to apply findings to nursing practice or to use the findings to conduct further research.

Research team. A group that collaborates to conduct a research project, from determining the initial research question through communicating the results.

Research rigor. Striving for excellence in research, which involves discipline, scrupulous adherence to detail, and strict accuracy.

(Continued)

Scientific inquiry. The process of analyzing data critically that have been gathered systematically about a particular phenomenon.

Scientific method. A systematic research process that involves the following steps: selecting and defining the problem, formulating research questions or hypotheses or both, collecting data, analyzing data, and reporting results.

Triangulation. Use of quantitative and qualitative methods to collect data about a particular phenomenon.

Ways of knowing. An assortment of methods used to acquire new knowledge, including tradition, authority, trial and error, and intuition.

Understanding nursing research is more than learning a method of inquiry. Perhaps above all, **nursing research** is a process that allows nurses to ask questions that are aimed at gaining new knowledge to improve patient care. Whether nurses practice in an acute-care facility, long-term rehabilitation setting, or community agency, quality care is expected to reflect assimilation of knowledge into practice. In addition, nurses are responsible for assuming an active role in developing a body of nursing knowledge. Nurses must examine how research can best be incorporated into their everyday practice. In this chapter the value of nursing research is discussed, and the application of the scientific method in nursing is described. The role of the research consumer and guidelines for participating in research are also addressed.

The Importance of Research in Nursing

The challenges confronting the health-care system compel practitioners in all specialties to justify their clinical decisions. The discipline of nursing is no exception. Nurses participate in research activities to develop, refine, and extend **nursing science**, which is a unique body of nursing knowledge. Nursing research is systematic inquiry designed to develop knowledge about issues of importance to nursing.[1] As an academic and professional discipline, clinical practice is an integral part of nursing's activities, along with educating clinicians and administration of nursing services. Therefore, research in nursing encompasses systematic inquiry into each of these areas. Nurses who base their clinical decisions on scientifically documented information act in a professionally accountable manner and help define the identity of nursing and promote excellence in practice through knowledge development.

Evidence-Based Practice

The terms "clinical decisions" and "actions based on research findings" mean that nurses engage in evidence-based practice (EBP). Such practice is informed by the best available evidence as it relates to patient care. Evidence-based nursing practice relies on evidence from research and refers to clinicians making an effort to integrate research findings into clinical thinking and decision making.[2,3]

In applying the best research evidence available, nurses improve the practice of nursing. By asking questions such as "What is the best evidence for a particular intervention?" or "How do nurses provide best practice?" or "What are the highest achievable outcomes for the patient, family, and nurse?", nurses work with other members of the health-care team to use existing evidence to improve practice. Nurses likewise need to question current nursing practices and use evidence to make appropriate changes and make care more effective. A more detailed discussion of EBP is in Chapter 3.

Nursing is a discipline with its own body of knowledge that focuses on knowing and understanding individuals and their health experiences. No other discipline is as concerned with the individual and how health is experienced. By designing relevant research, nurse scientists contribute to the development of specific nursing knowledge that aids problem-solving in patient care.

The importance of nursing research is an established reality; it is no longer necessary to justify its value. Instead, nurses must focus on improving their understanding of the research process and fostering the development of research designs that provide the information needed to explain, change, and expand nursing practice.

What Is Research?

Research is a systematic inquiry into a subject that uses various approaches (quantitative and qualitative methods) to answer questions and solve problems. The goal of research is to discover new knowledge and relationships and find solutions to problems or questions.[2] Research is sometimes referred to as synonymous with problem-solving. This is incorrect because research deals with discovering or generating new knowledge, whereas problem-solving refers to using current knowledge. Previous research generates knowledge used in problem-solving. If use of existing knowledge is found to be inadequate, problems can be posed as research questions in need of scientific investigation. New knowledge is then applied to deal with future problems.

What is knowledge? Knowledge is information acquired in a variety of ways. **Ways of knowing** are various methods used to acquire new knowledge. For example, you may say that you *know* your friend John, *know* that Earth rotates around the sun, *know* how to give an injection, and *know* pharmacology. These are all examples of knowing: being familiar with a person, comprehending the facts, acquiring a psychomotor skill, and mastering a subject matter.[4] Knowledge can be gained from a variety of sources such as tradition, authority, trial and error, personal experience, intuition, logical reasoning, and use of the scientific method.[1] Use of the scientific method is of primary concern to nursing as a science. As consumers of research, nurses need to know how information is gathered and organized in a research or scientific context.

The Scientific Method

Achieving the research goal of discovering new knowledge and relationships requires understanding the scientific method. Students hearing the word *science* often think of laboratories, experiments, intellectual skills, and mathematics. They believe scientists are individuals with a tremendous amount of knowledge, drawing on years of experience. While this might be somewhat true, science is a method of knowing and acquiring new knowledge.

Scientific inquiry is a process in which observable, verifiable data are systematically collected from our surroundings through our senses to describe, explain, or predict events.[1] The **scientific method** involves selecting and defining a problem, formulating research question(s) or hypotheses or both, collecting data, analyzing data, and reporting results. Two characteristics that are unique to the scientific method and not associated with other ways of knowing are objectivity and the use of empirical data.[1,2] **Objectivity** is defined as an ability to distance the research process as much as possible from the scientist's personal beliefs, values, and attitudes. The scientific approach is applied in such a way that other scientists will have confidence in the conclusions. The term **empirical data** refers to documenting objective data through direct observation. Findings are grounded in reality rather than personal bias or the subjective belief of the researcher.

The scientific method involves testing of ideas, hunches, or guesses. For example, a nurse may have an idea that patients who receive preoperative teaching will have a healthier postoperative recuperative period. A physician might guess that people who are more internally controlled will lose more weight than those who are externally controlled. Both examples are only guesses or hunches. A systematic, planned approach to data collection, analysis, and evaluation is necessary to see if such guesses or hunches hold up. The value of using the scientific method is that the method can be replicated by other researchers.

Replication is the ability of researchers to repeat a study using the same variables and methods or slight variations of them. Replication is an important concept in research. An essential characteristic of a research study is that it should be replicable so that research findings can be verified. Repeating a study increases the extent to which the research findings can be generalized, providing additional evidence of validity.

Nursing research is the systematic application of the scientific method to the study of phenomena of interest to the nursing profession. For example, systematic investigation of patients and their health needs is of primary concern to nursing. The results of such an investigation add to the body of knowledge that is unique to nursing. A major difference between scientific research and nursing research is the nature of the material studied. Nursing research primarily involves studying people, and people do not behave consistently, as do chemicals in a laboratory. In a laboratory setting, it is much easier to explain, predict, and control the situation. Rigid controls that are imposed and maintained in a laboratory setting are impossible to achieve in the practice setting. Likewise, ethical considerations do not allow the full range of experimental techniques with people.

Scientific inquiry is sometimes referred to as **quantitative research**. The notion of objective observations made by the researcher, along with the ability to generalize the findings to other populations, constitutes a scientific approach. Quantitative methods are well developed and have been used extensively and effectively in nursing research. Quantitative research methods emphasize measurement, testing of hypotheses, and statistical analysis of data.[1,2] Quantitative nursing research uses traditional quantitative approaches such as experiments, questionnaires, and surveys to advance nursing science. When the research question addresses an individual's subjective experience, different methods must be used to study that type of phenomenon.

Qualitative research is an approach to structuring knowledge that uses methods of inquiry that emphasize verbal descriptions and the meaning of the experience for the individual.[5] Qualitative research methods emphasize understanding of phenomena from the individual's perspective. Participant observation, in-depth interviews, case studies, ethnographies, and narrative analyses are the tools used to gain new knowledge in qualitative research. Regardless of the methods used, researchers have the responsibility of conducting a study with rigor and skill. **Research rigor** is the striving for excellence in research that involves discipline, scrupulous adherence to detail, and strict accuracy.[4]

Triangulation refers to the use of both quantitative and qualitative methods to collect data about a particular phenomenon.[5] The term can also refer to various combinations of research designs or instruments used in the same study. A combination of psychosocial instruments, interviews, and observations can be used to describe a particularly complex phenomenon. The two approaches are complementary and provide an accurate representation of reality.

Research and the Entry-Level Nurse

The scope of research activities for which nurses are responsible is clearly articulated in a publication of the American Association of Colleges of

Nursing titled *Position Statement on Nursing Research*[6] and *Position Statement on Education for Participation in Nursing Research,* published by the American Nurses Association.[7] Expectations and research competencies of graduates at each level of nursing education are discussed. Suggested research activities for nurses at various educational levels are presented in Table 1.1. These guidelines provide direction for nurses so that they may initiate research activities that can be carried out individually or in collaboration with other nursing professionals.

The role of the researcher is classified on a continuum by the degree of participation in research studies. At one end of the continuum are

---

| TABLE 1.1 | Research Training of Nurses at All Educational Levels |

Baccalaureate Degree in Nursing

1. Read, understand, interpret, and apply research findings from nursing and other disciplines into clinical practice.
2. Understand basic elements of evidence-based nursing practice.
3. Work with others to identify potential nursing research problems that need to be investigated.
4. Collaborate on research teams.
5. Share research findings with colleagues.

Master's Degree in Nursing

1. Evaluate research findings.
2. Develop and implement evidence-based practice guidelines.
3. Identify practice and systems problems requiring study.
4. Collaborate and assist others in initiating research.

Practice-Focused Doctoral Programs

1. Translate scientific knowledge into complex clinical interventions tailored to meet individual, family, and community health and illness needs.
2. Use advanced leadership knowledge and skills to evaluate the translation of research into practice and collaborate with new researchers/scientists on new health policy research opportunities.
3. Focus on evaluation and use of research rather than the conduct of research.

Research-Focused Doctoral Programs

1. Pursue intellectual inquiry and conduct independent research for the purpose of extending nursing knowledge.
2. Plan and launch independent programs of research.

Postdoctoral Programs

1. Establish programs of research with formal mentorship from senior researchers/scientists.

Source: Adapted from: American Association of Colleges of Nursing: Position Statement on Nursing Research. American Association of Colleges of Nursing, Washington, DC, 2006.

nurses who are consumers of research. The role of the **research consumer** requires the ability to read and evaluate research reports. Nurses are increasingly expected to maintain at least this level of involvement with research. Developing skills to read and understand research critically takes time and repeated practice and requires knowledge of the research process. At the other end of the continuum are nurses who conduct research and actively participate in the design and implementation of a study. As members of a **research team,** nurses can collaborate on the development of an idea and actually participate in the design and production of a study. Today, nursing research is undertaken by many nurses with advanced degrees who are working in the clinical setting. Several research-related activities, in which nurses may participate to gain a fundamental understanding of research, are listed in Table 1.2.[2]

Participation in research activities is shared by nurses at all levels and requires knowledge of the research process and the ability to determine what constitutes good research. Developing the skill of reading and evaluating research reports allows nurses to feel confident that the findings of a study are accurate, will provide an improvement in nursing practice, and have meaning in nurses' own working lives.

Guidelines for Scientific Integrity

Every nurse scientist has the responsibility of promoting the integrity of nursing science. In this pursuit, nurse scientists are guided by principles that include respect for the integrity of knowledge, collegiality, honesty, trust, objectivity, and openness. These principles are universal and relevant for each phase of the research process. The nature of nursing and the problems of interest to nurse scientists allow a variety of methods that are appropriate for investigating nursing problems. Although

---

TABLE 1.2	**Expand Your Knowledge of Research–Extension Activities**

- Participate in or set up a journal club in a practice setting in which nurse colleagues discuss research articles.
- Attend research presentations at professional conferences of interest to you.
- Help develop an idea for a research study.
- Review a completed research proposal and offer your clinical expertise and mentorship, if possible.
- Assist in data collection research, for example, distributing questionnaires to patients or observing and recording patients' behaviors.
- Collaborate on the development of an idea for a research project in your field.
- Participate on a hospital or university institutional review board that examines the ethical aspects of a proposed study.

different methods may highlight specific issues and questions, the underlying principles of scientific integrity remain the same.

The Midwest Nursing Research Society developed *Scientific Integrity Guidelines*,[8] which include data access and management and publication practices. Principles that guide the actions of researchers with respect to data access and management are presented in Table 1.3.

TABLE 1.3	**Scientific Integrity Guidelines**

Data Access

1. All coinvestigators on a team have access to data, as agreed on at the beginning of the research project, and all assume responsibility for safeguarding data confidentiality.
2. Without violating subject information confidentiality, scientists should provide data to the journal editor, if requested, to enable a more complete evaluation of manuscripts.
3. Following publication of results, scientists may be expected to provide sufficient information to enable other qualified scientists to replicate the study.
4. Different considerations apply before publication. Research materials and data are considered privileged until they are formally disseminated. Disclosure or sharing of data prior to peer review and publication may violate confidentiality.
5. Sharing of results with the news media should only be done following completion of peer review.
6. Any discoveries/inventions from research leading to patents are governed by policies of the institution.
7. Investigators are encouraged to provide other researchers, including graduate students, with access to their data for purposes of secondary analysis.

Data Management

1. Specific teams should develop and agree on procedures appropriate for the project.
2. Data are collected according to stated protocol.
3. Potential sources of bias in design and conduct are identified and minimized by researchers.
4. Scientists have the responsibility to ascertain that data are reported accurately, including the decision rules used for collecting and analyzing data.
5. If an error is discovered, it is corrected and made public.
6. The principal investigator is responsible for ensuring that data are of high quality and that steps are taken to prevent intentional withholding or selective reporting of data that may be contrary to investigator expectations.
7. It is recommended that original data be preserved for a period of 5 to 7 years or longer, as there is reasonable expectation that the original data will continue to be the basis of ongoing research, publication, or both. Exceptions involving considerations for human subjects may be negotiated with the institutional review board.

Source: Adapted from: Midwest Nursing Research Society. Guidelines for Scientific Integrity, ed. 2. Midwest Nursing Research Society, Wheat Ridge, CO, 2002.

Scholarly Publications and Practices

Disseminating research findings is an integral part of the research process. Scholarly publications are documents that communicate to other professionals the methods and achievements used in academic study and research investigation. The growth of and support for nursing research are reflected by the impressive number of journals devoted to the publication of nursing research studies. These research journals (with their abbreviated titles from Index Medicus) include *Advances in Nursing Science (Adv Nurs Sci), Applied Nursing Research (Appl Nurs Res), Journal of Nursing Scholarship (J Nurs Scholarship), Nursing Science Quarterly (Nurs Science Q), Nursing Research (Nurs Res), Research in Nursing and Health (Res Nurs Health), Scholarly Inquiry for Nursing Practice (Scholarly Inquiry Nurs Pract),* and *Western Journal of Nursing Research (West J Nurs Res).*

In addition to research journals, the consumer of research can find a wealth of relevant scientific knowledge in many of the specialty journals. Some of the more common specialty journals include *American Journal of Maternal Child Nursing (Am J Maternal Child Nurs), Association of Operating Room Nurses Journal (AORN J), The Diabetes Educator (Diabetes Educ), Heart & Lung (Heart Lung),* and *Oncology Nursing Forum (Oncol Nurs Forum).* Authorship in any type of journal indicates responsibility for the published work and significant contribution to the conception and execution of the paper. A list of guidelines that refer to intellectual honesty and responsibility in publication practice is presented in Table 1.4.[8]

TABLE 1.4	**Guidelines for Authorship of Published Papers**

1. Authors contribute substantially to the published work. This involves assuming responsibility for two or more of the following areas: conception and design, execution of the study, analysis and interpretation of data, and preparation and revision of the manuscript. Others, who provide financial, technical, information, or other kinds of support, may be acknowledged but may not be considered authors.
2. Decisions about conferring and ordering of authorship need to be made in advance, based on the foregoing considerations. Order may be reassessed if contributions change.
3. Status of individuals, such as trainees/students or their rank per se, should not be a determining factor in authorship decisions.
4. It is important to realize that the principal investigator, when directing a team on sponsored projects, assumes overall responsibility for all publications resulting from the project, regardless of his or her authorship status, unless negotiated otherwise.
5. All authors should review the final manuscript and take responsibility for the work.

(Continued)

TABLE 1.4	Guidelines for Authorship of Published Papers—cont'd

6. Duplicate and fragmented publications should be avoided. When the same or substantially similar content is reported in two or more publications, authors should notify editors, who should inform reviewers.

7. Authors should provide additional information requested by editors (e.g., raw data, delineation of authors' contributions, assurances that appropriate regulatory guidelines have been met in the conduct of research).

8. When parties disagree on authorship matters, they are encouraged to seek consultation from colleagues.

Source: Adapted from: Midwest Nursing Research Society. Guidelines for Scientific Integrity, ed. 2. Midwest Nursing Research Society, Wheat Ridge, CO, 2002.

Promoting Nursing Research

Nursing organizations have responded to the need for support of research activities. In 1986, the National Center for Nursing Research (NCNR) was established under the Health Research Extension Act and the auspices of the American Nurses Association. The purpose of the NCNR was to conduct a program of grants and awards supporting nursing research and training, to promote health, and to further the prevention and mitigation of the effects of disease. In 1993, the NCNR was awarded the status of an institute in the structure of the National Institutes of Health (NIH) and was renamed the National Institute of Nursing Research (NINR).

The National Nursing Research Agenda was launched in 1987 to provide structure for selecting initiatives and developing the knowledge base for nursing practice. Senior nurse researchers around the country were invited to the Conference on Nursing Research Priorities (CORP #1) in Washington, D.C., in 1988 to help identify research priorities. During CORP #2, held in Washington, D.C., in 1992, key nurse scientists from all areas of nursing practice identified research priorities through the year 1999. The research agenda emphasized linking research to practice, along with providing nurse researchers with an opportunity to interact among themselves and with researchers from other disciplines. NINR research priorities selected from both conferences and research opportunities for the 21st century are presented in Table 1.5.

Most recently, the NINR published the 2011 strategic plan, titled *"Bringing Science to Life."*[9] Dr. Patricia Grady (NINR director) envisions this new strategic plan as a blueprint for increasing nursing science's contributions to health-care research. The focus of research priorities is on health promotion and disease prevention; improving quality of life through self-management, symptom management, and caregiving; eliminating health disparities; and taking the lead in addressing end-of-life research.

| *TABLE 1.5* | **Nursing Research Priorities as Defined by the National Institute of Nursing Research (NINR)** |

First Conference on Nursing Research Priorities (1988)

- Low Birthweight: Mothers and Infants
- HIV Infection: Prevention and Care
- Long-Term Care for Older Adults
- Symptom Management: Pain
- Nursing Informatics: Enhancing Patient Care
- Health Promotion for Older Children and Adolescents
- Technology Dependency Across the Life Span

Second Conference on Nursing Research Priorities (1992)

- Community-Based Nursing Models
- Effectiveness of Nursing Interventions in HIV/AIDS
- Cognitive Impairment
- Living with Chronic Illness
- Biobehavioral Factors Related to Immunocompetence

NINR Research Priorities (2000–2002)

- Chronic Illnesses
- Quality and Cost-Effectiveness Care
- Health Promotion and Disease Prevention
- Management of Symptoms Adaptation to New Technologies
- Health Disparities
- Palliative Care at the End of Life

NINR Research Priorities (2004–2006)

- Setting Directions for End-of-Life Research
- Develop strategies to improve decision making and treatment at the end of life.
- Validate instruments and refine methodologies to address complex issues of end-of-life research.
- Develop interventions to improve palliative care and enhance quality of life for the dying patient, along with supporting family and informal caregiver.
- Explain factors related to end of life among underserved groups.
- Support development of informatics tools that will facilitate integration and analysis of data from end-of-life studies.
- Increase efforts to expand end-of-life research through research training, interdisciplinary programs, supplemental awards, small grants, and center grants.

Continuing Areas of Research (2006–2010)

- Promoting Health and Preventing Disease
- Improving Quality of Life (e.g., Self-management; Symptom Management; Caregiving)
- Eliminating Health Disparities
- Setting Directions for End-of-Life Research

The mission of the NINR is to promote and improve the health of individuals, families, communities, and populations. NINR supports and conducts clinical and basic research training on health and illness across the life span. The research focus encompasses health promotion and disease prevention, quality of life, health disparities, and end-of-life issues. NINR seeks to extend nursing science by integrating the biological and behavioral sciences, employing new technologies to research questions, improving research methods, and developing the scientists of the future.[10]

NINR accomplishes its mission by supporting grants to universities and other research organizations as well as by conducting research intramurally in Bethesda, Maryland. In addition, NINR supports research training and career development in the area of nursing research. Examples of NINR-supported research include the following.[9,10]

- **Cancer.** It is possible to predict which cancer patients are likely to experience nausea during chemotherapy and to prevent or ease this unpleasant side effect and improve adherence to the life-saving treatments.
- **End of Life.** Family members involved in making a decision to withdraw support experience extremely high stress levels, which are reduced in the presence of an advance directive.
- **Feeding Tubes.** An inexpensive bedside test equals costly x-rays in accurately determining incorrect insertion or dislocation of feeding tubes used to provide nutrition fluids.
- **Care of AIDS Patients in Hospital Units.** Care of AIDS patients in dedicated units that have higher nurse-patient ratios and closer involvement of nurses and physicians with specialized AIDS experience significantly lowers mortality rates and increases satisfaction with care.
- **Diabetes.** Teens who typically have trouble controlling their diabetes are able to improve control after training in coping skills, particularly in difficult social situations.
- **Cardiovascular Disease.** A highly effective cardiovascular risk reduction program about nutrition and exercise that is fun and easy to follow was tested for grade school children and was found to help them establish positive health habits.
- **Pain.** Certain pain relievers for acute pain are more effective in women than in men, underscoring the importance of gender when considering analgesics.
- **Transitional Care.** Researchers developed a model for the transition from hospital to home care that has been tested in a variety of patient populations. A modification of this model, applied to prenatal and infant care, reduces infant hospitalizations and deaths, resulting in lower overall health costs.

WEB LINKS

The following Web sites offer students some helpful information on research, funding possibilities, and network opportunities.

Agency for Healthcare Research and Quality
    http://www.abcpr.gov/
American Academy of Nursing
    http://www.nursingworld.org/aan
Centers for Disease Control and Prevention
    http://www.cdc.gov/
Council for the Advancement of Nursing Science
    http://www.nursingscience.org
Eastern Nursing Research Society
    http://www.enrs-go.org/
Midwest Nursing Research Society
    http://www.mnrs.org/
National Institutes of Health
    http://www.nih.gov/
National Institutes of Nursing Research
    http://www.nih.gov/ninr/
Sigma Theta Tau International
    http://www.nursingsociety.org/
Southern Nursing Research Society
    http://www.snrs.org/

SUMMARY OF KEY IDEAS

1. Nurses are responsible for assuming an active role in developing a body of nursing knowledge.

2. Evidence-based practice (EBP) allows nurses to use the best research evidence available in making clinical decisions.

3. Nursing has its own unique body of knowledge that represents the knowing, experiencing, and understanding of phenomena related to providing patient care.

4. The scientific method is an approach to gaining new knowledge that is a systematic collection of empirical data.

5. Replicating a study increases the extent to which research findings are verified by providing additional evidence of the validity of the findings.

6. The role of the research consumer includes the ability to read and critique research reports.

7. Key nursing research journals include *Advances in Nursing Science, Applied Nursing Research, Image: Journal of Nursing Scholarship,*

Nursing Research, Nursing Science Quarterly, Research in Nursing and Health, Scholarship Inquiry for Nursing Practice, and *Western Journal of Nursing Research.*

8. Nurses are responsible for promoting the integrity of nursing science by respecting the integrity of knowledge, collegiality, honesty, trust, objectivity, and openness when conducting research.

LEARNING ACTIVITIES

1. Select back issues of a research journal and identify several quantitative and qualitative studies. Did each study satisfy the definition of research as stated in this chapter? Why or why not?

2. Did any of the studies combine both quantitative and qualitative approaches? If yes, were both approaches necessary? Why or why not?

REFERENCES

1. Gillis, A, and Jackson, W: Research for Nurses: Methods and Interpretation. FA Davis Company, Philadelphia, 2002, pp 7–10, 23–28.
2. Polit, DF, and Beck, CT: Essentials of Nursing Research: Methods, Appraisal, and Utilization, ed. 6. Lippincott Williams & Wilkins, Philadelphia, 2006, pp 3–29.
3. Brown, SJ: Knowledge for Health Care Practice: A Guide to Using Research Evidence. WB Saunders, Philadelphia, 1999, pp 3–4.
4. Burns, N, and Groves, SK: The Practice of Nursing Research: Conduct, Critique, and Utilization, ed. 4. WB Saunders, Philadelphia, 2001, pp 11–14, 38–39.
5. Morse, JM, and Field, PA: Qualitative Research Methods for Health Professionals, ed. 2. Sage Publications, Thousand Oaks, CA, 1995, pp 16–19.
6. American Association of Colleges of Nursing: Position Statement on Nursing Research. American Association of Colleges of Nursing, Washington, DC, 2006.
7. American Nurses Association: Position Statement: Education for Participation in Nursing Research. American Nurses Association, Washington, DC, 1994.
8. Scientific Integrity Committee of the Midwest Nursing Research Society: Guidelines for Scientific Integrity, ed. 2. Midwest Nursing Research Society, Wheat Ridge, CO, 2002.
9. National Institute of Nursing Research: Strategic Plan 2011: Bringing Science to Life. National Institutes of Health, U.S. Department of Health and Human Services, Bethesda, MD, 2011.
10. National Institute of Nursing Research. About NINR: Mission statement, accessed May 2008, www.ninr.nih.gov/AboutNINR/NINRMissionand StrategicPlan

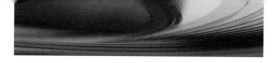

CHAPTER

2

UNDERSTANDING THE RESEARCH PROCESS AND ETHICAL ISSUES IN NURSING RESEARCH

JAMES A. FAIN, PHD, RN, BC-ADM, FAAN

LEARNING OBJECTIVES

By the end of this chapter, you will be able to:
1. Identify the basic components of the research process.
2. Distinguish between basic and applied research and between experimental and nonexperimental research.
3. Understand human rights as they apply to undertaking research involving human participants.
4. Define informed consent and its key elements.
5. Explain the role of institutional review boards in safeguarding the rights of subjects participating in a study.
6. Explain how to evaluate the ethical implications of a research report.

GLOSSARY OF KEY TERMS

Anonymity. A condition in which the identity of subjects remains unknown, even to the researcher, to protect subjects participating in a study and to promote objective results.

Applied research. A type of study designed to gather knowledge that has direct clinical application.

Basic research. A type of study designed to develop the knowledge base and extend theory without direct focus on clinical application.

Confidentiality. Protecting data that are gathered or learned from patients by not disclosing information without their permission.

Correlational research. A type of nonexperimental study designed to examine the relationship between and among variables.

(Continued)

Cross-sectional research. A study that collects data at a particular point in time and does not require follow-up.

Descriptive research. A type of nonexperimental study designed to provide a knowledge base when little is known about a phenomenon; used to describe variables rather than to test a predicted relationship.

Experimental research. A study in which the researcher manipulates and controls one or more variables and observes the effect on one or more other variables.

Human rights. The protection of subjects participating in a research study; includes the right to freedom from injury, the right to privacy and dignity, and the right to anonymity and confidentiality.

Longitudinal research. A study that follows a cohort of subjects and collects data over time.

Nonexperimental research. A descriptive study that does not exhibit a great amount of control over variables.

Prospective research. A study that examines data collected in the present.

Retrospective research. A study that examines data collected in the past.

Risk-benefit ratio. The relationship between potential harm to subjects and potential positive outcomes gained by participating in a research study; an evaluation used by subjects to make voluntary informed consent.

Vulnerable research participant. Those persons who are relatively or absolutely incapable of protecting their own interests and unable to provide meaningful informed consent.

The ability to read and evaluate research findings is important for nurses when practice is evidence based. Learning about components of the research process helps nurses become consumers of research and helps them develop the ability to determine the quality and merit of research reports. The purpose of this chapter is to provide an overview of the research process and the various types and methods of research. Specific components of the research process are examined in succeeding chapters. This chapter includes a discussion of the accountability of researchers in maintaining ethical standards at all phases of the research process.

The Research Process

The research process involves decision making in order to consider various alternatives and to decide what methods will answer particular research question(s) or test hypotheses. The term "research" is derived from an earlier word that means to go around, to explore, and to circle. Many major decisions that researchers make are conceptual. Ideally, the chosen methodology follows these conceptual decisions logically and coherently. The research process is also flexible. There is no one correct answer to the research question but rather multiple possibilities from which researchers must choose, all with their own strengths and weaknesses.

Polit and Beck[1] describe 18 steps associated with the research process, while Gillis and Jackson[2] identify 7 steps. The use of the word "steps" can be misleading. The word implies finishing one activity or task before moving on to the next. Steps in the research process, however, tend to vary in their sequence and number, depending on the purpose of the study and the researcher's style. Therefore, it is more useful to think of steps as guidelines.

The research process is actually circular. When conducting a study, researchers may need to go back and forth to rethink and reconceptualize the problem several times. For example, researchers continually review the literature to keep up with the most current information and to refer to other research reports to get ideas for sampling, operational definitions, and research designs. Available instrumentation for measurement also influences the way that researchers think about the problem, even though conceptualization precedes the selection of measures. Another example of the circular nature of research is the use of the results of one study to create questions for the next study. Researchers may find at the end of a study that they have asked the wrong question(s). This observation does not necessarily mean that the time and energy put into the study were wasted. Refining questions is an important part of the process. Sometimes researchers cannot determine the correct question without first researching an incorrect question.

The intent of the research process is not to present a set of rules but rather to describe the general thinking of researchers who plan the study. Although many different research models exist, the research process actually consists of standard elements (Fig. 2.1); the order may vary, and the steps may overlap in different research situations. General steps associated with the research process include the following:

1. Selecting and defining the problem.
2. Selecting a research design.
3. Collecting data.
4. Analyzing data.
5. Using the research findings.

Each of these steps is discussed in detail in later chapters; a brief overview of the process follows.

Step 1

This step involves selecting and defining an area of research that provides an opportunity to advance nursing knowledge. Through a review of related literature, the researcher determines a rationale for conducting the study, a justification of the need to investigate the

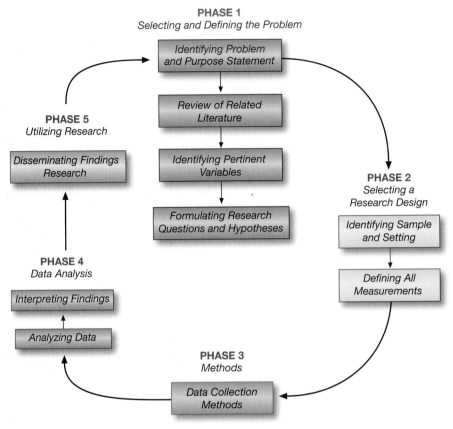

Fig 2•1 Model of research process.

problem, and a theoretical framework for interpreting the results (see Chapter 5). Research questions, hypotheses, or both, are proposed in step 1 (see Chapter 6).

Step 2

In step 2, the researcher designs the study and plans the methods of subject selection, testing, and measurement (Chapters 7 and 8) to ensure that all procedures are clearly defined. The choice of the research design is based on how the research problem is conceptualized. These planning tasks act as guides to help with the selection of appropriate methods for analyzing the data.

Step 3

In step 3, the researcher implements the plans that were designed in steps 1 and 2. Data collection is usually the most time-consuming part of this phase (Chapter 9). After the data have been collected and recorded, the researcher must organize the information into an appropriate form for analysis.

Step 4

Step 4 involves analyzing, interpreting, and making valid conclusions about the data. Statistical procedures are applied to summarize the quantitative data in a meaningful way (Chapter 10). During this step, research hypotheses will be either supported or not supported. Analysis of results leads to new questions that stimulate further study.

Step 5

In this final step of the research process, researchers have the responsibility of sharing their findings with other colleagues. Research findings that are not disseminated to other colleagues are of little value to anyone. Reporting of research can take many forms, including journal articles, abstracts, oral presentations, and poster presentations. The research process culminates with interpreting the findings and communicating any new knowledge gained from the research (Chapter 13).

Types of Research

The research process provides a general strategy for gathering, analyzing, and interpreting data to answer research questions or test hypotheses. Classification of research is based on the purpose of a study (see Chapter 4) and amount of control used (see Chapter 11). One such classification is basic versus applied research.

Basic Versus Applied Research

Basic research is often referred to as pure or fundamental research. The major purpose of basic research is to obtain empirical data that can be used to develop, refine, or test a theory without immediate concern for direct application to clinical practice. Basic research closely resembles the work done in laboratories and is associated with scientists. Researchers who study how blood cells function, for example, or who examine the structure and function of parts of the brain, are conducting basic research to better understand those structures. Although the information gained from basic research may be useful later in the development of a particular treatment or drug, the sole purpose of the study is to advance knowledge in a given subject area.

Applied research, as the name suggests, is conducted to gain knowledge that can be used in a practical setting. This type of research is usually performed in actual practice conditions, on subjects who represent the group to which the results will be applied. Regardless of the type of problem studied, research findings contribute to some modification of present practices.

Excerpt 2.1 displays findings from an applied research study that determined if there was a difference between upper arm and forearm blood pressure measurements (BPMs) among adults and examined the relationship of participants' characteristics to the BPM differences. Through the use of a noninvasive automatic inflatable BP device, two BPMs at the upper arm and two BPMs at the forearm were obtained for 106 participants in the study. Such knowledge is pertinent for nurses to understand differences between the two sites.

Most clinical nursing research falls into the category of applied research; nursing has not, for the most part, been involved in basic research. Although the difference between basic and applied research appears to be distinct, a continuum exists between the two extremes. In many cases, one must have basic knowledge to be able to interpret the findings of applied studies. Many studies provide clinical applications as well as new knowledge that contributes to a theoretical understanding of basic behavior.

Experimental Versus Nonexperimental

Another classification of research is experimental versus nonexperimental. **Experimental research** refers to a study in which the researcher manipulates and controls one or more variables and observes the effect of manipulation on other variables.[1,2] The notion of manipulation and control refers to the researcher having the ability to administer a treatment (sometimes referred to as an intervention) to some participants in a study and not administering (or administering an alternative treatment) to

---

EXCERPT 2.1

Example of Findings From an Applied Research Study

Discussion

Findings confirm prior research that has indicated that upper arm BPMs tend to be lower than forearm BPMs and extend present knowledge by identifying for whom upper arm and forearm BP readings have the greatest difference. The largest difference in upper arm and forearm BPMs was for men and adults who were middle-aged or obese. Most other investigators have found individual variability in participants but have not reported personal characteristics associated with higher readings. Only Palatini and associates (2004) assessed the difference between upper arm and forearm mean BPMs in men and women and found a greater difference for men in the diastolic mean BPM.

Obese adults, who are more likely to have their BPMs taken on the forearm when the standard cuff size does not fit the upper arm, have the greatest difference between upper arm and forearm BPMs.

Source: Domiano, KL et al: Comparison of upper arm and forearm blood pressure. Clin Nurs Res 37:241, 2008.

others. For example, a nurse might be interested in examining the impact of a preoperative teaching program with respect to use of pain medication. One group of participants (experimental group) is instructed how to cough and breathe deeply as well as set expectations for the immediate postoperative period, whereas a second group is given a standard brochure with preoperative instructions. Both groups are measured on the amount of pain medication administered during the first 8 hours postoperatively. In this case, the experimental research design tests whether a preoperative teaching program has an impact on pain medication usage. Experimental research is carried out using several types of designs (e.g., experimental and quasi-experimental). See Chapter 11 for a more detailed discussion of experimental research designs.

Nguyen, Nilsson, Hellstrom, and Bengtson's[3] study is an example of an experimental design. The study evaluated the effect music had on pain and anxiety in children undergoing lumbar punctures. An experimental design tested 40 children (ages 7 to 12) with leukemia, followed by interviews with 20 of the participants. Participants were randomly assigned to a music group ($n = 20$) or control group ($n = 20$). The primary outcome associated with the study was pain and anxiety scores. Secondary outcomes included heart rate, blood pressure, respiratory rate, and oxygen saturation. Ten children in each group were chosen consecutively to have an interview according to a predetermined schedule. Interviews were carried out after informed consent was obtained and in connection with completion of the lumbar puncture procedure to avoid impact of memory bias. The interview guide included three open-ended questions.

Nonexperimental research refers to studies that are more descriptive or exploratory in nature. The researcher is interested in describing what already exists. Descriptive studies answer the question "What is this?" Nonexperimental research is sometimes classified as descriptive or correlational. In **descriptive research** a particular situation or event that already exists is described systematically. No attempt is made to explain or predict what the situation might be in the future or how it might be changed. Descriptive research uses questionnaires, surveys, interviews, or observations to collect data. Sample subjects chosen represent the population at large. For example, Hilton,[4] in a nonexperimental, descriptive study, investigated the intake of folic acid among women between the ages of 18 and 24. A convenience sample of 42 female college students enrolled in a small liberal arts college in western North Carolina was invited to participate and fill out a survey. With the literature suggesting a link between folic acid intake and the incidence of neural tube defects in newborns, the focus of the study was to determine whether young women consume the recommended daily allowance of folic acid. There was no attempt to examine relationships or make predictions.

Correlational research examines the relationship between and among variables. The research collects data on at least two variables for the same group of individuals and calculates a correlation coefficient between the measures. A high number of research studies in nursing are classified as descriptive correlational designs.

Greene and colleagues[5] explored relationships among metabolic control, self-care behaviors, and parenting styles among adolescents with type 1 diabetes. The study was descriptive in that sociodemographic data, along with scores on the parenting practices report, metabolic control (A1C), and overall diabetes self-care, were reported on adolescents with type 1 diabetes. The study was correlational in nature because researchers examined the relationship of parenting style with metabolic control (A1C) and diabetes self-care behaviors.

Classification of Research by Time Dimension

"Retrospective" and "prospective" characterize a particular time perspective. **Retrospective research** examines data collected in the past, typified by review of medical records. In these records, events have already occurred and variables have already been measured. In Excerpt 2.2, data were collected using an existing database to identify whether parental advice for home care by telephone triage pediatric nurses led to a change in location of care from the emergency department (ED) or medical doctor's office to the home setting for children ages 12 to 24 months with an uncomplicated febrile illness.

Prospective research examines data collected in the present. Prospective studies are more reliable than retrospective studies because of the

---

EXCERPT 2.2

Use of an Existing Database as a Retrospective Approach to Research

Methods
Research Design
This was a descriptive correlational study that investigated whether parents with a child who has an uncomplicated febrile illness followed home-care advice given by pediatric triage nurses. This study was undertaken through a retrospective analysis of parents' calls to a nurse-run telephone triage center. Data were collected from the Children's Careline database using the individual call records of children ages 12 to 24 months with an uncomplicated febrile illness as the primary problem. These parents or guardians were all given the same home-care advice.

Source: Light, PA, Hupcey, JE, and Clark, MB: Nursing telephone triage and its influence on parents' choice of care for febrile children. J Pediatr Nurs 20:424, 2005.

potential for greater control of data collection. For example, Martin et al[6] designed a prospective study of patients undergoing an elective cardiac surgical procedure designed to assess the relationship between perioperative complications and health-related quality of life (HRQL) at 1 year after elective open heart surgery. In addition, authors assessed the association between HRQL scores at 1 year after open-heart surgery and intermediate-term survival.

Cross-Sectional Versus Longitudinal Research

Cross-sectional research collects data at one point in time with no follow-up. The result is a measurement of what exists today, with no attempt to document changes over time in either the past or the future. In Excerpt 2.3, pain perception in elderly subjects who were cognitively impaired was assessed using a cross-sectional approach. In this study, the authors chose to assess pain once, with all subjects being tested at the same time. There was no attempt to monitor these subjects over time.

Longitudinal research follows a cohort of subjects and collects data at different intervals over time. In Excerpt 2.4, the authors state that data were collected over 9 months. The various data collection points were not identified. An advantage of longitudinal research is the ability to collect data on the same individuals over time. However, there are

---

EXCERPT 2.3

Example of Cross-sectional Research

Design and Setting

This cross-sectional study used face-to-face scripted interviews and chart review. Residents were selected regardless of their length of time in the institution, physical condition, or pain history.

Participant Selection

Participants were randomly selected by using a list of bed numbers without regard to length of stay or admission date. Inclusion criteria for the study were English-speaking residents, older than 65 years, who were not comatose. Both university and agency human subjects internal review boards approved the study.

Procedure

A scripted interview format was used to obtain cognitive functioning and pain data. The Short Portable Mental Status Questionnaire (SPMSQ) was administered to evaluate and classify level of cognitive impairments. After administration of the SPMSQ, each resident was asked if he or she had any pain. If after 30 seconds there was no response, the question was asked, "Do you hurt anywhere?"

Source: Manz, BD, et al: Pain assessment in the cognitively impaired and unimpaired elderly. Pain Manag Nurs 1:106, 2000.

EXCERPT 2.4

Example of Longitudinal Research

Research Methods

This study was designed to evaluate the feasibility of implementing the DSM intervention in a rural area with African American participants. For this purpose, a longitudinal, quasi-experimental study using a one-group pretest-posttest design was conducted from February 1999 to November 1999. Specific aims were to (1) evaluate the effects of dietary self-management education on physiological outcomes, diabetes self-management, and costs of care; (2) assess adherence to intervention sessions; (3) assess the ability to recruit an African American sample; and (4) assess the ability to retain rural African Americans in the study.

Source: Anderson-Loftin, W, et al: Culturally competent dietary education for southern rural African Americans with diabetes. Diabetes Educ 28:245, 2002.

several practical difficulties associated with longitudinal research. Loss of subjects at different points is a major problem. In addition, longitudinal research studies can be threatened by testing effects because subjects are tested repeatedly.

Researchers make decisions as to whether they will conduct retrospective or prospective studies based on either causes in the past (retrospective) or present causes for future effects (prospective). In addition, researchers may look for descriptions of events and things that occurred in the past (retrospective), may follow individuals into the future to describe events as they occur (prospective), or may describe what exists today (cross-sectional).

Ethical Issues in Nursing Research

For many nursing students, the first personal contact with research will be when they invite patients to participate in a study or when they help with data collection. With nursing studies dealing primarily with human participants, there is a concern for protecting individuals from any harmful effects that might result from participation in a study. As nurses engage in various research activities, it is important that the profession operate from a sound ethical knowledge base. For example, adequate protection of research subjects may cause a delay in the proposed schedule or a change in the research design. Regardless, maintaining the safety and human rights of human participants must be the priority at all times.

Developing Professional Guidelines

To help you, nursing has developed guidelines to ensure the protection of human participants while research is conducted. The basic documents that have been used to develop guidelines are based on the articles of the Nuremberg Code (1947)[7] and the Declaration of Helsinki (1964).[8] The articles of the Nuremberg Code serve as a standard against which to measure the individual rights of subjects participating in experimental and clinical research.

Historical Events That Helped Shape Guidelines for Human Participant Protection

Before World War II, few guidelines were available to ensure the protection of human participants participating in research. Although Germany was the most scientifically and technologically advanced country during World War II, the Nazi Party exploited people's trust in the medical community and public health by performing unethical experiments on populations they discriminated against. For example, in one series of experiments, Air Force pilots were placed in vacuum chambers that could duplicate the low air pressure and anoxia (lack of oxygen) at altitudes over 65,000 feet. The German Air Force was interested in understanding if pilots could survive at extremely high altitudes, only to find that over 40 percent of the pilots died as a result of anoxia and ruptured lungs. The German Air Force was also involved in investigating survival times after pilots parachuted into cold water. Pilots were immersed for hours in tubs of ice water; others were fed nothing for days but saltwater. Still others were kept outside at subfreezing temperatures for hours. Finally, at several concentration camps, Polish women were shot and slashed on the legs. Wounds were stuffed with glass, dirt, and various bacteria cultures and sewn shut. The infected wounds were then treated with experimental anti-infective agents. In all instances, no attempts were made to relieve the tremendous suffering caused by these experiments. It was not uncommon for one out of every four individuals to die as a result of their involvement in the experiments.[9]

Nuremberg Code

As a result of the horrifying acts and unethical medical research experiments conducted by Nazi doctors in the name of science, the Nuremberg Trials took place. Several U.S. judges who presided over the final judgment in the Nuremberg Trials were instrumental in developing the Nuremberg Code. The code was developed in 1947 to address protection of human participants and basic principles of ethical behavior. Sections of the Nuremberg Code are presented in Table 2.1. Articles within the code emphasize adequate protection of subjects from risk or harm, the right to withdraw from experimentation, and adequate qualifications of those conducting research.[7]

Declaration of Helsinki

In 1964, the World Medical Association met in Finland and developed guidelines for physicians conducting research. In addition to reiterating

TABLE 2.1	Sections of the Nuremberg Code[7]

1. The voluntary consent of the human subject is absolutely essential.
2. The experiment should be such as to yield fruitful results . . . and not random or unnecessary.
3. The experiment should be based on . . . [prior knowledge] and the anticipated results should justify the experiment.
4. The experiment should . . . avoid all unnecessary physical and mental suffering and injury.
5. No experiment should be conducted where there is a prior reason to believe that death or disabling injury will occur, except where the experimental physicians also serve as subjects.
6. The degree of risk should never exceed . . . the importance of the problem to be solved.
7. Proper preparations should be made and adequate facilities provided to protect subjects against possibilities of injury, disability, or death.
8. The experiment should be conducted only by scientifically qualified persons.
9. During the course of treatment, the human subject should be able to bring the experiment to an end.
10. During the course of treatment the scientist must be prepared to terminate the experiment if he or she has probable cause . . . that a continuation of the experiment is likely to result in injury, disability, or death to the experimental subject.

aspects of the Nuremberg Code, the Declaration of Helsinki outlined two categories of research: research that has a therapeutic value for subjects and research that does not have direct therapeutic value for subjects.

The essence of the Declaration was the need for subjects to be informed of the benefits of the study before consenting to participate in the research. Subjects also were to be informed when their participation could be harmful or of little value to them.[8] The Declaration also allowed legal guardians to grant permission to enroll subjects in research and recommended written consent be given.

Even after the Nuremberg Code was established and informed consent laws were rewritten, protection of human participant rights was far from guaranteed. The Centers for Disease Control and Prevention conducted studies in the rural South to determine the prevalence of syphilis among blacks while exploring the possibilities of treatment. Tuskegee, a town in Macon County, Alabama, was found to have the highest incidence of syphilis among six counties.

The Tuskegee Syphilis Study

In 1932, the U.S. Public Health Service (USPHS) began an experiment in Tuskegee, Alabama. The study included 400 black sharecroppers diagnosed with syphilis and 200 black men who did not have syphilis. The study, known as the Tuskegee Syphilis Study, began in 1932 and ended in 1972. The study design called for the selection of black men with syphilis who were between 25 and 60 years of age. Subjects were randomly assigned into two groups, 400 men with untreated syphilis and 200 men without syphilis. As the study began, difficulties arose in recruiting subjects. Consequently, the men were told they were ill and would be offered free treatment. The USPHS did not inform subjects that they were part of a research study on syphilis. Instead, they were told they were being treated for "bad blood."

In 1933, the USPHS decided to continue with the study and treat subjects with mercurial ointment, a noneffective drug. This occurred in the face of findings in every textbook that clearly advocated treating patients who had syphilis, even in the disease's latent stages. By 1936, first reports were out that men with syphilis developed more complications than did the control group. By 1946, the death rate for men with untreated syphilis was twice as high as for the control group. In 1955, it was likewise reported that more than 30 percent of those autopsied had died directly from advanced syphilitic lesions of the cardiovascular or central nervous system.[10,11] After the study ended, those men who had syphilis, along with their wives and children who had contracted the disease, were given free antibiotics and lifetime medical care. However, the damage to their health, as well as their trust in the medical research community, was beyond repair. In a formal White House ceremony in 1997, President Clinton apologized to subjects and their families who participated in the Tuskegee Study and called for a renewed emphasis on research ethics.

The Willowbrook Study

The Willowbrook State School on Staten Island, New York, was the focus of unethical research from the 1950s to 1970. The purpose of the Willowbrook Study was to determine the period of infectivity of infectious hepatitis. Subjects were mentally handicapped children who were given either intramuscular or oral doses of hepatitis B virus. If parents wished to admit their child to the school, they were required to sign their child on as a study participant. Parents gave consent for the administration of the hepatitis B virus, but they were not told of the serious consequences, such as flu-like symptoms, skin rashes, and liver damage. During the 20-year investigation, Willowbrook closed its doors to new admissions because of overcrowding, yet the research ward continued to admit new residents. Administrators at Willowbrook believed they were conducting ethical research in a category called "natural experiments." The question whether the Willowbrook experiment was an ethical "study in nature" has been debated for years. The belief was that if there was no cure or treatment for a particular disease, then observing its course with the informed consent of participants is a study of nature.[11]

The Crisis at Johns Hopkins University

In April 2001, a 24-year-old healthy volunteer and technician at Johns Hopkins Asthma and Allergy Center consented to participate in a study. The purpose of the study was to gain a better understanding of the pathophysiology of asthma, specifically the mechanism of airway hyper-responsiveness. The study was based on the hypothesis that in normal individuals, lung inflation protects the airways from obstruction through a neural mechanism that might be lacking or impaired in people with asthma.[12]

The protocol involved healthy subjects inhaling a ganglionic blocker, hexamethonium. If ganglionic blockage suppressed the protective effects of deep inspiration on the airways, it would suggest that neural mechanisms helped the airways stay open. Hexamethonium was chosen because it blocks neurotransmission. The drug had been used to treat hypertension, but it was removed from the U.S. market in 1972 after the Food and Drug Administration (FDA) found it was ineffective.[12]

In the consent form, hexamethonium was described as "a medication that has been used during surgery, as part of anesthesia; that is capable of stopping some nerves in your airways from functioning for a short period." The section on risks stated that hexamethonium "may reduce your blood pressure and make you feel dizzy, especially when you stand up." The consent document was later criticized as having "failed to indicate that inhaled hexamethonium was experimental and not approved by the FDA" and because it was referred to as "medication."[12]

The 24-year-old volunteer was the third subject to receive hexamethonium. Mild shortness of breath and cough developed in the first subject, resolving over a period of about 8 days. The second subject received hexamethonium while the first subject still had symptoms. The 24-year-old volunteer inhaled 1 gm of hexamethonium on May 4, 2001, and developed a cough. On May 9, the volunteer was hospitalized with fever, hypoxemia, and abnormalities on a chest x-ray. By May 12, progressive dyspnea had developed, and the volunteer was transferred to the intensive care unit. On June 2, the volunteer died as a result of progressive hypotension and multiorgan failure.[12]

The crisis at Johns Hopkins University led to several reviews of clinical research. These reviews were conducted by internal and external review committees convened by the university, the FDA, and the U.S. Office for Human Research Protections. After the death of the volunteer, Johns Hopkins temporarily suspended all studies involving healthy volunteers.

Other Scandals Regarding Unethical Research Studies

Beecher,[13] a well-known Harvard anesthesiologist, describes a series of unethical research studies conducted at major medical institutions across the country. The article makes it clear how widespread the problems really were. All of these studies reinforce the important need for institutional review boards (IRBs) to review studies conscientiously and for researchers to act ethically. Rothman[14] cautions researchers not to take advantage of subjects in particular social predicaments because they will become accomplices to the problem, not observers of it. As laid out here, the reader should be struck by the very recent examples of experiments gone terribly wrong, as well as the horrifying examples from Nazi Germany.

Developing Guidelines for Clinical Nursing Research

The articles of the Nuremberg Code and Declaration of Helsinki are prototypes for the development of guidelines for conducting research in nursing. The American Nurses Association (ANA) and American Association of Colleges of Nursing (AACN) have developed two documents that provide such direction. In a position statement from the ANA titled *Education for Participation in Nursing Research* and a position statement from AACN titled *Nursing Research*,[15,16] general research competencies expected of graduates from associate, baccalaureate, and graduate degree programs in nursing are outlined (see Chapter 1). In *Human Rights Guidelines for Nurses in Clinical and Other Research*,[17] the principles in the Nuremberg Code are emphasized and directed toward voluntary participation of subjects, protection of human participants, and informed consent. This document focuses on the rights of participants who are involved in research, along with ethical issues within clinical nursing research settings. A summary of this document is presented in Table 2.2. Adhering to these guidelines reduces the chance of violating the rights of subjects. Key points addressed in the document are summarized in Figure 2.2.

Protecting Human Rights

The guidelines presented in Table 2.2 provide nurses with principles intended to safeguard human rights. The researcher must consider these guidelines at every stage of the research process, from selecting and defining the problem, to selecting a research design and collecting data, to interpreting and publishing the results. **Human rights** involves the protection of human participants participating in research; the term refers to the following three rights outlined in the ANA guidelines:[11]

1. Right to freedom from injury
2. Right to privacy and dignity
3. Right to anonymity and confidentiality

Right to Freedom From Injury

A basic responsibility of all researchers is to protect participants from harm while they are participating in a study. Participants have the right not to incur physical or emotional injury as a result of participating. If there is a possibility that any injury could occur, subjects need to know

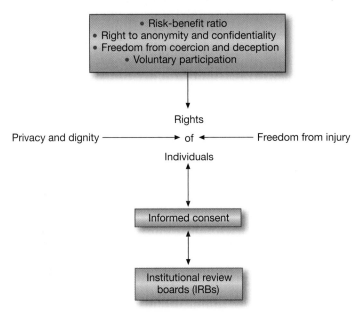

Fig 2•2 American Nurses' Association guidelines for protecting human rights.

TABLE 2.2	**Summary of Guidelines for Protecting the Rights of Human Subjects**

1. If research participation (medical, nursing, or other) is a condition of employment, nurses must be informed in writing of the nature of activity involved in advance of employment, and if this is not done, nurses must be given the opportunity to not participate in research.
   Potential risks to others must be clarified in advance of research as must ways to identify risks and counteract potential harm.
2. *Freedom from risk of injury or harm.* Researchers must estimate risk and benefit involved, and subjects must be informed of any potential mental or physical risk as well as personal benefit. Participants must be informed of procedures or activities that extend beyond personal need. Nurses must carefully monitor sources of potential risk of injury and protect subjects who are particularly vulnerable as a result of illness or members of captive groups (e.g., prisoners, students, institutionalized patients, and the poor).
   Right to privacy and dignity. All proposals, instruments, and procedures involved in the research activity must be discussed with prospective subjects and others participating in the project so that they may make an informed decision about whether to participate.

TABLE 2.2	Summary of Guidelines for Protecting the Rights of Human Subjects—cont'd

Right to anonymity. The researcher must describe to prospective subjects the methods that protect the identity of subjects and the information that will be obtained under privileged conditions.

3. Guidelines for protecting human rights apply to all individuals involved in a research activity. The use of subjects with limited civil freedom can usually only be justified when there is a predicted benefit to them or others in similar circumstances.

4. Nurses have an obligation to protect human rights and a professional responsibility to support research that broadens the scientific knowledge base of nursing for the practice and delivery of service.

5. Voluntary informed consent to participate in research must be obtained from all prospective subjects or their legal representatives.

6. Nurses have an obligation to serve on institutional review boards to review the ethical implications of proposed and ongoing research. All studies that involve gathering data from humans, animals, or charts should be reviewed by health-care professionals and community representatives.

Source: Adapted from American Nurses' Association: Human Rights Guidelines for Nurses in Clinical and Other Research. American Nurses' Association, Kansas City, MO, 1985, used with permission.

an estimate of the extent of such injury before giving their consent. Providing participants with an estimate of the potential risks in relation to the potential benefits is called the **risk-benefit ratio.** Two factors emerge when attempting to ensure the right to freedom from injury:

1. Ability of the benefit to justify participants' exposure to involved risks
2. The participants' vulnerability

The risks to participants must be justified by the potential benefit to the individual (in the case of clinical research) or to society (in the case of knowledge produced). In short, *the benefits should exceed the risks.* Even then, however, a cancer patient's risks of increased side effects from multiple chemotherapeutic agents may not always be justified by advancing society's knowledge of cancer treatment.

The risk-benefit ratio remains a primary objective standard by which we can judge the ethics of certain research procedures. Calculating this ratio involves naming and weighing the benefits, as well as considering the following:

1. How important is the research?
2. How serious are the risks to human participants involved in the research?

In any case, if potential for harm exists, whether physiological or psychological, the researcher must explain how the risks will be minimized. Participants must be fully aware of the risks along with benefits associated with the study.[9]

Vulnerable Research Participants Needing Protection

Federal regulations impose additional requirements upon institutional review boards when protecting the welfare of particularly vulnerable subjects. **Vulnerable research participants** are those persons who are relatively or absolutely incapable of protecting their own interests and unable to provide meaningful informed consent. The ability to provide informed consent means a person has the mental capacity to understand the information provided, to appreciate how it is relevant to their particular circumstance, and to make a reasonable decision about participation in the study.

The Office for Human Research Protections (OHRP) is the agency responsible for setting policies and regulations regarding the protection of the rights, welfare, and well-being of subjects participating in research. A list of vulnerable research subjects needing protection is provided in Table 2.3. In general, special regulations allow IRBs to approve research that is of minimal risk or that will benefit subjects directly. In addition, research involving persons whose mental capacity to consent is questionable requires careful consideration to ensure that each person is provided additional safeguards for his or her safety and welfare. Refer to the OHRP Web site (www.hhs.gov/ohrp) for specific policies and regulations supporting research involving vulnerable subjects.

Right to Privacy and Dignity

The type of data collected may be highly sensitive in regard to the subjects' privacy and dignity. Many questionnaires or surveys require

TABLE 2.3	Vulnerable Research Subjects

Children
Cognitively impaired
Elderly
Human fetuses
Mentally incapacitated
Neonates
Prisoners
Sedated or unconscious (comatose) patients
Students and employees
Terminally ill patients

subjects to provide data such as income, marital status, personal activities, opinions and beliefs, and attitudes. In addition, the use of cameras, one-way mirrors, tape recorders, diaries, and patient records may easily be construed as an invasion of privacy. Participant observation is frequently used as a method to collect data in qualitative research studies. Such an approach may not be clearly understood by subjects. In all instances, the researcher is obligated to make sure that subjects clearly understand all procedures, the type of data being collected, and the data collection methods, so that they can make an informed decision about participating in a study.

Right to Anonymity and Confidentiality

Closely related to protecting privacy and dignity is the right of subjects to remain anonymous and to be assured of confidentiality. The researcher must plan carefully to consider handling, storage, and reporting of data. **Anonymity** refers to keeping participants nameless[9] and limiting access to information that is gathered about subjects. Anonymity can be facilitated by using code numbers for subjects' identity to prevent others from linking reported information with them. A master code list should be kept locked up, with access to the data limited to those who are intimately involved in the research. In anonymity, even the researcher cannot link the data to the subject.

Confidentiality refers to protecting data by not divulging information that is gathered or learned in caring for a patient without that individual's permission to do so.[9,15] This right is extremely important when the information may carry a stigma, such as a diagnosis of HIV or AIDS, evidence of domestic violence, or a prison record.

Ensuring the Protection of Human Rights

Several procedures can be used to ensure protection of human rights, such as procedures for obtaining informed consent and review of study protocols by an ethics committee, often referred to as an institutional review board.

Key Elements of Informed Consent

A basic responsibility of researchers is to ensure that potential subjects understand the implications of participating in a research study and recognize that they have the freedom to decide whether they want to participate. The idea that individuals have the right to decide for themselves is referred to as the principle of self-determination, which is central to the process of informed consent.

Key elements of informed consent are (1) providing potential subjects with sufficient information about participating in a research study and (2) assuring them that participation is voluntary and can be withdrawn at any time without negative consequences. The language is kept simple to make sure that all subjects understand the meaning of informed consent.

Participants give informed consent before participating in a study by signing a written consent form, which is also signed and dated by the researcher and a witness. The researcher discusses the proposed research study with subjects to provide feedback in response to their questions, concerns, or both. Consent forms should be divided into sections with headings. Medical jargon should be avoided for purposes of clarity and readability; sentences should be short, margins should be reasonably wide, and the pages should not be overcrowded with too much text. An example of a consent form is shown in Figure 2.3. The following information should be conveyed to potential subjects:

1. Title of the study
2. Personnel engaged in the study (e.g., principal investigator, coinvestigator(s), research assistants)
3. Invitation to participate in the study (e.g., "You are invited to participate in a research study"; not "requested," "chosen," or "eligible")
4. Reason the particular person is being invited to participate
5. Clear description of the purpose of the study
6. Detailed description of procedures of the study (e.g., descriptions of what will actually occur; how much time is required of the subject; whether hospitalization will be required and whether it will always, sometimes, or never be required as part of the subject's standard care; how much and how often blood will be drawn, if applicable)
7. Potential risks to subjects, including psychological, social, and physical risks (e.g., explanation of steps that will be taken to protect against risks; estimation of likelihood of occurrence, severity, and duration of potential risks, if applicable)
8. Potential benefits of the study (e.g., identification of desired benefit to society, the risk-benefit ratio, statement of whether there are direct subject benefits)
9. Economic considerations (e.g., whether subjects will incur any additional expenses as a result of participation)
10. Confidentiality considerations (e.g., explanation of steps that will be taken to ensure the confidentiality of information that is obtained during the course of the study, such as who will have access to the data and when the data and specimens will be destroyed)
11. Freedom of subjects to ask questions and withdraw from the study at any time without penalty

Some research subjects may be unwilling or unable to sign a consent form. For example, the elderly may be wary of signing forms, and other

**University of Massachusetts Medical Center
Committee for the Protection of Human Subjects in Research
Consent to Participate in a Research Project**

Title: Patient Empowerment Program for People with Diabetes
Principle Investigator: James A. Fain, PhD, RN, BC-ADM, FAAN

Research Subject's Name _____ Date: _____

PURPOSE
You are invited to volunteer for a research study. You have been chosen to take part in this study because you have diabetes. The main objective is to see if a program that helps develop skills and self-awareness in the areas of goal setting, problem solving, stress management, coping, and motivation would be beneficial to patients with diabetes. The purpose of this study is to try to find an effective way to prepare patients with diabetes to make decisions.

It is important for you to know that your participation is entirely voluntary. You may decide not to take part in or quit the study at any time, without any penalty. You will be told about any new information or changes in the study that might affect your participation.

To take part in this study you must agree to participate in an outpatient educational program. The program will take place weekly for 2 hours and last a total of six (6) weeks. Each session will involve a brief presentation of key concepts related to the topic; completion of self-assessment worksheets; and small group discussions. You will be encouraged to bring a spouse, family member, or friend to each session.

PROCEDURES
If you agree to participate in this study, you will be invited to an orientation session where a discussion about the program along with sample worksheets will be presented. You will be asked to complete several questionnaires along with giving us permission to access your medical records to obtain the most recent glycosylated hemoglobin level which was performed as a routine procedure during your treatment at the diabetes clinic. In addition, at the end of 6 weeks, you will be asked to complete the questionnaires a second time along with giving us permission to access once again your glycosylated hemoglobin levels. Questions throughout the program will focus on exploring life satisfactions, coping with diabetes, addressing daily stresses, and setting priorities.

Not everyone in the study will initially participate in the program. You will either be assigned to attend the program (experimental group) or not attend (comparison group). At the conclusion of the program, all those individuals who did not attend the program will be asked to complete the questionnaires a second time. After that time, the program will be provided for all those individuals who did not initially participate in the program.

RISKS
We can foresee few risks that might occur if you decide to participate in this study. A minor risk is the possibility that certain questions regarding anxiety, stress, and feelings toward diabetes may arouse psychologically distressing emotions. If this is the case, you will be able to speak to a member of the research team or staff within the clinic.

BENEFITS
There is no promise or guarantee of any medical benefits to you resulting from your participation in this study. However, you might have a better insight into your own values, goals, and needs as they relate to living with diabetes. In addition, your participation may help others with diabetes in the future as a result of knowledge gained from this research.

ALTERNATIVES
Your standard treatment will be the same whether or not you decide to be in the study. However, the educational program is not presently available for study.

COSTS
There will be no additional cost to you from being in this research study. Patients will not be charged for any materials used in this research study.

CONFIDENTIALITY
Your research records will be confidential. In all records of the study you will be identified by a code number and your name will be known only to the researchers. Your name will not be

Fig 2•3 Example of an adult consent form. *(Continued)*

University of Massachusetts Medical Center
Committee for the Protection of Human Subjects in Research
Consent to Participate in a Research Project (continued)

used in any reports or publications of this study. Once again, your participation in this study is entirely voluntary. You may withdraw from the study at any time.

Please feel free to ask any questions you may have about the study or about your rights as a research subject. If other questions occur to you later, you may contact James A. Fain, PhD, RN, BC-ADM, FAAN, the Principle Investigator, at (508) 856-5661. If at any time during or after the study, you would like to discuss the study or your research rights with someone who is not associated with the study, you may contact the Administrative Coordinator for the Committee for the Protection of Human Subjects in Research at UMMC, (508) 856-4261. Consent to Participate in the Research Project, H-2895 entitled "Patient Empowerment Program for People with Diabetes."

Subject's Name _____

P.I. Name _____

The purpose and procedures of this research project have been explained to me and I understand them. I have been told about all the predictable discomfort, risks, and benefits that might result, and I understand them. I agree to participate as a subject in this research project. I understand that I may end my participation at any time.

_____   Date: _____
Subject's Signature

NAME: (print) _____

Relationship to Subject: _____

Witness Signature: _____

Date: _____

NAME: (print) _____

Fig 2•3—cont'd

individuals may have certain physical handicaps preventing them from being able to sign. The researcher needs to decide the best way possible to document permission. In some cases, an audiotaped or videotaped recording may be used to present information and obtain verbal consent. In the case of children, a parent or legal guardian must sign the consent form. Children (individuals under 18 years of age) are not considered legally competent to provide informed consent. When children are involved in a study, the researcher should obtain informed consent of the parent or legal guardian as well as assent of the child. Assent of a child refers to a child's affirmative agreement to participate in a research study. Failure of the child to object, however, cannot be construed as assent. An example of a child's assent form is shown in Figure 2.4.

University of Massachusetts Medical Center
Committee for the Protection of Human Subjects in Research
Consent to Participate in a Research Project entitled:

Multidimensional Sense of Humor in School-Aged Children:
A Pilot Study

_____   _____
Child's Name (print)   Date

Parent/Guardian Consent: The purpose and procedures of this research project, the predictable risks, and the benefits that my child may experience have been explained to me. Alternatives to my child's participation in this study have also been discussed. I have read and understand this consent form. I voluntarily consent to my child's participation in this study. I understand that my child and I may end our participation at any time.

_____   _____
Parent/Legal Guardian Signature   Date

_____   _____
Parent/Legal Guardian Signature (print)   Date

Child Assent: My parent/legal guardian has explained this study to me. We have Dr. Fain's telephone number and can call Dr. Fain at any time if we have any further questions. I have decided to do this study even though I know I do not have to.

_____
Child's Signature

Fig 2•4 Examples of child's assent form.

Institutional Review Boards

In addition to ensuring that subjects give voluntary informed consent to participate in a study, most institutions and funding agencies have a mechanism for reviewing research proposals. As mentioned earlier, IRBs are review groups responsible for ensuring that researchers do not engage in unethical behavior or conduct poorly designed research studies.

The major responsibility of an IRB is to review research proposals at convened meetings to ensure that federal guidelines are followed. Proposals submitted to IRBs are reviewed in detail. The IRB ensures that the researcher is not violating rights of human participants. Lawyers, lay persons, and clergy often serve on IRBs to deal with nonscientific issues. Feasibility of conducting a study, however, is outside the realm of the IRB. The IRB also reviews the procedures for selecting subjects, ensuring voluntary informed consent, clearly written descriptions, and confidentiality. The decision to approve, modify, or disapprove a proposal must be made by a majority of IRB members.

Some categories of research may qualify for an expedited review, such as when the use of noninvasive procedures is routine or if a study consists of surveys, interviews, or studies of existing records, provided that the data are collected in such a way that subjects cannot be identified and the study does not deal with sensitive issues. In the case of an expedited review, the chairperson and at least one other member of the IRB review the proposal. The advantage of an expedited review is that it is usually completed in less time than that required for a full IRB review.

Evaluating Evidence for the Protection of Human Rights

Most research reports provide only a sentence or two concerning review by an appropriate committee. Excerpt 2.5 displays an example of what is usually written in research reports regarding protection of human rights. Without a detailed explanation of data collection procedures, a number of issues can be raised as to the ethical acceptability of a given study. The information presented in Table 2.4 can help the researcher evaluate the protection of human rights in research reports. Nurses at all levels typically find themselves involved in carrying out research activities. As patient advocates, nurses must make an effort to verify the nature of a study and whether the study has been reviewed by an IRB. When human rights are violated, the nurse must report the concern to both the researcher and the IRB. Similarly, the nurse should not assume that the rights of subjects have been adequately addressed unless the exact nature of protection has been specified. It is incorrect to assume that the rights of subjects and the process of informed consent have been handled adequately unless the procedures are clearly articulated.

Training Program: Protecting Human Research Participants

The National Institutes of Health (NIH) require that all individuals receiving a NIH award must successfully complete an educational program reviewing issues (e.g., key historical events, ethical principles, informed consent, role of institutional review boards) that impact guidelines on human participant protection in research.

TABLE 2.4	Guidelines for Evaluating the Protection of Human Rights in Research Reports

Criteria for Evaluation	Comments
1. Is the research problem a significant one for nursing? Is the design scientifically sound?	If an answer to the problem will not benefit subjects or contribute to nursing knowledge, it may not be ethical to involve subjects.
2. Is the research designed to maximize benefit to human subjects and minimize risk?	If subjects are exposed to undue risk and the benefit or knowledge generated is minimal, ethical problems exist.
3. Is the selection of subjects ethically appropriate to study the research problem?	It is ethically inappropriate to use captive subjects when they are not members of groups that would benefit from the results.
4. Is there evidence of voluntary, informed consent?	Any evidence of subject coercion to participate and lack of information about the study purpose and subject participation violate human rights.
5. Is there evidence of subject deception?	Deception should be avoided if at all possible. The researcher must inform subjects about any deception and the reason for that deception, prior to subjects' consent. Subjects must be debriefed about any deception at end of study.
6. Have subjects been invited to consent when under high stress?	Consent under stress should be avoided if possible. Invitations to participate should be timed so as to not add to periods of stress (e.g., immediately before surgery or other complex procedures). Timing invitations well in advance is preferred.
7. Is informed consent given by a legal guardian or representative of a subject incapable of giving his or her own consent?	This type of consent must be done in the case of minors or subjects who are physically or mentally incapacitated.
8. Is there evidence in the research report by which individual subjects can be identified?	The researcher must take precautions that publication of the setting and data collection and analysis will protect the anonymity of subjects.
9. Is there evidence of an independent ethics review by a board or committee?	An ethics review should be mentioned in the research report.

EXCERPT 2.5

Example of Human Participants Approval from the Hospital Institutional Review Board (IRB)

Protection of Human Subjects

The institutional review board of the hospital approved this study and gave permission to use the data from the database for data collection. The institutional review board waivered informed consent because only call records were being examined and confidentiality of each caller was maintained by using a coding system for the calls. The researcher was the only person with access to the coding system, which involved assigning a number from 1 to 110 to each subject.

Source: Light, PA, Hupcey, JE, and Clark, MB: Nursing telephone triage and its influence on parents' choice of care for febrile children. J Pediatr Nurs 20:424, 2005.

The NIH Office of Extramural Research has developed an online tutorial titled *Protecting Human Research Participants (PHRP)* for individuals involved in the design and/or conduct of research involving human participants. This tutorial satisfies NIH educational requirements. Upon successfully completing the tutorial, a certificate of completion can be printed as documentation of compliance with the requirement. Such a certificate from NIH may also be applicable to other institutions requiring education in the area of protection of human participants. Refer to NIH Office of Extramural Research, Protecting Human Participants Web site (http://phrp.nihtraining.com) to register for the tutorial.

WEB LINKS

The following Web site offers students some helpful information on the Code of Ethics for Nursing and the American Nurses Association (ANA) Position Statement on Ethics and Human Rights.

American Nurses Association
  http://nursingworld.org

SUMMARY OF KEY IDEAS

1. The research process is a decision-making process.

2. The five general phases of the research process are selecting and defining the problem, selecting a research design, collecting data, analyzing data, and using research findings.

3. Research studies are classified based on the purpose of the study and degree of control.

4. Basic research refers to investigations conducted to develop, refine, or test theory.

5. Applied research refers to investigations conducted to generate knowledge that will have a direct impact on clinical practice.

6. Ethical principles relevant to nursing research were originally derived from the Nuremberg Code and Declaration of Helsinki.

7. The ANA has developed two documents that provide direction for nurses engaged in research activities: *Guidelines for the Investigative Function of Nurses* and *Human Rights Guidelines for Nurses in Clinical and Other Research.*

8. The basic rights of human participants include the right to freedom from injury, the right to privacy and dignity, and the right to anonymity and confidentiality.

9. Informed consent includes the elements of adequate disclosure (providing subjects with enough information for them to make a voluntary decision), comprehension (ensuring that participants understand the information provided), and freedom from coercion.

10. IRBs or institutional review boards, are responsible for reviewing research proposals and commenting on the rights of human participants.

LEARNING ACTIVITIES

1. Choose two research articles of interest to you.

    a. Does the researcher examine a problem that is relevant to nursing science?

    b. How would you classify the type of research conducted?

2. Choose a research article in which people were participants. Consider the issue of protecting human rights.

    a. How were human participant rights alluded to in the article?

    b. What information would you need to help you assess the adequacy of the protection of human rights?

    c. If you were to conduct a similar research study, what steps would you take to protect the rights and ensure the safety of the human subjects?

3. Identify several key points in the Tuskegee Syphilis Study, Willowbrook Study, and Crisis at Johns Hopkins University that raise ethical issues.

REFERENCES

1. Polit, DF, and Beck, CT: Essentials of Nursing Research: Methods, ed. 6. Lippincott Williams & Wilkins, Philadelphia, 2006, pp 51–65.
2. Gillis, A, and Jackson, W: Research for Nurses: Methods and Interpretation. FA Davis Company, Philadelphia, 2002, pp 13–14.
3. Nguyen, TN, Nilsson, S, Hellstrom, AL, and Bengtson, A: Music therapy to reduce pain and anxiety in children with cancer undergoing lumbar puncture: A randomized clinical trial. J Pediatr Oncol Nurs 27:146, 2010.
4. Hilton, JJ: Folic acid intake of young women. J Obstet Gynecol Neonatal Nurs 31:172, 2002.
5. Greene, MS, et al: Metabolic control, self-care behaviors, and parenting in adolescents with type 1 diabetes. Diabetes Educ 36:326, 2010.
6. Martin, LM, et al: The association between early outcome, health-related quality of life, and survival following elective open-heart surgery. J Cardio Nurs 23:432, 2008.
7. Katz, J: Experimentation With Human Beings. Russell Sage Foundation, New York, 1972, pp 289–290.
8. World Medical Association: Human experimentation code of ethics of the World Medical Association, Declaration of Helsinki. Br Med J 2:177, 1964.
9. Getz, K, and Borfitz, D: Informed Consent: The Consumer's Guide to the Risks and Benefits of Volunteering for Clinical Trials. Thomson Healthcare Inc., Boston, 2002, pp 70–121.
10. Brandt, AM: Racism and research: The case of the Tuskegee Study. Hastings Center Report 8:21, 1978.
11. Gillis, A, and Jackson, W: Research for nurses: Methods and interpretation. FA Davis Company, Philadelphia, 2000, pp 322–348.
12. Steinbrook, R: Protecting research subjects: The Crisis at Johns Hopkins. N Engl J Med 346:716, 2002.
13. Beecher, HK: Ethics and clinical research. N Engl J Med 274:1354, 1996.
14. Rothman, DJ: Were Tuskegee and Willowbrook studies in nature? Hastings Center Report 12:5, 1982.
15. American Association of Colleges of Nursing: Position Statement on Nursing Research. American Association of Colleges of Nursing, Washington, DC, 2006.
16. American Nurses Association: Position Statement: Education for Participation in Nursing Research. American Nurses Association, Washington, DC, 1994.
17. American Nurses' Association: Human Rights Guidelines for Nurses in Clinical and Other Research. American Nurses' Association, Kansas City, MO, 1985.

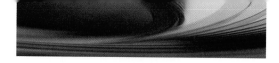

CHAPTER

3

UNDERSTANDING EVIDENCE-BASED PRACTICE

JAMES A. FAIN, PhD, RN, BC-ADM, FAAN

LEARNING OBJECTIVES

By the end of this chapter, you will be able to:
1. Define evidence-based practice (EBP).
2. Distinguish between evidence-based medicine (EBM) and evidence-based nursing (EBN).
3. Define *meta-analysis*.
4. Identify several reasons for the delay in using research findings in nursing practice.
5. List some limitations associated with EBP.
6. Identify steps associated with the process of EBP.
7. Describe some of the more commonly used electronic databases in EBM.
8. Discuss the level of evidence associated with appraising research studies.
9. Participate in the process of retrieval, appraisal, and synthesis of evidence to improve patient outcomes.
10. Integrate evidence, clinical judgment, and patient preferences in planning, implementing, and evaluating outcomes of care.

GLOSSARY OF KEY TERMS

ACP Journal Club. The ACP (American College of Physicians) Journal Club summarizes and interprets the best evidence of one recent study or review article from traditional journals, based on the criteria provided by the practitioner.

Agency for Healthcare Research and Quality (AHRQ). The AHRQ has promoted EBP through the establishment of 12 Evidence-Based Practice Centers (EPCs).

Background questions. Questions focusing on basic or general knowledge about a condition and/or disorder.

Cochrane Database of Systematic Reviews. One of the most popular databases is The Cochrane Library, which reviews and summarizes individual clinical trials and systematic reviews from more than 100 medical journals.

(Continued)

Evidence-based medicine (EBM). The conscientious, explicit, and judicious use of current best evidence in making decisions about the care of individual patients. The practice of EBM means integrating individual clinical expertise with the best available external clinical evidence from systematic research.

Evidence-based nursing (EBN). The conscientious, explicit, and judicious use of theory-derived, research-based information in making decisions about care delivery to individuals or groups of patients and in consideration of individual needs and preferences.

Foreground questions. Questions focusing on specific knowledge to inform clinical decisions or actions.

InfoPOEMS. Info-POEMS (Patient-Oriented Evidence that Matters) is a database similar to the ACP Journal Club; it reviews and provides commentary on recent articles.

Knowledge-focused triggers. Ideas that emerge from staff when they read, listen to research presentations, or encounter EBP guidelines by federal agencies or specialty organizations.

MD Consult. A database that provides full-text access to textbooks, journal articles, practice guidelines, patient education handouts, and drug awareness.

Meta-analysis. A statistical method that takes the results of many studies in a specific area and synthesizes their findings to draw conclusions regarding the state of the science in the area of focus.

National Guideline Clearinghouse. This Clearinghouse provides a collection of evidence-based clinical practice guidelines.

PICO model. Four components (P—Patient/Population/Problem; I—Intervention; C—Comparison; O—Outcome) that provide structure when writing clinical questions.

Problem-focused triggers. Ideas that emerge from staff in the context of clinical practice by examining quality improvement data, risk surveillance data, benchmarking data, or a recurrence of a clinical problem.

Research utilization. The process by which knowledge generated from research becomes incorporated into clinical practice.

Nurses use a variety of sources of information in making care decisions around certain treatments, therapies, and interventions. Unfortunately, many of these sources of information may have been derived from a textbook or journal article or perhaps from a conversation with a respected colleague or professor. To a lesser extent, information may have come from scientific research findings. Although nurses have advocated research-based practice for years, this goal has been difficult to achieve. During the past decade, there has been a renewed call for health-care professionals to base their care on the best research evidence available. The evidence-based practice (EBP) movement is consistent with nursing's goal of providing research-based care to patients. This chapter provides an overview of EBP, along with a discussion of an assortment of evidence-based tools.

Evidence-Based Practice: What Is It?

Evidence-based practice was derived from the principle that health-care professionals should not center their practice on tradition or experience, but rather on scientific research findings. The concept of EBP originated within the field of medicine; it was initially termed **evidence-based medicine (EBM)**. Evidence-based medicine was originally defined by Sackett and colleagues[1] as the conscientious, explicit, and judicious use of current best evidence in making decisions about the care of individual patients. EBM means integrating individual clinical expertise with the best available external clinical evidence from systematic research.

The concept of EBM has been expanded and applied across all health-care areas under the term "evidence-based health care (EBH)" or evidence-based practice. Both terms refer to the critical appraisal of research findings and decisions regarding whether, and how, to use findings in the care of patients.

Ingersoll[2] differentiated **evidence-based nursing (EBN)** from EBM by suggesting that EBN is the conscientious, explicit, and judicious use of theory-derived, research-based information in making decisions about care delivery to individuals or groups of patients and in consideration of individual needs and preferences. EBN *deemphasizes* ritual, isolated, and unsystematic clinical experiences, ungrounded opinions, and tradition as a basis for practice. Instead, EBN stresses the use of research findings.[3]

Characteristics of Evidence-Based Practice

Important features or characteristics of EBP exist. First, EBP is a problem-solving approach that considers the context of the nurse's current clinical experience.[3] Clinical experience refers to the nurse's ability to use his or her clinical skills and past experience to identify each patient's unique health state and diagnosis, the individual risks, and benefits of potential interventions.[4]

Second, EBP brings together the best available research evidence by combining research with knowledge and theory.[3] Use of the best evidence from patient-centered clinical research allows accuracy and precision of diagnostic tests; the power of prognosis markers; and the efficacy and safety of therapeutic and preventive regimens.[4] Finally, EBP allows patient values to be heard. If they are to serve the patient, the unique preferences, concerns, and expectations each patient brings to a clinical encounter are integrated into clinical decisions.

Evidence-Based Practice Versus Research Utilization

The terms "EBP" and "research utilization" are often used synonymously. While there are similarities between both terms, there is a distinct difference. **Research utilization** is the process by which knowledge generated from research becomes incorporated into clinical practice.[5] The process involves critical analysis of research findings along with implementation and evaluation of changes in practice. Research utilization emphasizes translating empirically derived knowledge into real-world applications.[6] It is often thought of as a subset of EBP focusing on application of research findings.[7]

The purpose of research utilization is the application of available knowledge to improve patient outcomes. While the approach to conducting research is planned and organized, research utilization compiles the results of several studies and applies the new knowledge to clinical practice.[5] However, research findings are not always incorporated into clinical practice. Some nurses never read about or hear of research findings; others do not feel empowered to make changes in practice. In other situations, researchers may not publish research findings or make the findings available to nurses.

As nurses begin to read and attempt to integrate research findings into pratice, most utilization efforts tend to be informal. However, the goal is to formalize research utilization to disseminate research findings and help nurses develop research-based policies, procedures, and clinical practice guidelines. Strategies to ensure research-based practice are important components of the research utilization process.[5] Between 1975 and 1995, several models or approaches to research utilization were developed to help disseminate nursing research. Many of the earlier models were funded projects focusing on adoption of clinical innovation with hopes of developing research-based protocols and clinical practice guidelines. Table 3.1 lists several nursing research utilization models.[5] For a more in-depth discussion of each model refer to the corresponding reference.

EBP is a broader term that not only includes the definition of research utilization, but also integrates clinical expertise with the best available

TABLE 3.1	Nursing Research Utilization Models	
Date	**Model**	**Reference**
1975–1977	Western Interstate Commission for Higher Education (WICHE)	Krueger, JC: Utilization of nursing research: The planning process, J Nurs Adm 8:6, 1978.
1975–1981	Conduct and Utilization of Research in Nursing (CURN)	Jorsley, JA, Crane, J, Crabrtree, MK: Using Research to Improve Nursing Practice: A Guide. Grune & Stratton, New York, 1983.
1976–1985	The Nursing Child Assessment Satellite Training (NCAST)	King, D, Barnard, KE, Hoehn, R: Disseminating the results of nursing research. Nurs Outlook 29:164, 1981.

TABLE 3.1	Nursing Research Utilization Models—cont'd	
Date	**Model**	**Reference**
1976	Stetler/Marram Model	Stetler, CB, Marriam, G; Evaluation of research findings for applicability in practice. Nurs Outlook 24:559, 1976.
1989	American Association of Critical Care Nurses (AACN)	Mitchell, PH, et al: American Association of Critical Care Nurses Demonstration Project: Profile of excellence in critical care nursing. Heart Lung 18:219, 1989.
1994	Stetler	Stetler, CB: Refinement of the Stetler/Marram model for application of research findings to practice. Nurs Outlook 42:15, 1994.
1994	Iowa Model of Research in Practice	Titler, MG, et al: Infusing research into practice to promote quality care. Nurs Res 43:307, 1994.

evidence from systematic research.[7] Clinical expertise refers to the proficiency and judgment nurses acquire through clinical experience and clinical practice. The best clinical evidence can inform, but never replace, clinical expertise. It is clinical expertise that decides whether the evidence applies to the individual patient and how it is integrated into a clinical decision.

EBP begins by asking the question, "What is the best possible evidence available to solve a clinical problem?" While findings from rigorous research studies are considered the best possible evidence, EBP draws on other sources of systematically generated evidence integrating it with clinical expertise, patient preferences, and existing resources.[6,8] Because the more rigorous research studies are more likely to inform nurses, randomized control trials (RCTs) have become the "gold standard" for judging the strength and quality of the evidence. In some instances, questions/problems within the four major categories associated with EBP (therapy, treatment, diagnostic tests, and prognosis) may not require RCTs, or RCTs have not been conducted. Nurses then are to refer to the next best available evidence. When nurses use research findings and the best available evidence as their foundation for clinical decision making, the outcome is EBP.

The Research–Practice Gap

The research–practice gap refers to that period from when knowledge is produced to when it is practiced by health-care professionals.[8] Although the concept and movement of EBP continue to gain popularity, there is still a delay in using nursing research findings in practice. Several reasons[3,9] for this delay are listed in Table 3.2.

Limitations of Evidence-Based Practice

Several limitations associated with the science and practices of EBM have been identified. Three limitations that are universal to science include a shortage of coherent, consistent scientific evidence; difficulties in applying any evidence to care of individual patients; and barriers to any practice of high-quality medicine.[4] Limitations unique to the practice of EBM include a need for developing skills in researching and appraising the research, the limited amount of time in practice to master such skills, and scarce resources to access the evidence.[4]

Steps Associated With Evidence-Based Practice

All nursing research utilization models presented in Table 3.1 provide guidelines or steps on how to design and implement research utilization projects. Over time, several of these models were revised and began the process of using evidence to guide practice. One such model was the Iowa Model of Research in Practice. In 2001, Titler's[10] revised model was renamed the Iowa Model of Evidence-Based Practice to Promote

TABLE 3.2	Reasons for the Delay in Using Research Findings in Nursing Practice

1. Nurses in practice do not know about research findings.
2. Nurses in practice are often not clear about who will benefit from the research findings or about the risks involved.
3. Nurses in practice do not usually associate with those individuals (i.e., scientists, academic researchers) who produce knowledge. There is often a lack of dialogue between researchers and clinicians.
4. Nurse researchers and nurse clinicians use different languages.
5. Nurses in practice lack the skills to locate and read research reports.
6. Research is often reported in language of statistics instead of being reported in clinically meaningful terms.
7. Nurses and nurse managers do not develop opportunities for acceptance and introduction of innovation.

Quality Care and included steps on how to carry out processes and activities of EBP. Steps associated with guiding the process of EBP include selecting a topic and formulating a question, forming a team, tracking down the best possible evidence, and appraising the evidence critically.

Selecting a Topic and Formulating a Clinical Question

The Iowa Model of Evidence-Based Practice to Promote Quality Care was designed with the assumption that ideas for EBP start with a stimulus or trigger. The selection of a topic can be either a knowledge-focused trigger or problem-focused trigger.[10] **Knowledge-focused triggers** are ideas generated when staff read, listen to scientific papers at research conferences, or encounter EBP guidelines by federal agencies or specialty organizations.[11] Examples of knowledge-focused triggers may include pain management, prevention of skin breakdown, assessment of nasogastric tube placement, and patency of arterial lines. **Problem-focused triggers** are identified by staff in the context of clinical practice by examining quality improvement data, risk surveillance data, benchmarking data, or a recurrence of a clinical problem.[11] Examples of problem-focused triggers may include increased incidence of deep vein thrombosis and pulmonary emboli.

Most clinical problems are first identified by clinicians who ask, "*Why do we do it this way?*" "*Is there a better way to do this?*" "*What was the rationale for making that decision?*" "*Could it be done better, more efficiently, and more effectively?*" Questions or problems may also arise when new knowledge or technology emerges.

Questions in practice may crop up from central issues involved in caring for patients. Clinical questions, just like researchable problems, need a specific focus. For example, quality improvement studies may indicate that patients' pain is poorly controlled on medical surgical units. Before beginning to track down the best evidence possible, the specific nature of the question must be determined. Perhaps the problem is related to a specific age group (young, middle-aged, or elderly) or the nurses' attitudes toward pain. Narrowing the focus to address the assessment and management of pain in older adults, for example, makes tracking evidence more feasible.

A list of issues related to writing clinical questions is presented in Table 3.3.[4] This listing is neither exhaustive nor mutually exclusive. In formulating a clinical question it is important to decide what type of question to ask. Melnyk and Fineout-Overholt[12] refer to type of question as either background or foreground. **Background questions** are asked because of the need for basic or general knowledge about a condition and/or disorder.[12] Background questions include two essential components: a question (who, what, where, how, why) and a verb. Most background questions are answered by checking a textbook and tend to be opinion based rather than evidence based. Examples of background include such questions as What causes migraines?; What

TABLE 3.3	Issues to Consider When Writing Clinical Questions

1. Clinical findings: Gathering and interpreting findings from a patient's history, physical signs, symptoms, and laboratory data.
2. Etiology: Understanding the reason or cause of disease.
3. Clinical manifestations: Knowing symptoms or behaviors of disease and how to use such knowledge in classifying patients' illnesses.
4. Differential diagnosis: Considering possible causes of disease by comparing illnesses that share features of the presenting illness, but differ in other ways.
5. Diagnostic test: Selecting and interpreting diagnostic tests to confirm or dismiss a diagnosis.
6. Prognosis: Predicting the clinical course and end of disease over time.
7. Therapy: Selecting particular treatments to offer patients based on cost and what is most effective.
8. Prevention: Reducing the chance or occurrence of disease by identifying and modifying risk factors along with appropriate screening.
9. Experience and meaning: Gaining an understanding or meaning of everyday experiences from the patient's perspective.
10. Self-improvement: Keeping up to date by improving clinical skills and being more clinically efficient.

Source: Adapted from Sackett, DL, et al: Evidence-Based Medicine: How to Practice and Teach EBM, ed. 2. Churchill Livingstone, Edinburgh, 2000, pp 1–35.

is the best diagnostic test for a kidney stone?; and How often should women over the age of 40 have mammograms?

Foreground questions ask for specific knowledge to inform clinical decisions or action.[12] Foreground questions include four components: P–Patient/Population; I–Intervention; C–Comparison; and O–Outcome. These components are referred to as the **PICO model**, providing structure when formulating a clinical question. Examples of foreground include questions such as How should you treat acute bronchitis in children under the age of two? and Should patients with whiplash injury wear a cervical collar? Table 3.4 displays examples of how foreground questions might be constructed using the PICO model.

Forming a Team

Once the clinical question has been identified, the next step is to select appropriate members to compose the team. A well-balanced team is critical to the success of EBP efforts. Be sure members of the team are familiar with the problem along with interested stakeholders in the delivery of care. For example, a team working on pain management should be interdisciplinary and include various health-care professionals: nurses, pharmacists, physicians, and psychologists. In addition, administrative types (e.g., chief nursing officers, managers, directors, supervisors) who may directly or indirectly interfere with efforts of the team need to be included in EBP implementation and kept informed every step of the way.

TABLE 3.4	Constructing Foreground Clinical Questions: PICO Model

Patient	Intervention (or cause)	Comparison (optional)	Outcome
In patients with acute bronchitis	do antibiotics		reduce sputum production, cough or days off?
In children with cancer	what are the current treatments		in the management of fever and infection?
Among family members of patients undergoing diagnostic procedures	does standard care,	listening to tranquil music or audiotaped comedy routines,	make a difference in the reduction of reported anxiety?
In menopausal women	does taking calcium plus vitamin D		prevent fracture?

In some circumstances, it may be important to seek participation from individuals outside your immediate department so as to be connected to larger organizational goals.

Tracking Down the Best Evidence

Once the clinical question has been identified and the team formed, the next step is to obtain related articles. As you begin to track down the best evidence, it is a good idea to start searching broadly rather than beginning specifically. Identify the indexes, journals, databases, and other sources of which you are aware, and spend some time pursuing them. Textbooks will not be helpful, although you may find some useful information about the pathophysiology of a disease. Textbooks are not appropriate for establishing the cause, diagnosis, prognosis, prevention, or treatment of a disorder. Perhaps the reference lists from textbooks could help identify other potential resources.

As you begin to launch your search, you might consider working with the librarian at your institution. Share your clinical questions with the librarian. He or she will be able to point you in the right direction and provide some consultation. It is important for you to work with the librarian and participate in computerized searching that needs to be conducted. Your understanding of the topic and clinical experience are extremely valuable when working with the librarian.

Collaborating and networking with other nurses is another way to track down the best evidence. Perhaps such a strategy may involve using the Internet to access a discussion group. Posting a query about a topic may produce information and answers from other nurse colleagues. In addition, collaborating with nurses within one's specialty organization or at other clinical agencies may prove valuable.

Evidence Databases

Current best evidence from specific research studies can be found in a number of electronic databases. The best of these is Evidence-Based Medicine Reviews (EBMR) from OVID Technologies (www.ovid.com). EBMR combines several electronic databases, including MEDLINE, HealthSTAR, CANCERLIT, AIDSLINE, Best Evidence (BE), and the Cochrane Database of Systematic Reviews. Several of these databases are also available separately on CD-ROMs and the Internet.

MEDLINE is the largest biomedical research literature database and is available on CD-ROM and the Internet. MEDLINE comprises information from several print indexes, including Index Medicus, Index to Dental Literature, and International Nursing Index. MEDLINE indexes published research in allied health, biological sciences, information sciences, physical sciences, and the humanities. Because of its large size (over 10 million references), it is challenging to get exactly what you want. More specialized clinical research databases are available and easier to use (i.e., the Cochrane Database of Systematic Reviews).

HealthSTAR indexes published literature on health services, technology, administration, and research. The focus in this database is on both clinical and nonclinical aspects of health-care delivery. In addition to journals, HealthSTAR indexes material from books, book chapters, government documents, newspaper articles, and technical reports.

CANCERLIT indexes cancer literature, including journal articles, government reports, technical reports, meeting abstracts and papers, and monographs.

AIDSLINE indexes published literature on HIV infections and AIDS. It focuses on the biomedical, epidemiological, oncological, health-care administration, and social and behavioral sciences literature. AIDSLINE indexes literature from journal articles, monographs, meeting abstracts and papers, newsletters, and government reports.

The Cochrane Library is an electronic library designed to make available the evidence needed to make informed health-care decisions. The program presents the growing body of work of the Cochrane Collaboration and others interested in EBM. Currently, the library maintains four databases:

1. The Cochrane Database of Systematic Reviews
2. The Database of Abstracts of Reviews of Effectiveness
3. The Cochrane Controlled Trials Register
4. The Cochrane Review of Methodology Database

The **Cochrane Database of Systematic Reviews** is one of the most popular databases in The Cochrane Library; the database reviews individual clinical trials and summarizes systematic reviews from over 100 medical journals. When searching the Cochrane Review of Methodology Database, explicit selection criteria are needed. Each review includes the same predefined sections (i.e., description of study, methodological qualities of included studies, results, discussion, implications for practice). The Cochrane Review of Methodology Database provides an efficient method of interpreting the results of many studies.

There are several ways a researcher pulls together the accumulated information on a topic. Results of many studies are synthesized to produce new knowledge by a statistical method called meta-analysis. **Meta-analysis**, sometimes referred to as quantitative synthesis, is not a research design; rather, it is a method that takes the results of many studies in a specific area and synthesizes their findings to draw conclusions regarding the state of the science in the area of focus.[13] Instead of individual subjects being the unit of analysis, individual *studies* are the unit of analysis. Information is extracted about the strength of the relationship of the independent and dependent variables of each study. This information is quantified and an average score is computed across all studies.

Other Resources on Evidence-Based Health Care

ACP Journal Club. The **ACP Journal Club** is published by the American College of Physicians—American Society of Internal Medicine (http://www.acponline.com). The ACP Journal Club summarizes and interprets the best evidence of one recent study or review article from traditional journals, based on the criteria provided by the practitioner. Use of the ACP Journal Club is important when you need to know quickly about one study or review. Such a resource provides the best evidence from high-quality studies, selected from a variety of journals.

InfoPOEMS. **InfoPOEMS** (Patient-Oriented Evidence that Matters) is published by the *Journal of Family Practice* (http://www.infopoems.com). InfoPOEMS is a database similar to the ACP Journal Club in that it reviews and provides commentary on one recent article.

National Guideline Clearinghouse. The **National Guideline Clearinghouse** (http://www.guideline.gov) provides a collection of evidence-based clinical practice guidelines, without providing an integrative review. The Clearinghouse provides recommendations on a given topic from more than one organization, and often several (e.g., American Medical Association, Agency for Healthcare Research and Quality). These guidelines may reflect the bias of the particular author.

MD Consult. MD Consult (http://www.mdconsult.com) provides full-text access to textbooks, journal articles, practice guidelines, patient education handouts, and drug awareness information. Use MD Consult when you need to find some quick background information on a particular topic in a variety of formats. MD Consult provides current information, such as medical news, what patients are reading, clinical topics, and weekly updates from several journals.

Agency for Healthcare Research and Quality. The **Agency for Healthcare Research and Quality (AHRQ)** (http://www.ahcpr.gov) was formerly known as the Agency for Health Care Policy and Research (AHCPR). AHRQ has promoted EBP through the establishment of 12 Evidence-Based Practice Centers (EPCs). These centers are responsible for developing evidence guidelines and technology assessments on various clinical topics including diagnosis of sleep apnea, depression, acute sinusitis in children, and treatment of attention-deficit/hyperactivity disorder.

Many computerized databases are user friendly and have a great deal of help incorporated into their programs to help you with what you are looking for, while teaching you to be a better researcher. Basic tips associated with searching some of the databases listed above are provided in Table 3.5.

TABLE 3.5   Tips on Searching Databases

1. Basic/background information
   MD Consult
   National Guidelines
   MEDLINE/reviews
2. Short critiques or recent studies/reviews
   MEDLINE/abstracts
   InfoPOEMS
   Best evidence
3. Common well-studied topics
   MEDLINE/reviews
   InfoPOEMS
   Best evidence
   Cochrane
4. Practice guidelines/algorithms
   National Guidelines
   Cochrane
   MD Consult
   MEDLINE/guidelines
5. Uncommon/specific/current topic
   MEDLINE

Appraising the Evidence Critically

After completing the search on a particular topic, it is important to read and critically appraise the resulting evidence before being applied in practice. General strategies when reading research articles include skimming the report and then reading it more thoroughly. It is often helpful to collaborate with someone with more research expertise. When nurses first start reading research, they may feel hesitant and unsure about their abilities. Inexperienced research readers often use their common sense and clinical expertise to critique the design and identify problems and issues.

Various hierarchies of evidence have been developed and used over time. Several different approaches to grading evidence or use of a rating scale have been proposed. While there is no general consensus among researchers and/or associations about what constitutes different grades and/or levels of evidence, most hierarchies rank randomized control trials (RCTs) as the strongest. For many years, the focus on "effectiveness of health-care interventions" has been the main reason RCTs have been ranked as the strongest level of evidence.[14] Effectiveness is concerned with whether an intervention works as intended and achieves the desired outcomes.[14] Thus, it can be argued that multi-center RCTs provide the best possible evidence for the effectiveness of an intervention with results being generalizable to different populations, settings, and circumstances. A general hierarchy of research evidence is presented in Table 3.6. Refer to Sackett et al[4] for a detailed discussion of levels of evidence and grades of recommendation. An example of levels of evidence as proposed by The Joint ACCP/AACVPR Pulmonary Rehabilitation Guidelines Panel[15] is presented in Table 3.7.

Ethical Concerns Around EBP

In practicing EBM it is important for all health-care professionals to share research findings and research evidence with patients and their families as part of the decision-making process regarding care and treatment.[9] Information must be shared in ways that invite patients to participate in these decisions. Presentation of information should include whether there is a great deal of evidence in support of a certain

TABLE 3.6	Hierarchy of Research Evidence
• Meta-analysis of randomized clinical trials	STRONGEST Evidence
• Individual randomized clinical trials	
• Individual cohort study	
• Outcomes research	
• Individual case-control study	
• Case studies	
• Expert opinion	WEAKEST Evidence

TABLE 3.7	The Joint ACCP/AACVPR Pulmonary Rehabilitation Guidelines Panel: Summary of Hierarchy of Evidence

Strength of Evidence

A. Scientific evidence provided by well-designed, well-conducted, controlled trials (randomized and nonrandomized) with statistically significant results that consistently support guideline recommendation

B. Scientific evidence provided by observational studies or by controlled trials with less consistent results to support guideline recommendation

C. Expert opinion that supports guideline recommendation because available scientific evidence did not present consistent results or because controlled trials were lacking

Type of Evidence

I. Evidence from systematic review or meta-analysis of all relevant randomized controlled trials (RCTs) or EBP clinical practice guidelines based on systematic reviews or RCTs

II. Evidence from at least one well-designed RCT

III. Evidence from well-designed controlled trials without randomization

IV. Evidence from well-designed case-control and cohort studies

V. Evidence from systematic reviews of descriptive and qualitative studies

VI. Evidence from single descriptive or qualitative studies

VII. Evidence from opinion or authorities and/or reports of expert committees[12]

Source: Adapted from: ACCP/AACVPR: Special report: Pulmonary rehabilitation, Joint AACP/AACVPR evidence-based guidelines. Chest 112:1363, 1997.

treatment and/or therapy, what benefits are likely to be realized and which ones are more in doubt, and what are the likely adverse outcomes versus uncommon ones. You need not feel obligated to present findings and evidence independent of your appraisal of them. You should feel free to express your informed views regarding the meaning of findings, particularly as they apply to the patient with whom you are talking.[9]

WEB LINKS

The following Web sites offer students some helpful information on the best evidence for health care, including clinical information and practice guidelines.

Agency for Healthcare Research & Quality
  http://www.ahrq.gov
The Cochrane Collection
  http://www.cochrane.org
National Guideline Clearinghouse
  http://www.guidelines.gov

SUMMARY OF KEY IDEAS

1. Evidence-based medicine (EBM) is a movement that has developed to assist health-care professionals to base their care on the best research evidence possible.

2. Evidence-based nursing (EBN) eliminates the attention to the type of research design and incorporates the use of theory-derived and research-based information.

3. Research utilization is the process by which knowledge generated from research becomes incorporated into clinical practice.

4. A delay in using nursing research findings in clinical practice still exists today.

5. The practice of EBM is focused on several steps, including selecting and formulating clinical question(s), forming a team, tracking down the best evidence, and appraising the evidence critically.

6. Use of the PICO model provides structure when framing a clinical question so that an appropriate literature review can be performed.

7. Best evidence from research studies is found in a number of electronic databases. The best of these is Evidence-Based Medicine Reviews (EBMRs) from OVID Technologies, which includes the Cochrane Database of Systematic Reviews.

8. Meta-analysis is a statistical technique that takes the results of many studies in a specific area and synthesizes their findings to draw conclusions regarding the state of the science in the area of focus.

9. It is important for health-care professionals to share research evidence and findings with patients and their families with professional sensitivity and responsibility.

LEARNING ACTIVITIES

1. Obtain a copy of a research-based practice guideline developed by one of the Evidence-Based Practice Centers through the Agency for Healthcare Research and Quality (AHRQ). Complete the Appraisal of Evidence Form for a Practice Guideline.

Synopsis
What does the guideline address?

What population of patients is the guideline intended for?

What are the key decision points addressed by the guideline?

What process was used to develop the guideline?

Credibility Profile

Is the guideline based on a comprehensive meta-analysis or integrative review?

Is the scientific basis for each recommendation provided?

Are the key decision points addressed?

At each decision point, was the full range of actions evaluated?

Is the discussion of the way the panel reached decisions convincing that all evidence was considered in an impartial manner?

Are the guidelines current?

Was the panel that developed the guidelines made up of people with the necessary skills, expertise, and backgrounds?

Are the recommendations credible?

Applicability Profile

Does the guideline address a problem, decision, or situation seen in practice?

Is the guideline being used in whole or in part?

Are the recommended courses of action acceptable and feasible to you and your patients?

To follow the guideline, what will you have to do differently?

Do you have the resources, skills, and equipment to implement this guideline accurately and safely?

Should you adopt this guideline in its entirety?

Should you adopt parts of it?

How will you know if your patients are benefiting from your use of the guideline?

REFERENCES

1. Sackett, DL, et al: Evidence-based medicine: What it is and what it isn't. Br Med J 312:71, 1996.
2. Ingersoll, GL: Evidence-based nursing: What it is and what it isn't. Nurs Outlook 48:151, 2000.
3. McEwen, M, and Wills, EM: Theoretical Basis for Nursing. Lippincott Williams & Wilkins, Philadelphia, 2002, pp 356–358.
4. Sackett, DL, et al: Evidence-Based Medicine: How to Practice and Teach EBM, ed. 2. Churchill Livingstone, Edinburgh, 2000, pp 1–35.
5. Nicoll, LH, and Beyea, SC: Research utilization. In Fain, JA (ed): Reading, Understanding, and Applying Nursing Research: A Text and Workbook. FA Davis Company, Philadelphia, 1999, pp 262–264.
6. Polit, DF, and Beck, CT: Essentials of Nursing Research: Methods, Appraisal, and Utilization, ed. 6. Lippincott Williams & Wilkins, Philadelphia, 2006, p 458.
7. Titler, MG: Developing an evidence-based practice. In LoBiondo-Wood, G, and Haber, J (eds): Nursing

Research: Methods, Critical Appraisal, and Utilization, ed. 6. Mosby-Year Book, St. Louis, 2006, pp 440–441.

8. Wood, MJ: The state of evidence-based practice. Clin Nurs Res 17:71, 2008.

9. Brown, SJ: Knowledge for Health Care Practice: A Guide to Using Research Evidence. WB Saunders, Philadelphia, 1999, pp 15–19, 188–196, 241.

10. Titler, MG, et al: The Iowa model of evidence-based practice to promote quality. Crit Care Nurs Clin North Am 13:497–509, 2001.

11. Titler, MG: Developing an evidence-based practice. In LoBiondo-Wood, G, and Haber, J (eds): Nursing Research: Methods, Critical Appraisal, and Utilization, ed. 6. Mosby-Year Book, St. Louis, 2006, pp 445–446.

12. Melnyk, BM, and Fineout-Overholt, E: Evidence-Based Practice in Nursing and Healthcare: A Guide to Best Practice. Lippincott Williams & Wilkins, Philadelphia, 2005.

13. LoBiondo-Wood, G, and Haber, J: Nonexperimental designs. In LoBiondo-Wood, G, and Haber, J (eds): Nursing Research: Methods, Critical Appraisal, and Utilization, ed. 6. Mosby-Year Book, St. Louis, 2006, pp 253–254.

14. Evans, D: Hierarchy of evidence: A framework for ranking evidence evaluating healthcare interventions. J Clin Nurs 12:77, 2003.

15. ACCP/AACVPR: Special report: Pulmonary rehabilitation, Joint AACP/AACVPR evidence-based guidelines. Chest 112:1363, 1997.

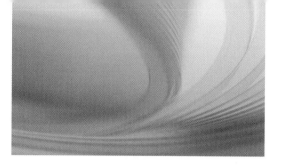

PART 2

Planning a Research Study

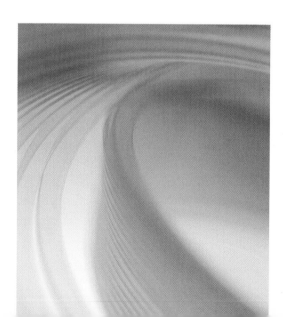

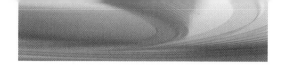

CHAPTER

4

SELECTING AND DEFINING A PROBLEM

James A. Fain, PhD, RN, BC-ADM, FAAN

LEARNING OBJECTIVES

By the end of this chapter, you will be able to:

1. Distinguish between a problem statement and the purpose of a study.
2. Identify several characteristics of a good problem statement.
3. Identify a problem statement in a journal article.
4. Cite different sources of ideas for selecting a research problem.
5. Describe the purpose of a literature review.
6. Identify the characteristics of a relevant literature review.
7. Differentiate between primary and secondary sources.
8. Compare advantages and disadvantages of print and computer database sources for searching the literature.

GLOSSARY OF KEY TERMS

Electronic databases. Bibliographic files that can be accessed by the computer through an online search (i.e., directly communicating with a host computer over telephone lines or the Internet) or by CD-ROM (compact discs that store bibliographic information).

Empirical literature. Data-based literature that presents reports of completed research; also called scientific literature.

Literature review. A critical summary of the most important scholarly literature on a particular topic. Scholarly literature can refer to research-based publications and conceptual or theoretical literature.

Operational definitions. Explanations of concepts or variables in terms of how they are defined for a particular study.

Primary source. Source reported by the person(s) who conducted the research or developed the theory; refers to original data or firsthand facts.

Problem statement. A statement of the topic under study, outlining all relevant variables within the study, providing justification for the choice of topic, and guiding the selection of the research design.

Purpose statement. A statement that describes why the study has been created.

(Continued)

Refereed journals. A journal that determines acceptance of manuscripts based on the recommendations of peer reviewers.

Replication. The duplication of research procedures in a second study to determine whether earlier results can be repeated.

Scientific literature. A data-based literature presenting reports of completed research.

Secondary source. Source reported by person(s) other than the individual(s) who conducted the research or developed the theory; usually represents a comment, summary, or critique of another's work.

Theoretical literature. Conceptual articles presenting reports of theories, some of which underlie research studies, and other non–research-related material.

Selecting and defining a research problem begins with identifying a potential problem and ends with at least one hypothesis or research question. The process is based on a thorough review and critical analysis of the literature. As the problem is identified, the researcher refines it until it is amenable to empirical investigation. This process entails much time and thought. This chapter focuses on the formulation and evaluation of problem statements and on how a researcher conducts a literature review.

Problem Statement

Formulating and defining the problem is the first and most important step in the research process. The **problem statement** provides direction for the research design and is typically stated at the beginning of a research report or journal article. The opening sentences describe the problem and focus on what is being studied. The problem statement justifies the study by citing background information about the problem and its contributions to practice, theory, or both. In other words, the problem statement makes a case for conducting the study and provides the basis for generating a variety of research purposes. When the problem statement is effectively written, the remaining steps of the research process fall into place.

The problem statement is the foundation of the research design. Problem statements consist of several paragraphs identifying a significant researchable problem, citing significant literature sources to justify the research study, and stating the goals of the study. Complete problem statements are usually not found in most journal articles owing to page limitations.

Excerpt 4.1 presents a problem statement that has been published in a journal article. Within the first few sentences, authors identify an area of research (e.g., how women with breast cancer can find meaning in their lives throughout the recovery process) and outline pertinent variables.

EXCERPT 4.1

Example of a Problem Statement

According to the American Cancer Society (ACS), breast cancer is the number one cancer diagnosed in women today; one in eight women will have breast cancer during their lifetime. In a report titled, "Cancer Facts and Figures 2007–2008," the ACS estimated that 240,510 women were newly diagnosed with breast cancer in 2007 and that more than 40,000 women of all ages will die from breast cancer. Breast cancer represents a pivotal change in any woman's life regardless of her age. Women fear the diagnosis of breast cancer more than they fear myocardial infarction, although myocardial infarction is more likely to kill them.

The experience of breast cancer can create many challenges for a woman; it also can be a catalyst for change and growth. Currently, there is a 90% 5-year survival rate for white women and a 76% survival rate for African American women; 20-year survival rates are greater than 50%. Self-transcendence can help women face the challenges of breast cancer and attain a sense of spiritual well-being across the course of the disease and for the remainder of their lives. Coward (1998) found that women who have been diagnosed with breast cancer eventually have an increased sense of well-being, have a purpose in life, and develop interconnectedness with others. According to Coward and Reed (1996), through self-transcendence, women with breast cancer can be healed and find meaning in their lives throughout the recovery process.

Spiritual well-being and spiritual practices employed by women recovering from breast cancer have not been described in the literature. Knowledge of the spiritual well-being and practices of women recovering from breast cancer is important for holistic nursing care. Nurses can assist women to understand dimensions of spiritual well-being and engage in spiritual practices that lead to enhanced self-transcendence.

Source: Thomas, JC, et al: Self-transcendence, spiritual well-being, and spiritual practices of women with breast cancer. J Holist Nurs 28:115–122, 2010.

Characteristics

By definition, the problem statement describes a problem in need of investigation. A basic prerequisite of a research problem is that it must be researchable. A researchable problem is one that researchers can investigate by collecting and analyzing data. By using the scientific method, the researcher attempts to make conclusions based on data or information concerning key concepts in the problem. To collect these data, the researcher must create operational definitions.

Operational definitions are clear-cut statements of how variables are measured. These definitions are important if quantitative research is to be meaningful. For example, the concepts of self-transcendence, spiritual well-being, and spiritual practices are addressed in Excerpt 4.1. To render these concepts operational, the researcher provides measurable definitions that are valid reflections of the concepts. In most journal articles, the operational definitions are found in the "Methods" section under the subheading of "Instruments" or "Data Collection."

Ethical and philosophical problems are not researchable. These types of problems elicit a range of opinions with no right or wrong answers. For example, prolonging the dying process with inappropriate measures; caring for patients/families who are misinformed; or not considering the patient's quality of life. Research can be used to assess how people feel about such problems but cannot resolve them. Debating these issues, however, may elicit further knowledge that might be useful.

Another characteristic of a problem statement concerns whether the problem is significant enough to warrant a study. The problem should have the potential for contributing to and extending the scientific body of nursing knowledge. Haber[1] has identified several criteria that serve as a guideline for selecting research problems (Table 4.1).

Once the problem has been identified, the feasibility of the study needs to be considered. Despite how researchable or significant a problem may be, the following variables must also be considered to determine whether a problem is appropriate for study: availability of subjects, time and money constraints, researchers' expertise, cooperation of others, available resources, and any ethical considerations. Access to faculty advisors or experienced researchers can help a beginning researcher decide a problem's feasibility.

Purpose Statement

The purpose of the study is a single statement that identifies why the problem is being studied. The **purpose statement** specifies the overall goal and intent of the research while clarifying the knowledge to be gained. The purpose of the study, seen more commonly in journal articles, is stated objectively and indicates the type of study to be conducted.

In some journal articles, the purpose statement is found at the end of the final paragraph reviewing the literature. In other journal articles, a

TABLE 4.1	Guidelines for Selecting Research Problems

- Clients, nurses, the medical community, and society will potentially benefit from the knowledge derived from the study.
- Results will be applicable to nursing practice, education, and/or administration.
- Results will be theoretically relevant.
- Findings will lend support to untested theoretical assumptions, challenge an existing theory, or clarify a conflict in the literature.
- Findings will potentially formulate or alter nursing practices or policies.

separate paragraph is devoted to the purpose statement. In Excerpt 4.2, two examples of purpose statements are displayed. One purpose statement is stated prior to the literature review (Background) while the other purpose statement is placed at the end of the problem statement. Note that both purpose statements are setting the stage for a different type of research design.

EXCERPT 4.2

Example of Two Purpose Statements

The incidence of diabetes has reached an epidemic level in the United States, with the disease affecting nearly 9% of the population. The prevalence of diabetes increased more than 60% in the decade from 1990 to 2001 (CDC, 2005), and the disease was the sixth leading cause of death in the United States in 2002. The majority of people with diabetes have type 2 diabetes, which is characterized by insulin resistance and relative insulin deficiency. Although autoimmune destruction of beta cells is not a factor, the insulin secretory response is inadequate to compensate for insulin resistance.

Latinos, the fastest growing minority group in the United States, are among the hardest hit by the diabetes epidemic. The prevalence of diabetes in Latinos is approximately 10%, 1.7 times the rate seen in non-Latino whites. The prevalence rate increases with age, and whereas approximately 21% of all people above 60 years will have diabetes, of Latinos age 50 years or older, 25%–30% have diabetes.

Self-management of diabetes is crucial to achieving glycemic control, and tight glycemic control decreases the incidence of microvascular complications. Glycemic control is assessed by monitoring glycosylated hemoglobin (HbA1C), which reflects the average level of glycemia over the preceding 3 months.

Self-management strategies, such as weight loss and diet changes to limit episodes of hyperglycemia after meals, are foundational for glycemic control. Making the necessary dietary changes is particularly challenging as it generally requires modification of food preferences that have been established over the course of a lifetime and may be culturally bound.

Some researchers have suggested that Latinos have difficulty in achieving adequate glucose control, leading to the stereotyping of Latinos as noncompliant. However, several studies have suggested that culturally tailored diabetes interventions aimed at improving self-managing skills may result in improved glycemic control. Specific cultural modifications in these studies included the use of promoter (lay peer educators) and bilingual nurses and dietitians, the incorporation of Mexican American dietary preferences and cultural beliefs, low-literacy materials, and content delivery in Spanish. The purpose of the study was to test the feasibility and examine the effects of a culturally tailored intervention for Mexican Americans with type 2 diabetes.

Source: Vincent, D, Pasvogel, A, and Barrera, L: A feasibility study of a culturally tailored diabetes intervention for Mexican Americans. Biological Res Nurs 9: 130–141, 2007.

(Continued)

EXCERPT 4.2

Example of Two Purpose Statements—cont'd

Advances in medical technology are contributing to longer life expectancies, making care of the elderly an important global health issue. The prevalence of depressive symptoms in the elderly around the world is varied, but tends to be high. For example, the prevalence of depressive symptoms ranged from 26% to 40% among community-dwelling older persons in Europe and 12.8% to 55% among community-dwelling and institutional older adults in Taiwan.

Common risk factors identified for depressive symptoms are poor perceived health, poor cognitive status, and impaired ability to perform activities of daily living. Another strong predictor of depression in older persons is the level of social support. Due to lack of family support and poverty, residents of public elder care homes may be vulnerable to depression. However, the major concern of these institutions is to provide living arrangements for elderly residents, so their health issues may be underestimated. The purpose of this study was to explore self-care management strategies and risk factors for depressive symptoms among residents of public elder care homes in Taiwan.

Source: Tsai, Y: Self-care management and risk factors for depressive symptoms among Taiwanese institutional older persons. Nurs Res 56:124, 2007.

Brink and Wood[2] suggest that the purpose statement can be written in one of three ways: as a declarative statement, as a question, or as a hypothesis. Choosing which form to use depends on the researcher's knowledge of previous research findings. The purpose statement should include information about what the researcher intends to do (describe, identify, observe); information about the setting (where the researcher plans to collect data); and information about the subjects.

In Excerpt 4.2, both purpose statements were written as declarative statements. In the first example, the purpose of the study was to test the feasibility and examine the effects of a culturally tailored intervention for Mexican Americans with type 2 diabetes. This purpose statement contains information about what the researcher intends to do (test/evaluate effects of a tailored intervention), the setting of the study (diabetes education program), and the subjects of the study (Mexican Americans with type 2 diabetes).

Sources and Selection of Research Problems

Selecting a problem can be a difficult step in the research process. Students may spend many hours or days asking themselves, "How am I going to identify a significant problem that is appropriate to study?" The difficulty is not a lack of problems; the possibilities are endless.

Rather, the difficulty is learning how and where to find researchable problems, which can be an overwhelming task.

Nursing Practice

Research problems come from a variety of sources. However, the most meaningful ones are usually those derived from nursing practice or the investigator's own experience. Burns and Grove[3] acknowledged that nursing practice offers an important source of clinically relevant research problems. Nurses can develop observational and analytical skills that maximize each opportunity for discovering important questions and problems.

As an example of research derived from nursing practice, Domiano and colleagues[4] examined the practice of taking blood pressure measurements (BPMs). The upper arm is the primary site to use when taking a BPM. However, under certain circumstances it may not be possible to use the upper arm when taking BPMs. The forearm is then a commonly used alternative. A review of literature reveals that in a majority of studies, the forearm BPM has been higher when compared to upper arm BPM. Study findings may, however, be misleading because of different populations and individual characteristics being studied. The effect of individual characteristics on upper arm versus forearm differences has not been well documented and needs further study.

Literature Review

Another source for research problems is the literature. Examining the literature can generate ideas for possible areas of research. Examples of many kinds of problems that have been observed by other researchers can be found in research studies reported in various nursing and related journals. Additional questions and problems identified from published studies can provide the opportunity to expand on the work of others.

Theory

Investigating problems derived from theory can provide meaningful contributions to nursing knowledge. Researchable problems based on theory are less likely to involve a clinical problem; they are usually concerned with more general and abstract explanations of phenomena.[3]

Reading theories developed in nursing and other disciplines can provide research problems through a deductive process. The researcher reads theoretical schemata and conceptual frameworks that have been published in existing literature and asks whether a particular theory, such as stress and coping, adaptation, or family theory, might explain certain patterns observed under specified conditions. As an example of generating research problems based on theories or conceptual models, Heinrich[5] conducted a descriptive correlation study of men with HIV disease. The purpose of the study was to examine the relationship among hope, social support, uncertainty in illness, and spirituality and their effects on the perceived health of HIV seropositive men. The proposed conceptual model was based on theoretical propositions and empirical findings and tested by path analysis.

Selecting a problem based on theory may be a bit complex for beginning researchers, which is not to say that a hunch based on experience will never lead to a theoretical problem. It is more probable, however, that such a problem will result in an applied research study.

Replication

Replication is the duplication of research procedures in a second study to determine whether earlier results can be repeated. Beck[6] provided strong evidence that implementing research findings into nursing practice has been seriously hampered by the lack of replication studies. Some researchers believe replication to be less scholarly or less important than original research. Yet, replication of certain studies provides an excellent opportunity for researchers to discover results that conflict with previous research or disconfirm some aspect of an established theory.[7,8]

Selecting a Research Problem

The first step in selecting a problem is to identify a general problem area related to your area of expertise. Examples of problem areas may include the following:

- Factors that affect the duration of breastfeeding in adolescent mothers
- Patients' psychosocial adjustment after a cardiac event
- Perceived effect of illiteracy on patients receiving prenatal care
- Roles of the family in post-traumatic stress syndrome
- Communication patterns between health-care providers and child-care workers

A great deal of reading is required, and many hours must be devoted to planning and conducting the study. The next step is to narrow down the general problem area to a specific researchable problem. A problem that is too general would involve reviewing many unrelated articles. The literature review would inevitably be unnecessarily increased, resulting in many more hours spent in the library. This, in turn, would complicate the organization of the results and the subsequent hypothesis development. A problem that is too general leads to a study with too many variables that produces results that may be difficult to interpret.

Review of Related Literature

Having identified a researchable problem, the researcher is usually excited about moving ahead with the project. Too often, the literature review is considered a tedious and time-consuming process. This notion may be due to a lack of understanding of the purpose and importance of the literature review, along with a feeling of uneasiness by researchers who are not sure exactly how to proceed.

Definition, Purpose, and Scope

The **literature review** involves identification and analysis of relevant publications that contain information pertaining to the research problem. The literature review serves several important functions that make it worth the time and effort. The major purpose of reviewing the literature is to discover what is already known about the problem. This knowledge not only helps the researcher avoid unintentional duplication, but also provides the understanding and insight necessary to develop a logical framework. In other words, the literature review provides the researchers with important information concerning what has been done and what needs to be done. The purpose of a literature review is summarized in Table 4.2.

Beginning researchers seem to have difficulty determining the depth of a literature review. Although they understand that all literature directly related to their problem should be reviewed, they often do not know when to quit. They have trouble determining which articles are "related enough" to their problem to be included in the literature review. Deciding how much of a literature search is enough is based on the researcher's judgment. These decisions become easier after the researcher has conducted several literature reviews.

TABLE 4.2 Purpose of a Review of Literature

- Determines what is known and not known about a subject, concept, or problem.
- Determines gaps, consistencies, and inconsistencies in the literature about a subject, concept, or problem.
- Discovers unanswered questions about a subject, concept, or problem.
- Describes the strengths and weaknesses of designs/methods of inquiry and instruments used in earlier work.
- Discovers conceptual traditions used to examine problems.
- Generates useful research questions or problems for the discipline.
- Determines an appropriate research design/method (instruments, data collection, and data analysis methods) for answering the research question.
- Determines the need for replication of a well-designed study or refinement of a study.
- Promotes the development of protocols and policies related to nursing practice.
- Uncovers a new practice intervention or gains support for changing a practice intervention.

Several guidelines can help the beginning researcher determine what is appropriate for the literature review. First, the researcher must avoid the temptation to include everything. A well-defined literature review is preferred to one that contains many articles that are just somewhat related to the problem. Second, well-researched areas usually provide substantial amounts of literature directly related to the problem. Third, a common misconception is that the significance of a problem is related to how much literature is available. This is not so. In some areas of study, a lack of research-based articles increases the value of the study. However, researchers should not assume there is no further need of research when a topic reveals many already-published studies. Although topics are usually well developed, additional research may be needed and even specified in a published article.

Searching for Relevant Literature

Once the problem has been identified, the search for appropriate literature can begin. Important considerations when beginning the literature search are as follows:

- How many years back should you go?
- What literature should you search?
- How many articles and books do you need for an adequate literature search?
- Do you go beyond the library resources for information?

To answer the foregoing questions, researchers need to acquaint themselves with the library and the process of searching through the literature. Deciding how much of the literature review is needed becomes a difficult task until part of the literature review has been accomplished. Locke, Spirduso, and Silverman[9] identified a retrieval system as the searching process by which researchers screen a variety of published literature (e.g., research reports, research reviews, theoretical speculation, and scholarly discourse). The retrieval systems in large health science libraries and smaller institutions may vary enormously. Each discipline also may have its own particular mechanisms for searching the literature. Locke, Spirduso, and Silverman[9] identified several rules that attempt to make any retrieval effort more efficient (Table 4.3).

Sources of Information

Nursing Journals

Major sources of information for literature reviews are contained in nursing and social science journals that serve as available sources of the latest information on clinical topics. Because books usually take longer to publish, journals are the preferred mode for communicating the latest results

TABLE 4.3 **Rules for Searching the Literature**

1. Begin by planning how you will conduct your literature review. Do not just go to the library and start searching the literature. Instead, first talk with faculty and other colleagues who have some familiarity with the problem area and find out what they think you should read. Gather the recommended articles, skim over them, and record full citations of those that seem appropriate. Review the reference list in each article to determine which citations are most directly related to the problem. Retrieving these citations should be your priority when you return to the library.

2. When you go back to the library, talk first with the reference librarian, who can identify the retrieval systems that are most likely to be appropriate for your research problem. Do not begin by starting to search for literature.

3. Plan to devote a considerable amount of time learning how each retrieval system works. Use computerized systems whenever they are available, but do not automatically assume that a manual search is without value.

4. Think of your retrieval efforts as consisting of a series of stages.
   a. Identification. Find and record citations that seem potentially relevant. This work is done with indexes, bibliographies, reference lists, and computers.
   b. Confirmation. Determine whether the items identified can be obtained. This is work done with library holdings of serials and books, reprint services, interlibrary loan, and microfiche files.
   c. Skim and Screen. Assess each item to confirm that it actually contains content to be reviewed. Much of this work can be accomplished without obtaining the actual resource item and spending time in the stacks. The most important retrieval skill is the ability to resist the temptation to stop skimming and screening and immerse yourself in reading.
   d. Retrieval. Acquire the literature by checking out books, copying articles from journals, ordering microfiche and reprints, and requesting interlibrary loans. Not everything must be (or should be) retrieved. There is a strong argument for not having every article at hand when you draft the literature review.
   e. Review. Read and study the literature.

5. Keep track of all words used to identify or describe what you have learned; these will become the key words used by indexing systems for accessing their holdings. Building a key word list is like acquiring a set of master keys to a large building.

6. Always take advantage of other people's work. Research reviews in your area should have the highest priority in your search plan, as should annotated bibliographies and the reference list at the back of every article and book you retrieve. What could be a better search strategy than reading the reviews of literature crafted by students who have worked on similar problems? Dissertation Abstracts International is the "Yellow Pages" of research retrieval.

(Continued)

TABLE 4.3	**Rules for Searching the Literature—cont'd**

7. Record a complete citation for every item you identify as being useful for your research problem. Keep a record of what you find by using index cards or a computer program that alphabetizes and sorts by key words. No frustration can match that of having to backtrack to the library for a missing volume or page number.

8. As you make notes during the skimming and screening stages, make sure that your notes are clearly your own and not those of another author. Write any quotes verbatim, and attach the proper page citation.

of a research study. Refereed journals are important sources of scholarly literature. A **refereed journal** uses a panel of reviewers to review manuscripts for possible publication. Reviewers are chosen by the editor for their expertise as clinicians, researchers, and/or administrators. The reviews are usually performed blind, meaning that the reviewers do not know the name(s) of the author(s). A list of nursing journals that contain research and conceptual articles is found in Table 4.4. **Empirical literature**, sometimes referred to as **scientific literature**, is data-based literature presenting reports of completed research. Conceptual articles refer to **theoretical literature**, in which reports of theories, some of which underlie research studies, and other non–research-related material are presented.[1]

Primary Versus Secondary Sources

Several sources of literature are available to help the researcher conduct a literature review. These sources are divided into two categories: primary

TABLE 4.4	**Appropriate Journals for Literature Reviews**

- *Advances in Nursing Science*
- *Applied Nursing Research*
- *Clinical Nursing Research*
- *Journal of Advanced Nursing*
- *Journal of Nursing Scholarship*
- *Journal of Professional Nursing*
- *Journal of Qualitative Research*
- *Nursing and Health Care*
- *Nursing Research*
- *Nursing Science Quarterly*
- *Research and Theory for Nursing Practice*
- *Research in Nursing and Health*
- *Scholarly Inquiry for Nursing Practice*
- *Western Journal of Nursing Research*
- *Worldview on Evidence-Based Nursing*

sources and secondary sources. A **primary source** is written by the person(s) who developed the theory or conducted the research. An appropriate literature review mainly reflects the use of primary sources. In historical research, a primary source is an eyewitness or an original document. A **secondary source** is a brief description of a study, written by a person(s) other than the original researcher. Often a secondary source represents a response to, or a summary and critique of, the original researcher's work. Excerpt 4.3 provides an example of a secondary source of information.

EXCERPT 4.3

Example of a Secondary Source

Morgan, W, Raskin, P, and Rosenstock, J: Comparison of fish oil or corn oil supplements in hyperlipidemic subjects with NIDDM. Diabetes Care 18:83, 1995. Commentary by James A. Fain, PhD, RN, BC-ADM, FAAN.

Advanced practice nurses need to interpret the results of this study with caution. Findings showed that subjects who used fish oil supplements had significantly lower total plasma triglycerides and plasma very low-density lipoproteins (VLDL) compared with subjects who received corn oil supplements. A major lipid problem in patients with NIDDM is hypertriglyceridemia. Several studies have shown that hypertriglyceridemia in NIDDM is exaggerated by high-carbohydrate diets regardless of the carbohydrate source (e.g., simple or complex). Experimental and clinical studies further suggest that partial replacement of complex carbohydrates with monounsaturated fats may improve the hypertriglyceridemia of NIDDM without raising LDL cholesterol or compromising glycemic control.

Studies also have shown that polyunsaturated fatty acids (PUFAs) can lower plasma cholesterol levels, particularly LDL cholesterol. PUFAs are divided into two types: omega-6 and omega-3. These fatty acids may also have a beneficial effect for patients with NIDDM who have a greater risk of developing cardiovascular disease. The major source of omega-3 fatty acids may be beneficial to individuals with NIDDM because of the ability of fatty acids to reduce serum triglycerides. However, large doses of fish oils are needed to produce such an effect that, in turn, can elevate glucose levels and increase insulin requirements. More clinical trials with larger sample sizes are needed to confirm these findings of this study.

Advanced practitioners need to be aware that several capsule forms of omega-3 are available to the public and not regulated by the FDA. Dietary supplementation with fish oil capsules is generally not recommended. Instead, patients should be encouraged to eat 6 to 8 ounces of fish per week. Although salmon, mackerel, and herring are good sources of omega-3, consumption of all kinds of fish should be encouraged because of its low fat content and proportion of PUFAs.

Source: Fain, JA: A comparison of fish oil or corn oil supplements in hyperlipidemic subjects with NIDDM [Commentary]. APN SCAN 3:18, 1995.

Databases, Indexes, and Abstracts

Several strategies for locating research references are available. Most nursing students have access to college and university libraries and assistance from a reference librarian. **Electronic databases**, bibliographic files that can be accessed by the computer, are available either through an online search (i.e., directly communicating with a host computer over telephone lines or the Internet) or by CD-ROM (compact disks that store bibliographic information).[10] Most electronic databases are available through computer searches and can be accessed using software programs such as OVID, PaperChase, and SilverPlatter. These programs are user friendly and menu driven and have on-screen support. With such advances in technology, the search for references on a particular topic is greatly enhanced.

Computer searches have traditionally been performed using centralized databases, such as Medical Literature On-Line (MEDLINE) (medicine, nursing, and hospital articles) offered by the National Library of Medicine. The Cumulative Index to Nursing and Allied Health Literature (CINAHL) is another useful database for nurses. CINAHL covers references to all English-language and many foreign-language nursing journals as well as books, book chapters, nursing dissertations, and selected conference proceedings in nursing and allied health. The database covers materials dating from 1982 to the present.[10] PsycINFO (psychology online); AIDSLINE (AIDS information on-line); CancerLit (cancer literature); ERIC (Educational Resources Information Center); and CHID (Combined Health Information Database) are commonly used databases that have existed since the 1960s. Examples of commonly used databases along with Internet resources[11] relevant to nursing are shown in Table 4.5. A computer-assisted literature search is most effective when the topic has been well defined.

Knowing how to search the literature is an essential skill. Consulting with the reference librarian is well worth the time and effort. Among the most important approaches to finding relevant literature are manual searches of indexes. Indexes provide bibliographic citations, including names, titles, journals, dates, and pages. Indexes are used to find journal sources (periodicals) of data-based and conceptual articles on various topics. Depending on the topic, several indexes exist, including Hospital Literature Index, which covers nonclinical aspects of health-care delivery such as health planning, financial management, cost containment, and utilization review. Each index contains several volumes. Another important index for nursing research is the International Nursing Index, published by the *American Journal of Nursing*. Examples of other frequently used indexes are shown in Table 4.5.

Abstracts are summaries of articles that appear in other journals. Because titles can be misleading, abstracts are especially useful for determining if a particular reference is relevant to an area of study before

TABLE 4.5	Common Databases and Internet Resources Relevant to Nursing

Print Databases

1. Cumulative Index to Nursing and Allied Health Literature (CINAHL) (formerly called Cumulative Index to Nursing Literature): Known to many as "red books"
2. International Nursing Index (INI): Published by the American Journal of Nursing Company in cooperation with the National Library of Medicine (NLM)
3. Nursing Studies Index: Developed by Virginia Henderson; includes nursing literature from 1900 to 1959
4. Index Medicus (IM): Oldest health-related index
5. Health and Psychosocial Instruments (HAPI)

Electronic Databases

1. AIDSLINE (AIDS and HIV coverage)
2. BIOETHICSLINE (Biomedical ethics coverage)
3. CINAHL
4. EBM—Cochrane, ACP, Journal Club
5. MEDLINE
6. MEDLINEPlus
7. PsychINFO
8. QOLID (Quality of Life Instruments Database)
9. Social Sciences Citation Index

Health-Related Internet Directories

1. Bureau of the Census (http://www.census.gov)
2. Centers for Disease Control and Prevention (http://www.cdc.gov)
3. Evidence-Based Nursing (http://www.bmjpg.com/dataebnpp.html)
4. Health Web (http://www.healthweb.org)
5. Healthy People 2010 (http://www.web.health.gov/healthypeople)
6. Medscape (http://www.medscape.com)
7. National Guideline Clearinghouse (http://guideline.gov)
8. National Library of Medicine (http://www.nlm.nih.gov)
9. National Center for Health Statistics (http://www.cdc.gov.nchswww)
10. National Institute of Nursing Research (http://www.nih.gov/ninr)

searching for it on the shelves. Several abstract journals that are appropriate for nursing literature include *Nursing Abstracts*, *Psychological Abstracts*, *Sociological Abstracts*, *Child Development Abstracts*, and *Dissertation Abstracts*.

Analyzing, Organizing, and Reporting

For beginning researchers, the hardest part of writing the literature review may be thinking about how difficult the task will be. More time may be spent worrying about the process than doing it. Analyzing, organizing, and reporting is made easier by following the steps outlined in Table 4.3. The researcher should begin by reading through the notes quickly, which refreshes the memory and may also reveal some references that no longer seem sufficiently relevant. The following steps are recommended for writing a literature review:

1. Identify the major ideas (usually two or three) that are related to the problem statement.
2. List the concepts either in descending order of importance or in terms of logical presentation. Determine whether one concept needs to be understood before another can be introduced.
3. Prepare an outline using the major concepts as major headings. The time put into the outline at this stage will save time later and increase the chances of having an organized literature review. The outline does not have to be extremely detailed to be useful (Table 4.6).
4. Divide each major heading into logical subheadings, if applicable. The need for further differentiation is determined by the problem. More complex problems require more subheadings (see Table 4.6).
5. In a sentence or two, summarize the major findings of each study. Include complete reference citations.
6. Write an introductory paragraph explaining the significance of the two or three major concepts.
7. At the end of each section, summarize the findings for each group of studies. Write a paragraph at the end of each major concept or topic that summarizes the key points, supports the cohesiveness of the subheadings, and establishes the relevance of the proposed problem.
8. Compile the entire literature review and scan it for coherence, continuity, and smoothness of transition from one topic to the next. Carefully check each citation for accuracy.

TABLE 4.6 **Outlining the Literature Review**

Research Question: What are the smoking behaviors of women after being diagnosed with lung cancer?
First-stage outline: Identify concepts that provide the rationale for the study.

- Smoking is related to lung cancer.
- Smoking behaviors are associated with sociodemographic variables.
  Second-stage outline: Develop subheadings for each major concept.

   I. Smoking is related to lung cancer.
     A. Incidence of women who smoke.
     B. Gender-specific differences in smoking.

TABLE 4.6	**Outlining the Literature Review—cont'd**

II. Smoking behaviors are associated with sociodemographic variables.
  A. Relationship of smoking behaviors among women of color and ethnic background.
  B. Relationship of smoking behaviors of women in young, middle, and older adulthood.

Third-stage outline: Add most important references that support each subheading.

I. Smoking is related to lung cancer.
  A. The percentage of women who smoke has decreased from 33% in 1974 to 23% in 1990. However, the rate of decline is slower in women than in men, and women are smoking at an increasingly earlier age (Centers for Disease Control, 1993; Grit, 1993; USDHHS, 1989). Even a family history of lung cancer does not deter some women from smoking (Horowit, Smaldone & Viscoli, 1988).
  B. Investigations of gender-specific differences in smoking and quitting behavior suggest that women have more difficulty quitting (Blake et al, 1989; Grit, 1982; Novotony et al, 1990; Orlandi, 1987). Women are more likely than men to have tried to quit or to have actually quit after diagnosis of lung cancer (Grit, Nisenbaum, Elashoff, and Holmes, 1991).

II. Smoking behaviors are associated with sociodemographic variables.
  A. In an analysis of smoking patterns of white, Hispanic, and black men and women with cancer, white women were noted to have the highest smoking prevalence (29.6% of current smokers) (Spit et al, 1990).
  B. Continued smoking was reported most frequently in women ages 20 to 34 years and less frequently in women ages 65 years and older. Middle-aged women (45 to 65 years), however, smoked the most cigarettes per day.

CRITIQUING REVIEWS OF THE LITERATURE

Identify a research study to critique. Read the study to see if you recognize any key terms discussed in this chapter. Remember that all studies may not contain all key terms. The following questions serve as a guide in critiquing literature reviews.

1. *Has the literature review been conducted in a thorough manner?* Is the problem introduced within the first couple of paragraphs?

Within the first few paragraphs, the reader should be oriented quickly to the major areas of study. It is important that author(s) state the area of study concisely, what literature will be considered, and why some literature may be omitted.

2. *Can you identify the most relevant articles on the topic of interest?* How far back (publication dates) were the articles chosen to be included in the literature review? Look over the reference list, and make an assessment that the literature chosen supports and explains the rationale for this particular study. Literature reviews can be somewhat misleading. The purpose is *not* to demonstrate a comprehensive understanding of the general area. Instead, author(s) should be placing the hypotheses and/or research questions in the context of previous work to support and explain knowledge that this study intends to fill.

3. *Have the author(s) used mostly primary rather than secondary sources?* In almost all instances, articles presented in nursing journals reflect original research written by those individuals who actually conducted the research (primary source). Use caution with secondary sources because the description of a study may not be entirely correct.

4. *Has evaluation of key articles been presented succinctly in terms of critical appraisal of methodology and interpretation of results?* Identify if the literature review is only a summary of past work, with a historical account of each study and important milestones that lead up to the present study. It is important to compare and contrast the contributions of key studies, while discussing the strengths and weaknesses in existing research studies and identifying important gaps in the literature.

5. *Is there a summary statement or overall evaluation of the literature?* All good literature reviews end with a summary statement (or paragraphs) of the state of the science on the topic just discussed.

WEB LINKS

The following Web sites offer students some helpful information on selecting and defining a research problem.

American Nurses Association/Online Journal of Issues in Nursing
　http://nursingworld.org/ojin
OVID
　http://www.ovid.com
PaperChase
　http://www.paperchase.com

SUMMARY OF KEY IDEAS

1. The problem statement presents the topic to be studied, along with a description of the background and rationale for its significance.

2. A good problem statement expresses a relationship between two or more variables and can be investigated by collecting and analyzing data.

3. The purpose of a study is expressed as a single statement or question that specifies the overall goal of the study.

4. Nursing practice and personal experiences are good sources of research problems. Ideas can also come from literature, nursing theory, and previous research.

5. A literature review involves identifying, obtaining, and analyzing literature that is related to the research problem.

LEARNING ACTIVITIES

Problem Statement I

Coronary heart disease (CHD) is the leading cause of death for women in the United States. Approximately 250,000 to 500,000 American women die of CHD annually (Cochrane, 1992; Rich-Edwards, Manson, Hennekens, & Buring, 1995; Steingart, et al, 1991; Wenger, 1985). However, most women are unaware of the risk associated with developing CHD relative to other diseases. For example, one of five women will die from CHD compared with one of nine women who will die from breast cancer (Rich-Edwards, et al, 1995; Steingart, et al, 1991). In fact, the mortality rate for women with CHD exceeds that for all neoplastic diseases combined.

Coronary heart disease has long been thought of as a man's disease (Rich-Edwards, et al, 1995). The fact that women have been underrepresented in nearly all randomized, controlled studies of CHD until recently both reflects and contributes to a mistaken belief that women are not significantly affected by CHD (Barry, 1992). Reasons for excluding women from such studies include fear of teratogenicity; increased variability caused by a woman's menstrual cycle, pregnancy, and menopause; increased cost; and the false belief that gender-specific effects are unlikely to significantly influence treatment outcomes (Annual Report/Women's Health Research, 1991).

Consequently, little is known about gender differences in the presentation, pathophysiology, and treatment outcomes for CHD. Research involving women with CHD is in its infancy; the scientific basis for care offered to women with CHD is based largely on data extrapolated from clinical trials in which most of the subjects were men (Cochrane, 1992). The lack of data about women with CHD raises yet more questions regarding gender differences.

Of particular concern is the poorer survival rate for women compared with men following a myocardial infarction (MI). This finding is based on data from landmark studies such as the Framingham Heart

Study and the Multicenter Investigation of the Limitation of Infarct Size or MILIS Trial (Tofler, et al, 1987; Wingate, 1993). The increased incidence of mortality among women who experience an MI may reflect their older age and more coexisting illness at onset, suboptimal or delayed treatment, or both (Wenger, Speroff, & Packard, 1993).

A delay in treatment of MI has extensive consequences because myocardial cell death with irreversible loss of cellular function begins to occur 20 to 40 minutes after the onset of myocardial ischemia. Early intervention and treatment can dramatically reduce the irreversible loss of myocardial tissue (Ayanian & Epstein, 1991; Maynard, 1992). Therefore, early intervention for MI is paramount.

Yet several studies show that women undergo less intensive or less invasive evaluations than men, despite equal or more severe symptoms (Wenger, et al, 1993). Tobin and colleagues (1987) found that 4 percent of women, compared with 40 percent of men, with abnormal radionuclide scan during exercise were referred for cardiac catheterization. Data from the Multicenter Survival and Ventricular Enlargement (SAVE) Trial showed that women with a confirmed MI were less likely than their male counterparts to undergo cardiac catheterization (Mark, Shaw, DeLong, Califf, & Pryor, 1994; Steingart, et al, 1991). Using data from Massachusetts and Maryland state insurance claims (11,865 discharge summaries from Massachusetts and 6894 from Maryland), the overall rate for coronary angiography referrals among patients hospitalized for known CHD was 15 percent to 28 percent higher for men than for women (Ayanian & Epstein, 1991).

Maynard and Weaver (1992) suggested that there is something about the characteristics of chest pain at the time of emergency room evaluation and during the first few days of hospitalization that make it difficult to arrive at the diagnosis of acute MI in women. In fact, the clinical presentation of women with ischemic-type sensations may differ from that of males; women may actually have a different constellation of symptoms associated with MI. Data from the Myocardial Infarction Triage and Intervention (MITI) Registry revealed differing associated symptoms. Women complained more often of fatigue, nausea, and upper abdominal pain than men, and more men than women experienced diaphoresis (Maynard, 1992). In addition, data from the Framingham Heart Study showed that more women than men experience silent ischemia (the absence of chest pain)—34 percent versus 27 percent, respectively.

The current practice of differentiating between typical versus atypical symptoms of MI based on data extrapolated from clinical trials in which most of the subjects were male could be problematic. The purpose of this study is to determine whether a relationship exists between the gender differences in the presenting symptoms of acute MI and the typical evaluation of women with CHD.

Problem Statement 2

Osteoporosis is an age-related skeletal disorder with multiple etiologies, characterized by decreasing bone mass and increasing bone fragility when there are no other identified diseases (Ockene, 1994; Lappe, 1994). Fifty percent of all American women older than 45 years develop osteoporosis; 75 percent are affected by age 90 years (McMahon, Peterson, & Schilke, 1992). One in four white women will have at least one fracture by age 65, resulting in 1.5 million fractures/year (Erickson & Jones, 1992). The current health-care cost of $7 to $10 billion/year related to fractures resulting from postmenopausal osteoporosis is expected to reach $31 to $62 billion/year by the year 2020 (Lappe, 1994).

The primary treatment of postmenopausal osteoporosis is building and maintaining peak bone density during the years of skeletal maturation. Peak bone mass is reached by age 30 years. The goal of early intervention in young women is to maximize the bone mass by affecting the risk factors for osteoporosis. Lappe (1994) identified the major risk factors for development of postmenopausal osteoporosis as genetic influences; metabolic and endocrine status; dietary factors; exercise patterns; and exposure to drugs, alcohol, and cigarettes.

Dietary intake of calcium and protein affects the body's ability to achieve peak bone mass by age 30 years. At birth the total skeleton contains 25 g of calcium and increases to 1000 g at maturity, all from dietary intake (El-Choufli, Nelson, & Kleerekoper, 1994). One study recommended that young women monitor dietary intake of calcium and use calcium supplements to achieve the recommended calcium intake of 1200 to 1500 mg/day for adolescents and young women (Erickson & Jones, 1992).

Physical activity and weight-bearing exercises influence bone density in the maturing skeleton through the process of mechanical loading on bones. This longitudinal force stimulates osteoblasts to increase production, thereby maximizing and strengthening bone mass. Decreased activity levels have resulted in increased urinary excretion of calcium, with resultant decreases in bone mass and skeletal growth (Rutherford, 1990). A study of gender and developmental differences in exercise beliefs and performance compared boys and girls in grades six, seven, and eight in two school districts (Garcia, et al, 1995). Findings showed that girls continue to be a high-risk group for inactivity and could develop lifelong sedentary habits, with increased risk for skeletal deterioration.

Several studies have been published related to osteoporosis and behaviors aimed at its prevention in perimenopausal and postmenopausal women. However, no data are available about younger women and osteoporosis. A study of 91 postmenopausal women revealed that these women did not perform adequate osteoporosis prevention behaviors (Ali & Bennet, 1992). This study investigated the relationship between knowledge of osteoporosis and osteoporosis prevention behaviors, perceptions of barriers and benefits to milk intake, and health-promoting behaviors such as exercise. Higher levels of knowledge were associated with more consistent health practices and greater milk intake. Older postmenopausal women generally had less knowledge about osteoporosis than did younger postmenopausal women.

The lack of published research about osteoporosis knowledge, beliefs, and prevention behaviors in women who are still young enough to affect their peak bone mass reflects a significant problem. This information is critical to the development of appropriate educational and health-maintenance programs for younger women. The purpose of this descriptive study is to assess the knowledge of osteoporosis risk factors and preventive behaviors among women between the ages of 16 and 22 years.

Activity

1. Evaluate problem statements 1 and 2 by identifying:
   a. What is being studied.
   b. The justification for the study.
   c. The focus of the study (statement of purpose).
   d. The population being studied.

2. Rank each problem statement on a scale of 1 to 5 (5 = Excellent, 4 = Very Good, 3 = Good, 2 = Fair, 1 = Poor) as to the:
   a. Clarity.
   b. Importance to nursing.
   c. Comprehensiveness.
   d. Logical presentation.

3. Select a topic of interest. Identify four articles related to one of the concepts within the topic, and complete an outline similar to the one in Table 4.6.

REFERENCES

1. Haber, J: Developing research questions and hypotheses. In LoBiondo-Wood, G, and Haber, J (eds): Nursing Research: Critical Appraisal and Utilization, ed. 6. Mosby, St. Louis, 2006, pp 46–79.
2. Brink, PJ, and Wood, ME: Basic Steps in Planning Nursing Research: From Question to Proposal, ed. 5. Jones & Bartlett, Boston, 2001, pp 69–82.
3. Burns, N, and Grove, SK: The Practice of Nursing Research: Conduct, Critique, & Utilization, ed. 4. WB Saunders, Philadelphia, 2001, pp 87, 90.
4. Domiano, KL, Hinck, SM, Savinske, DL, and Hope, KL: Comparison of upper arm and forearm blood pressure. Clin Nurs Res 17:241, 2008.
5. Heinrich, CR: Enhancing the perceived health of HIV seropositive men. West J Nurs Res 25:367, 2003.
6. Beck, CT: Replication strategies for nursing research. Image J Nurs Sch 26:191, 1994.

7. Martin, PA: More replication studies needed. Appl Nurs Res 8:102, 1995.

8. Taunton, R: Replication: Key to research application. Dimens Crit Care Nurs 8:156, 1989.

9. Locke, LF, Spirduso, WW, and Silverman, SJ: Proposals That Work: A Guide for Planning Dissertations and Grant Proposals, ed. 5. Sage Publications, Thousand Oaks, CA, 2007, pp 63–90.

10. Polit, DF, and Beck, CT: Essentials of Nursing Research: Methods, Appraisal, and Utilization, ed. 6. Lippincott Williams & Wilkins, Philadelphia, 2006, pp 134–138.

11. Gillis, A, and Jackson, W: Research for Nurses: Methods and Interpretation. FA Davis Company, Philadelphia, 2002, pp 79–84.

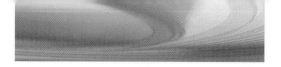

CHAPTER

5

APPLYING APPROPRIATE THEORIES AND CONCEPTUAL MODELS

JAMES A. FAIN, PHD, RN, BC-ADM, FAAN

LEARNING OBJECTIVES

By the end of this chapter, you will be able to:
1. Discuss the relationship between theory and research.
2. Describe the process of inductive and deductive reasoning.
3. Differentiate between the three types of theories (i.e., grand, middle-range, and practice).
4. Discuss the importance of borrowed theories.
5. Distinguish between a concept and a construct.
6. Suggest a theory or conceptual model for a topic of inquiry.

GLOSSARY OF KEY TERMS

Borrowed theories. Theories taken from other disciplines and applied to nursing questions and research problems.

Concepts. Symbolic statements describing a phenomenon or a class of phenomena.

Conceptual model. A set of abstract and general concepts that are assembled to address a phenomenon of interest. Sometimes referred to as theoretical framework or conceptual framework.

Constructs. Higher-level concepts that are derived from theories and that represent nonobservable behaviors.

Deductive approach. An approach to reasoning that generates theory by beginning with known facts, moving from the general to the specific. It is an approach used to test predictions and validate existing relationships.

Grand theories. Theories that are complex and broad in scope. Grand theories attempt to explain broad areas and include numerous concepts that are not well defined and that have ambiguous and unclear relationships.

(Continued)

Inductive approach. An approach to reasoning that involves collecting observations that lead to conclusions or hypotheses. This approach moves from specific observations to general statements that can be tested through research.

Metaparadigm. Refers to the primary or central phenomena that are of interest to a particular discipline.

Middle-range theories. Theories that look at a piece of reality and that contain clearly defined variables in which the nature and direction of relationships are specified.

Nursing theory. A specific and concrete set of concepts and propositions that accounts for or characterizes phenomena of interest to the discipline of nursing.

Practice theories. Theories that are more specific than middle-range theories and that produce specific directions or guidelines for practice.

Theory. An organized and systematic set of interrelated statements (concepts) that specify the nature of relationships between two or more variables, with the purpose of understanding a problem or nature of things.

Research is not conducted just to answer research questions or to test hypotheses; rather, it is conducted to develop through generating or testing of theory a body of knowledge unique to nursing. To build this knowledge effectively, the research process should be developed within some theoretical structure that facilitates analysis and interpretation of findings. When a study is placed within a theoretical context, it is theory that lets us speculate on the questions of why and how treatment works and what variables are related to one another. Thus, theory provides the structure for a research study, allowing the researcher to generalize beyond a specific situation and make predictions about what should happen in other, similar situations.[1] Research without theory results in disconnected information or data, which does not add up to an accumulated knowledge of nursing. This chapter provides a basic overview of theory as it relates to research and presents common terminology associated with the elements of theory. Criteria for evaluating theories and conceptual models will be described. Students interested in learning more about theories and conceptual models should pursue additional readings to acquire an in-depth understanding of the topic.

Overview of Theory

As researchers begin to explain and predict phenomena as a way of gaining knowledge, facts are collected through empirical investigations. As these facts accumulate, there is need for integration, organization, and classification in order to make the isolated facts meaningful. Researchers bring empirical findings into meaningful patterns that take the form of theories.

Defining theory is not an easy task because of the many fields of inquiry that contribute to the development of nursing knowledge.[2] At a basic level, **theory** is an organized and systematic set of interrelated statements (concepts) that specify the nature of relationships between two or more variables with the purpose of understanding a problem or nature of things.[3] Theories are organized and provide meaning to a complex collection of individual facts and observations. Theories pull together the results of observations, allowing researchers to make general statements about variables and the relationships among variables.

Theories serve several purposes in the development of science and clinical practice, depending on how we choose to use them. Theories summarize existing knowledge, giving meaning to isolated empirical findings. Theory provides a structure or framework that describes, explains, and predicts. It offers organization of nursing knowledge and provides a systematic means of collecting data to describe, explain, and predict nursing practice.[1]

The term "framework" refers to the conceptual underpinnings of a study. In a study based on a theory, the framework is usually referred to as the theoretical framework. In a study that has its roots in a specified conceptual model, the framework is often called the conceptual framework. These terms—"theoretical framework," "conceptual framework," and "conceptual model"—are often used interchangeably throughout the literature.[4]

Inductive Versus Deductive Approach to Discovering New Knowledge

The role that theory plays in clinical practice and research is best described by examining the relationship between theory and data. Figure 5.1 identifies the integration of inductive and deductive reasoning, starting from observations and moving up to concepts and theories. Researchers agree that the role of theory and data collection are essential features of the scientific method. There are two approaches to discovering or testing new knowledge. The researcher may move from observations to an idea (inductive approach) or from an idea to observations (deductive approach). Researchers who stress theory versus those who emphasize observations reflect a deductive theory-testing approach versus an inductive inquiry that is oriented toward discovery.

The **inductive approach** involves collecting observations that lead to conclusions or hypotheses. This approach begins with specific observations and moves to general statements that can be tested through research. Inductive reasoning underlies qualitative approaches to inquiry. In situations where conclusions are arrived at using very specific or limited data, generalizations of results can be erroneous.[5] Thus, study results can only be generalized to the sample in which data were collected.

The **deductive approach** generates theory by beginning with known facts moving from the general to the specific. It is an approach used to test predictions and validate existing relationships. Specific hypotheses

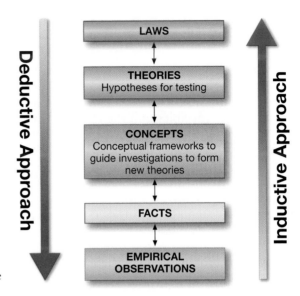

Fig 5•1 Integration of inductive and deductive reasoning.

can be deduced from a theory that serves as a more general statement of interrelated phenomena. Deductive reasoning helps to unveil existing relationships. As with inductive reasoning, inherent problems may exist with the deductive approach. Not all deductions can be verified, particularly when the methods of measurement are poor or undeveloped.

The validity of nursing knowledge generated through inductive and deductive reasoning depends on the accuracy of information or premises with which one is working. Conclusions are valid if the premises (statements) on which they are based are valid. Research is used to confirm or refute premises so nurses in practice may use them.[6]

Classification of Theories in Nursing

Theories unique to nursing help define how nursing is different from other disciplines. Fawcett[7] defines **nursing theory** as a specific and concrete set of concepts and propositions that claims to account for or characterize phenomena of interest to the discipline of nursing.

The term **metaparadigm** refers to the primary phenomena that are of interest to a particular discipline. The primary or central phenomena within nursing revolve around the concepts of person, environment, health, and nursing.[7] The first nurse scholar to disseminate writings on the central phenomena was Fawcett. The four concepts were not formalized as the metaparadigm of nursing until 1984. Definitions of each metaparadigm concept are displayed in Table 5.1.

Theories that deal with these four metaparadigm concepts are referred to as nursing theories. Nursing theories are classified according to the complexity and amount of abstraction in addressing person, environment,

TABLE 5.1	Nursing's Four Metaparadigm Concepts

1. The metaparadigm concept *person* refers to the individuals, families, communities, and other groups who are participants in nursing.
2. The metaparadigm concept *environment* refers to the person's significant others and physical surroundings, as well as to the setting in which nursing occurs, which ranges from the person's home to clinical agencies to society as a whole. The metaparadigm also refers to all the local, regional, national, and worldwide cultural, social, political, and economic conditions that are associated with the person's health.
3. The metaparadigm concept *health* refers to the person's state of well-being at the time that nursing occurs, which can range from high-level wellness to terminal illness.
4. The metaparadigm concept *nursing* refers to the definition of nursing, the action taken by nurses on behalf of or in conjunction with the person, and the goals or outcomes of nursing actions. Nursing actions are typically viewed as a systematic process of assessment, labeling, planning, intervention, and evaluation.

health, and nursing. Grand theory (macrotheory) describes a comprehensive conceptual framework; middle-range theory describes a framework that is relatively focused; and practice or prescriptive theory is smallest in scope.

Grand Theories

Grand theories are complex and broad in scope. They attempt to explain broad areas and include numerous concepts that are not well defined and that have ambiguous and unclear relationships. Because these theories are not grounded in empirical data, they are usually not useful as guides for nursing practice. In most instances, grand theories require further specification and partitioning of theoretical statements for them to be empirically tested and theoretically verified.

Use of a systems approach that focuses on the human needs for protection or relief from stress is central to the discipline of nursing. Gerstle, All, and Wallace[8] conducted an exploratory correlational study guided by the Neuman systems model to explore the impact of stressors on the quality of life of adult patients with chronic pain. Patients' perceptions of their health, functional status, and socioeconomic status, as well as psychological, spiritual, and familial aspects of life, were examined. The Neuman model views an individual as a system containing five components (i.e., physiological, psychological, developmental, sociocultural, and spiritual). Stability of the system is determined by its ability to cope with stressors. Based on Neuman's model, results revealed that a higher quality of life was associated with participants who were older, female, and employed, whereas a lower quality of life was associated with participants with a low income, higher treatment costs, and a lack of workers' compensation insurance. Other examples of grand theories developed by nurse theorists are presented in Table 5.2.

Middle-Range Theories

Middle-range theories were first introduced in the field of sociology[9] during the late 1960s. By the mid-1970s, middle-range theories were recognized as the latest step in knowledge development. Merton[9] describes **middle-range theories** as those that look at a piece of reality and contain clearly defined variables in which the nature and direction of relationships are specified.

Over the past 10 years, middle-range nursing theories have gained more popularity than grand theories because they are more specific, organized within a limited scope, contain fewer concepts/variables that are concrete and operationally defined, and have a stronger relationship with practice and research. Nursing has recognized middle-range nursing theories as appropriate for defining or refining the substantive component of nursing science and practice. The purpose of middle-range theories is to describe, explain, and predict phenomena; unlike grand theories, they are explicit and testable. Middle-range theories involve concepts and relationships that link practice and research, providing direction for everyday practice and research embedded in the discipline of nursing. Smith and Liehr[10] have published a text compiling 12 major middle-range theories. In reading each of the 12 middle-range theories, it is obvious that nursing has moved forward in the development of theoretical knowledge while presenting new opportunities for expanding the science of nursing through research and theory.

TABLE 5.2	Example of Grand Theories

- Faye G. Abdellah: Patient-centered approaches to nursing
- Virginia Henderson: The principles and practice of nursing
- Dorothy Johnson: The behavioral system model
- Imogene King: King's systems framework and theory of goal attainment
- Madeline Leininger: Cultural care diversity and universality theory
- Myra E. Levine: The conservation model
- Betty Neuman: The Neuman systems model
- Margaret Newman: Health as expanding consciousness
- Dorothea E. Orem: The self-care deficit nursing theory
- Rosemarie Rizzo Parse: The theory of human becoming
- Martha Rogers: The science of unitary and irreducible human beings
- Sister Callista Roy: The Roy adaptation model
- Jean Watson: Nursing—Human science and human caring: A theory of nursing

An example of a middle-range theory is Pender's Health Promotion Model. Kerr, Lusk, and Ronis[11] used Pender's Health Promotion Model (HPM) to identify factors that influenced Mexican American workers' use or nonuse of hearing protection devices (HPDs). Derived from social cognitive theory, the HPM is a useful middle-range theory. The HPM contains three major components: modifying factors, cognitive-perceptual factors, and health-related behavior use of HPDs. Modifying factors such as demographic characteristics and interpersonal influences are proposed as indirect influences on health-related behavior, exerting their influence through the cognitive-perceptual factors that directly affect behavior. Other examples of middle-range theories used in nursing are presented in Table 5.3.

Practice Theories

Practice theories, sometimes referred to as prescriptive theories, are important in developing a science of nursing practice.[3] Practice theories are more specific than middle-range theories and produce specific directions or guidelines for practice. These theories are aimed at providing knowledge about what nurses do in their practice, how they get to do what they do in practice, and what is affected (outcomes).[3] Practice theories can cover a particular element of a specialty, such as oncology nursing, obstetric nursing, or operating room nursing, or they may relate to another aspect of nursing, such as nursing administration or nursing education. Such theories typically describe elements of nursing care, such as cancer pain relief, or a specific experience, such as dying and end-of-life care. Practice theories contain few concepts and are easily understandable. They are usually narrow in scope, limited to specific populations, and explain a small aspect of reality.[1] Some examples of practice theories are presented in Table 5.4.

TABLE 5.3	**Example of Middle-Range Theories**

- Kathryn Barnard: Parent-child interaction
- Cheryl Beck: Postpartum depression theory
- Patricia Benner: Benner's model of skills acquisition in nursing
- Mary Burke and Margaret Hainsworth: Chronic sorrow
- Cheryl Cox: Motivation in health behavior (health self-determinism)
- Joan Eakes: Theory of chronic sorrow
- Elizabeth Lenz: Theory of unpleasant symptoms
- Ramona Mercer: Maternal role attainment
- Merle Mishel: Uncertainty of illness theory
- Nola Pender: Health promotion model
- Pamela Reed: Self-transcendence theory
- Cornelia Ruland and Shirley Moore: End-of-life care
- Sherri Ulbrich: Theory of exercise as self-care
- Janet Younger: Mastery of stress in mothers of preterm infants

TABLE 5.4	Example of Practice Theories

- Theories of caring, empowerment, and communication
- Theories of clinical inference and clinical decision making
- Theories of suctioning, wound care, rest, and learning
- Theory of end-of-life decision making

Borrowed Theories

As a practice profession, nursing often deals with phenomena that are not unique to nursing. A significant number of theories used as frameworks in nursing are based on theoretical work from other disciplines, such as sociology (e.g., sick-role theory); psychology (e.g., social-cognitive theory); or physiology (e.g., theory of pain perception). **Borrowed theories** are taken from other disciplines and applied to nursing questions and research problems. Knowledge gained from borrowed theories is useful provided the fit and relevance to nursing is clarified. In Excerpt 5.1, we see an example of a researcher expanding the theory of planned behavior (TPB) to help explain the influence of parents on adolescent behaviors and describe its application to adolescent sexual risk behaviors. Examples of borrowed theories are presented in Table 5.5.

EXCERPT 5.1

Example of Borrowed Theory Being Reconceputalized in a Nursing Study

The purpose of this article is to propose how one of the leading theories of health behavior, the theory of planned behavior (TPB), can be expanded to more explicitly incorporate the influences of parents on adolescent behavior. Although the TPB is known for its utility and predictive validity in understanding many health behaviors, the model pertains to the individual level. Influences outside the individual are not included; rather they are collectively relegated into the global category of "external influences." However, when addressing issues such as sexual risk behavior among adolescents, the exclusion of parental influences is a significant omission that limits the utility of the TPB.

In this analysis, TPB is expanded to incorporate a key influence from within an adolescent's most proximal environment: parents. Empirical evidence already exists to support the expanded model. The proposed expansion of the TPB indicates the conceptual underpinnings for family-based prevention programs to reduce HIV-related risk behaviors among adolescents.

Source: Hutchinson, MK, and Wood, EB: Reconceptualizing adolescent sexual risk in a parent-based expansion of the theory of planned behavior. J Nurs Schol 39:141, 2007.

TABLE 5.5	**Example of Borrowed Theories**

- Theories from sociology
- General systems theory
- Role theory
- Feminist theory
- Critical social theory
- Theories from the behavioral sciences (e.g., theory of planned behavior)
- Psychoanalytic theory
- Interpersonal theory
- Operant conditioning
- Human needs theory
- Person-centered theory
- Stress, coping, adaptation theory
- Theories from the medical sciences (e.g., homeostasis)
- Germ theory and principles of infection
- Theories of immunity and immune function
- Genetic principles and theories
- Pain management: Gate control theory

Concepts

Concepts are the building blocks of a theory. They are defined and understood within the theory of which they are part. Concepts are symbolic statements describing a phenomenon or a class of phenomena.[3] From birth, we begin to structure empirical impressions of the world around us in the form of concepts, such as "play," "food," or "mother," each of which implies a complex set of recognitions and expectations. Concepts vary in level of abstraction, from highly abstract (e.g., hope, love, empowerment, grief) to relatively concrete (e.g., pain, blood loss, temperature). Concepts are formulated in words that enable people to communicate their meanings about realities in the world.[3] Concepts develop within the context of experience and feelings so that they meet with our perception of reality. We supply labels to sets of behaviors, objects, and processes that allow us to identify and discuss them. A concept may be a single word (e.g., grief) or a phrase (e.g., maternal role attachment, health-promoting behaviors). Concepts may likewise have a theoretical or operational definition. In a theoretical definition, the concept is defined in relation to other concepts. A theoretical definition provides meaning to a term in the context of a theory. The operational definition identifies empirical indicators of the concept, which permits observation and measurement. An example of a theoretically and operationally defined concept is presented in Excerpt 5.2. Note how a theoretical definition of resilience is provided under the subheading Resilience (within the literature review), and the operational definition of resilience is provided under the subheading Methods (Measures).

Example of Theoretically and Operationally Defined Concept: Resilience

Resilience

Stewart and colleagues (1997) define resilience as the capacity of individuals to cope successfully with significant change, adversity, or risk; that the capacity changes over time; and that the capacity is enhanced by protective factors within the person and environment.

Methods

Measure

Resilience Scale (RS). Resilience, defined as beliefs in one's personal competence and acceptance of self and life that enhances individual adaptation, was measured by the Resilience Scale (RS). The RS is a 25-item self-report scale with a 7-point Likert response format. Possible scores ranged from 25 to 175, with higher scores indicating more resilience.

Source: Rew, L, Taylor-Seehafer, M, Thomas, NY, and Yockey, RD: Correlates of resilience in homeless adolescents. J Nurs Schol 33:33, 2001.

Higher-level concepts that are derived from theories and that represent nonobservable behaviors are called **constructs**. Examples of constructs are motivation, intelligence, anxiety, self-concept, achievement, and aptitude. What is observable is the behavior presumed to be a consequence of the hypothesized construct.

Conceptual Models

The term conceptual model is synonymous with such terms as conceptual framework and conceptual system. A **conceptual model** is defined as a set of abstract and general concepts that are assembled to address a phenomenon of central interest.[4,7] Conceptual models represent ideas or notions that have been put together in a unique way to describe a particular area of concern. The process may be likened to experiencing the world by looking through someone else's glasses or "walking in someone else's shoes." Because each person has different life experiences, wearing another's shoes changes the experience of events. Similarly, conceptual models put specific ideas or notions into a meaningful framework for viewing the world.[9] Conceptual models are loosely structured, as compared with theories, but provide a framework for communicating a particular perception of the world. In addition, conceptual models, like theories, can help facilitate the generation of hypotheses to be tested.

Discussion of Lazarus and Folkman's theory of stress and coping is shown in Excerpt 5.3. Note how the theoretical framework is a separate subheading within the Literature and Background section of the research

---

EXCERPT 5.3

Example of Theoretical Framework Linked to Nursing Problem

Literature Review and Background

Theoretical Framework for Growth in Parent Caregivers

Pediatric palliation is a stressful traumatic event for parent caregivers, yet a strength-based approach to understanding parents' experiences is also important. Folkman's (1997) revised theoretical framework of stress and coping and the conception of the construct of post-traumatic growth (PTG) of Tedeschi and Calhoun (1996, 2004) provide a lens for understanding both the positive and negative aspects of parental caregiving. Lazarus and Folkman (1984) originally proposed a cognitive theory of stress and coping in which an outcome, based on the appraisal of an event, could be either negative if the distress had not been resolved or positive if it had been resolved. In the revised model, Folkman recognized that positive emotion could in fact be present with or without resolution and could occur simultaneously with continuing distress. Tedeschi and Calhoun (1996) defined the concept of PTG and discussed its manifestations as experiencing new possibilities, enhanced relationships, enhanced strength, increased appreciation of life, and spiritual change. Their model attempted to explain the process involved in attaining PTG while acknowledging, similar to Folkman's model, that PTG can occur concurrently with continuing distress.

Purpose of the Study

Results reported in this article are from a secondary analysis of data obtained in a cross-sectional descriptive study. The primary study focused on the theoretical construct of PTG in the context of caregiving, with a particular focus on the factors that allow parent caregivers of children of life-limiting illnesses to not only survive but also grow from their experiences.

Source: Schneider, M, Steele, R, Cadell, S, and Hemsworth, D: Differences on psychosocial outcomes between male and female caregivers of children with life-limiting illnesses. J Pediatr Nurs 26:186, 2011.

---

study, with authors paying particular attention to making sure the framework relates back to nursing within the context of the problem being studied.

Conceptual Models of Nursing

Conceptual models of nursing not only provide direction for a study, but also present nursing in relation to the four central metaparadigm concepts (i.e., person, environment, health, nursing). Although some nurse researchers have used conceptual models of nursing that do not reflect all four concepts, the advantage of utilizing a nursing model is that the researcher views a study from a nursing perspective from the beginning. Within the nursing framework, each nursing model defines and relates the concepts in a unique manner. In essence, conceptual nursing models frame the way in which nursing will be viewed and the direction a research study will take.

CRITIQUING THEORIES AND CONCEPTUAL MODELS

Identify a research study to critique. Read the study to see if you recognize any key terms discussed in this chapter. Remember that all studies may not contain all key terms. The following questions[11] serve as a guide in critiquing theories and conceptual models.

1. *Was a theoretical framework clearly identified?* Discussion of the theoretical framework should be incorporated into several sections of the research report. First, the theoretical framework should be introduced and briefly described in the problem statement. Second, the framework should be described in more detail under its own heading, usually at the end of the literature review. Description of the theory should be from primary sources. Also, because theoretical frameworks are unfamiliar to many nurses, it is very important to read over the particular theory and become familiar with the concepts, relationships, and usefulness of the theory in extending nursing science. It will be difficult to determine if the theory was clearly stated, not knowing what the theory is all about.

2. *What type of theory (i.e., grand, middle-range, practice) was discussed?* Was the theory from nursing or another discipline? Look over the types of theories cited in Tables 5.2 to 5.5, and identify the theory stated in the research article. It is likewise important to examine the depth and extent of the literature review conducted. Has the author provided a sufficient amount of information to demonstrate the problem? Does the research contribute to the understanding of the phenomenon of interest? Is there a discussion related to the four metaparadigm concepts of nursing?

3. *Is the theory/framework consistent with a nursing perspective?* While the particular theory/framework does not have to originate from the discipline of nursing, it is important to consider its relevance to nursing. How the theory/framework relates to nursing within the context of the problem being studied needs to be articulated.

4. *Are concepts clearly and operationally defined in the study?* Concepts are selected for a theoretical framework based on their relevance to the phenomenon of interest. Thus, the problem statement, which describes the phenomenon of concern, will be a rich source of concepts for the framework. Each concept included in the framework needs to be defined conceptually and operationally in the methods section of the research report. This will explain how the framework influences or is reflected in the study's design, data collection strategies, and data analysis methods.

5. *Are study findings related to the theoretical rationale?* Findings of the study need to be discussed in terms of how they illustrate, support, challenge, or contradict the theoretical framework.

WEB LINKS

The following Web site offers students some general information on nursing theories.
General Information of Nursing theory
   http://currentnursing.com/nursing_theory

SUMMARY OF KEY IDEAS

1. A theory is a set of interrelated concepts that provide a view of reality for the purpose of describing, explaining, or predicting the phenomena of interest.

2. Nursing knowledge can be acquired through inductive and deductive reasoning.

3. The three types of theories (grand, middle-range, practice) are classified according to their level of abstraction.

4. Grand theories are global and attempt to describe and explain everything about a subject. Middle-range theories focus on a particular area of study and have clear propositions from which hypotheses can be derived. Practice theories are more specific and produce specific directions or guidelines for practice.

5. Knowledge gained from borrowed theories is useful, provided the fit and relevance to nursing are clarified. Concepts are the building blocks of theory.

6. A conceptual model is a set of abstract and general concepts that are assembled to address a phenomenon of interest.

7. Conceptual nursing models deal with the central phenomena of concern to nursing (i.e., person, environment, health, and nursing).

LEARNING ACTIVITIES

1. Select one of the theories cited in Table 5.1, and read one primary source of the theorist's original work. Review several research articles that cite the work of the particular theory, and answer the following questions:
   a. Do the research articles appear to use the theory appropriately?
   b. Are the studies consistent in their use of the theory?
   c. Did the studies contribute to the knowledge base of the theory? How?

2. Select one of the middle-range theories cited in Table 5.2, and read one primary source of the theorist's original work. Review several

research articles that cite the work of the particular theory, and answer the following questions.

a. Do the research articles appear to use the theory appropriately?

b. Are the studies consistent in their use of the theory?

c. Did the studies contribute to the knowledge base of the theory? How?

REFERENCES

1. McEwen, M, and Wills, EM: Theoretical Basis for Nursing. Lippincott Williams & Wilkins, Philadelphia, 2002, pp 23–68.
2. Chinn, PL, and Kramer, MK: Theory and Nursing: Integrated Knowledge Development, ed. 5. Mosby-Year Book, St. Louis, 1999, p 50.
3. Kim, HS: The Nature of Theoretical Thinking in Nursing, ed. 2. Springer Publishing Company, New York, 2000, pp 1–30.
4. Polit, DF, and Beck, CT: Essentials of Nursing Research: Methods, Appraisal, and Utilization, ed. 6. Lippincott Williams & Wilkins, Philadelphia, 2006, pp 153–174.
5. Liehr, P, and Smith, MJ: Theoretical framework. In LoBiondo-Wood, G, and Haber, J (eds): Nursing Research: Methods, Critical Appraisal, and Utilization, ed. 6. Mosby Elsevier, St. Louis, 2006, pp 111–125.
6. Gillis, A, and Jackson, W: Research for Nurses: Methods and Interpretation. FA Davis Company, Philadelphia, 2002, pp 10, 37–67.
7. Fawcett, J: Analysis and Evaluation of Contemporary Nursing Knowledge: Nursing Models and Theories. FA Davis Company, Philadelphia, 2000, pp 3–33.
8. Gerstle, DS, All, AC, and Wallace DC: Quality of life and chronic non-malignant pain. Pain Manag Nurs 2:98, 2001.
9. Merton, RK: Social Theory and Social Structure. The Free Press, New York, 1968.
10. Smith, MJ, and Liehr, PR: Middle Range Theory for Nursing, ed. 2. Springer Publisher Company, New York, NY, 2008.
11. Kerr, MJ, Lusk, SL, and Ronis, DL: Explaining Mexican American workers' hearing protection use with the health promotion model. Nurs Res 51:100, 2002.
12. Brockopp, DY, and Hastings-Tolsma, MT: Fundamentals of Nursing Research, ed. 3. Jones & Bartlett Publishers, Boston, 2003, pp 81–135.

FORMULATING HYPOTHESES AND RESEARCH QUESTIONS

James A. Fain, PhD, RN, BC-ADM, FAAN

LEARNING OBJECTIVES

By the end of this chapter, you will be able to:
1. Define a hypothesis.
2. Identify characteristics of a hypothesis.
3. Write different types of hypotheses.
4. Compare and contrast inductive versus deductive hypotheses, directional versus nondirectional hypotheses, simple versus complex hypotheses, and statistical (null) versus research hypotheses.
5. Describe the appropriate use of research questions.
6. Define independent, dependent, and extraneous variables.

GLOSSARY OF KEY TERMS

Complex hypothesis. A statement explaining and/or predicting relationships between two or more independent and dependent variables.

Deductive reasoning. A process that begins with a general picture and moves to a specific direction or prediction.

Dependent variable. A variable that is observed for changes or to assess the possible effect of a treatment or manipulation; may be the effect or outcome of an experimental procedure; also referred to as a criterion variable. Usually symbolized by the letter Y.

Directional hypothesis. A hypothesis that makes a specific prediction about the direction of the relationship between two variables.

Extraneous variable. A variable that is not controlled for in a study, which threatens the internal validity of the study.

Hypothesis. A statement about the relationship between the variables that are being investigated.

Hypothesis-generating study. A study that generates hypotheses by pulling together pieces of data from several descriptive/exploratory studies.

(Continued)

Independent variable. A variable that is manipulated and controlled by the researcher; also called a predictor variable. Usually symbolized by the letter X.

Inductive reasoning. A process that begins with details or specific observations and moves to a more general picture.

Nondirectional hypothesis. A hypothesis that does not stipulate in advance the direction and nature of the relationship between two variables.

Null hypothesis (H_0). A hypothesis stating that no relationship or difference exists between two variables. Also called statistical hypothesis.

Research hypothesis (H_1 or H_a). A hypothesis stating a relationship or difference between two variables. Also called an alternative, declarative, or scientific hypothesis.

Research question. A concise, interrogative statement written in the present tense that includes one or more variables.

Simple hypothesis. A statement explaining and/or predicting a relationship between one independent and one dependent variable.

Variable. A measurable characteristic that varies among the subjects being studied.

Hypotheses and research questions are formulated after the review of literature has been completed. The literature review identifies prior findings and provides a basis for understanding how the proposed study relates to previous knowledge. Hypotheses and research questions influence the study design, sampling techniques, and plans for data collection and analysis. Stating hypotheses and research questions requires the researcher to identify variables that are pertinent to the study. Determining how these variables are defined is important for purposes of measurement. This chapter focuses on the formulation of hypotheses and research questions; various types of variables are introduced and described.

Hypotheses

A **hypothesis** is a statement that explains or predicts the relationship or differences between two or more variables in terms of expected results or outcomes of a study. Researchers do not set out to prove hypotheses but rather to collect data that either support or refute them. A common misconception is that data must support the hypothesis for a study to be successful. Research studies do not have to prove anything to be considered worthwhile. Some of the most important findings have come from research in which the data did not support the hypothesis. A lack of support in research data forces the researcher to reevaluate the hypothesis.

Hypotheses serve several purposes. One purpose is to guide scientific inquiry for the advancement of knowledge. Researchers must go beyond mere gathering of isolated data and seek relationships and generalizations about the data. Another purpose is to provide direction for the research design and the collection, analysis, and interpretation of data. Hypotheses provide a basis for selecting the sample, the statistical analyses needed, and the relationships to be tested. For example, when the aim of a study is to explain certain relationships, the major emphasis is on linking the variables. Finally, hypotheses provide a framework for reporting the conclusions of a study; each hypothesis is tested separately, and conclusions relevant to each are stated.[1]

In a research study/report, hypotheses may be discussed under a separate subheading titled "Hypothesis." However, in many instances, hypotheses are not explicitly stated and may be inferred or implied after reading through the problem statement and purpose statement. Placement of hypotheses in a research study/report logically follows the literature review and theoretical framework.

Hypotheses are not always present in research studies/reports. In many instances, research studies/reports are guided by research questions. Descriptive or exploratory research studies usually do not have hypotheses. When there is lack of research on a particular topic, the intent of conducting the study focuses on describing rather than explaining phenomena. Thus, descriptive or exploratory research is important for laying the foundation for further study. The outcome of such studies allows the researcher to bring several pieces of data together so that hypotheses can be formulated for future studies. This is sometimes referred to as a **hypothesis-generating study**.

In some research studies/reports, research questions are present in addition to hypotheses. In many instances, the research questions may not directly pertain to the proposed outcomes stated in the hypothesis. Rather, the research questions may provide additional and sometimes serendipitous findings that enrich the study and provide direction for further study.[2]

Characteristics of Hypotheses

Nurses must know what constitutes good hypotheses to be able to read and critique research effectively. Good hypotheses state clearly and concisely the expected relationship (or difference) between two or more variables. Regardless of the specific format used to state a hypothesis, the statement includes the variables being studied, the population being studied, and the predicted outcomes. A general model for stating hypotheses is as follows: Subjects who receive X are more likely to have Y than subjects who do not receive X.

In the following examples, X represents the treatment (independent variable) or variable manipulated by the researcher and Y the observed outcome (dependent variable). Words and phrases such as "greater than," "less than," "positively," "negatively," and "difference" denote the direction of the proposed hypotheses.

Children ages 5 to 10 years old who are provided with prior information about their tonsillectomy will experience less postoperative anxiety than children of the same age who do not receive information.

Subjects = Children ages 5 to 10 years old
X = Provided with prior information
Y = Less postoperative anxiety

Nursing home residents exposed to 10 minutes of calming music experience less agitation than those who receive no such intervention.

Subjects = Nursing home residents
X = 10 minutes of calming music
Y = Less agitation

Children with a high sense of humor adjust better to having cancer than do those children with a low sense of humor.

Subjects = Children
X = Sense of humor (high versus low)
Y = Better adjustment to cancer

Patients who have had internal mammary artery grafting following coronary artery bypass surgery will experience greater chest pain or discomfort than patients who have had saphenous vein grafting.

Subjects = Patients
X = Internal mammary artery grafting following coronary artery
   bypass surgery
Y = Greater chest pain or discomfort

Excerpt 6.1 provides an example of two hypotheses from one study. In both examples, the population being studied (chemically dependent women); the treatment (subjects who participated in experiential and cognitive therapy groups versus those who did not); and the outcomes (higher levels of general and social self-efficacy) were presented.

All nouns in hypotheses or research questions should be defined first conceptually and then operationally. What if the characteristics of the subjects were not further defined in the article? How would you interpret the term "subjects"? People older than age 50 years? People 60 years and older? People 70 years and older? In applying research findings to practice, it is important to know how subjects are defined to be able to make a judgment about the applicability of the findings to a particular population. Similarly, a definition of "increased memory self-efficacy" should also be provided in this example. Later in this research report, an explanation of the intervention and memory self-efficacy is given, along with a description of the population being studied.

Variables identified in hypotheses must be operationally defined. This means specifying how the variables will be measured in terms of the

EXCERPT 6.1

Example of Two Hypotheses

To explore self-efficacy further with chemically dependent women, the following hypotheses were examined:

1. Chemically dependent women who have participated in experiential or cognitive therapy groups will have higher levels of general self-efficacy than will women who are chemically dependent but who have not participated in either therapy group.

2. Chemically dependent women who have participated in experiential and cognitive therapy groups will have higher levels of social self-efficacy than will women who are chemically dependent but who have not participated in either therapy group.

Source: Washington, OGM: Effects of group therapy on chemically dependent women's self-efficacy. Image J Nurs Schol 32:347, 2000.

instruments, scales, or both, that will be used. Research studies have been criticized for lack of a clear definition of the concepts and variables being studied. Concepts and variables need to be logically defined according to their relationship to the problem. The hypotheses presented in Excerpt 6.2 include a definition of the instruments that measure the dependent variables. In the first hypothesis, depression is measured by a score on the Center for Epidemiologic Studies Depression Scale (CES-D), with fatigue being measured by a score on the Piper Fatigue Scale (PFS). In the second hypothesis, transformational coping is measured by utilizing two subscales of the Jalowiec Coping Scale. Both examples illustrate the collection of data using quantitative instruments. Many statistical techniques can then be applied to measure interval and ratio variables.

A hypothesis must state an expected relationship between two variables. In the example, "If adults with chronic non-malignant pain (CNP) differ from one another, they will differ from one another in quality of life (QOL)," there is no proposed relationship to test. An expected relationship could be stated as follows: There is a higher perception of QOL in a group of adults with CNP who completed a pain management program compared with adults with CNP who have not completed a program.

A hypothesis that states several relationships among variables can be difficult to decipher. Limiting hypotheses to a single relationship between two variables adds clarity in terms of understanding the intended relationship and the conclusions that follow data analysis.

A well-stated hypothesis must be testable. Hypotheses are never proved right or wrong through testing. Hypotheses are either supported or not supported, based on the collection and analysis of data. Variables included in the hypothesis lend themselves to observation, measurement, and analysis. The predicted outcomes proposed in the hypothesis either will or will not be congruent with the actual outcome when the hypothesis

---

EXCERPT 6.2

Operational Definition of Variables Within Hypotheses

The purpose of this study was to examine the relationship between individual hardiness and caregiver strain, as measured by depression and fatigue in persons caring for functionally impaired older adults (high stress conditions), and to determine if use of transformational coping strategies mediates the relationship between hardiness and caregiver outcomes.

Hypotheses

1. Caregivers with higher individual hardiness will experience lower strain as measured by depression (Center for Epidemiological Studies Depression Scale—CES-D) and fatigue (Piper Fatigue Scale—PFS).

2. Caregivers with higher individual hardiness will use more transformational coping strategies (as measured by two subscales of the Jalowiec Coping Scale—Confrontive and Optimistic Scales) than caregivers with lower individual hardiness.

Source: Clark, PC: Effects of individual and family hardiness on caregiver depression and fatigue. Res Nurs Health 25:37, 2002, with permission.

---

is tested. Hypotheses advance scientific knowledge by confirming or not confirming relationships. Some studies may require more than one hypothesis.

Types of Hypotheses

Hypotheses are classified as simple versus complex, nondirectional versus directional, and statistical versus research.

Simple Versus Complex

A **simple hypothesis** states the relationship between two variables. Using a simple but clearly stated format makes it easier for readers to understand and formulate conclusions following data analysis. A **complex hypothesis** states the relationship between two or more independent variables and two or more dependent variables. Simple hypotheses are easier to test, measure, and analyze because nursing research involves human beings, who are complex. Many hypotheses in nursing research may be complex; however, the most important considerations for researchers to think about are the following:

What type of hypothesis is best for your study?
Is the study you are planning feasible?

If, for example, a complex hypothesis is appropriate, but you cannot collect the data to test it, then a simple hypothesis should be used instead. Several examples of simple and complex hypotheses are presented in Table 6.1.

TABLE 6.1	Simple and Complex Hypotheses

Simple Hypotheses

1. Subjects will have less discomfort following administration of the two-track intramuscular injection compared with administration by standard injection.

Independent variable = Type of injection administered (two-track versus standard)
Dependent variable = Discomfort

2. Patients with greater knowledge of diabetes will have significantly higher rates of adherence to the treatment regimen than will patients who have less knowledge about diabetes.

Independent variable = Amount of knowledge (greater versus lesser)
Dependent variable = Compliance adherence

3. Healthy young adults who consume 720 mL of ice water within 10 minutes will have a significant increase in systolic blood pressure as compared with healthy young adults who consume 720 mL of room-temperature water within 10 minutes.

Independent variable = Temperature of water (ice water versus room temperature)
Dependent variable = Systolic blood pressure

Complex Hypotheses

1. Newborns fed at 1, 2, and 3 hours of life (HOL) produce stool earlier, have lower serum indirect bilirubin levels, less observed jaundice at 48 HOL, and a lower percentage of weight loss than do infants initially fed at 4 HOL.

Independent variable = Time of feeding (1, 2, and 3 HOL versus 4 HOL)
Dependent variables = Time of stool, level of indirect bilirubin, presence/ absence of jaundice at 48 HOL, percentage of weight loss

2. Abdominal surgery patients who received preoperative teaching will have a decreased perception of pain and request fewer analgesics than patients undergoing abdominal surgery who receive structured postoperative teaching.

Independent variable = Timing of teaching (preoperative versus postoperative)
Dependent variables = Perception of pain, request for analgesics

3. Nurses who deliver nursing care using a primary nursing model will have an increase in patient satisfaction with nursing care, a decrease in absenteeism, and an improvement in their perception of the work environment as compared with nurses who deliver nursing care by the conventional method of team nursing.

Independent variable = Delivery of nursing care (primary versus team nursing)
Dependent variables = Patient satisfaction, absenteeism, perception of work environment.

Nondirectional Versus Directional

A **nondirectional hypothesis** states a relationship between variables, but it has no specific direction. Nondirectional hypotheses are used when past research provides conflicting results or when the direction of the relationship is unknown. Instead of writing nondirectional hypotheses, researchers may instead ask, "What is the relationship between X and Y?" A **directional hypothesis** states the direction of the relationship between variables. Such hypotheses are usually derived from conceptual models or findings from previous research. Directional hypotheses are clearer and more logical than nondirectional hypotheses. Using directional hypotheses, researchers are better able to indicate a direction of the relationship between the variables being studied as knowledge about that particular topic increases. Two examples of directional hypotheses are shown in Excerpt 6.3.

Statistical Versus Research

A **null hypothesis** (H_0), also referred to as a statistical hypothesis, states that no relationship (or difference) exists between two variables. Statistical hypotheses are usually used because they suit the statistical techniques that determine whether an observed relationship is probably a chance relationship or probably a true relationship. Excerpt 6.4 provides an illustration of a null hypothesis.

Because null hypotheses do not reflect the researcher's true expectations of a study's results, two hypotheses are often stated. This is done in various ways. A declarative research hypothesis may be used to communicate the researcher's true expectations, along with a statistical hypothesis to permit statistical testing. Another strategy is to state a research hypothesis, analyze the data (assuming a null hypothesis), and make inferences based on the target population identified in the research

---

EXCERPT 6.3

Example of Two Directional Hypothesis

The purpose of this study was to investigate a conceptual model in which depression was proposed to have direct negative effects on positive health practices as well as indirect negative effects through maternal-fetal attachment. Based on this framework, the following hypotheses were examined:

1. Women who have higher levels of depressive symptoms will have lower levels of maternal-fetal attachment.

2. Women who have higher levels of depressive symptoms will report fewer positive health practices.

Source: Lindgren, K: Relationship among maternal-fetal attachment, prenatal depression, and health practices in pregnancy. Res Nurs Health 24:203, 2001, with permission.

EXCERPT 6.4

Example of Null Hypothesis

Hypothesis

There will be no significant difference in the weights of children obtained while being held by an adult on adult scales compared with the weights of children obtained using infant scales.

Source: Vessey, JA, and Stueve, DL: A comparison of two techniques for weighing young children. Pediatr Nurs 22:327, 1996, with permission.

---

hypothesis. Given that few studies are really designed to verify the nonexistence of a relationship, it seems logical that most studies should be based on research hypotheses.

A **research hypothesis**, also referred to as an "alternative (H_1 or H_a)," "declarative," or "scientific" hypothesis, states that a relationship or difference exists between variables. Such hypotheses indicate what the researcher expects to find as a result of conducting a study. Research hypotheses can be simple or complex, directional or nondirectional. In each of the three hypotheses illustrated in Excerpt 6.5, the authors state that a difference exists between variables. The three hypotheses are directional, with authors predicting that two variables in each of the three hypotheses will be in a particular direction based on information previously confirmed in the literature. Factors such as the nature of pregnancy and delivery, paternal presence during childbirth, and parental satisfaction with the experience are believed to contribute to successful adjustment.

Another way to categorize hypotheses is according to how they are derived. Hypotheses can be derived inductively or deductively. **Inductive reasoning** is a process that begins with details or specific observations and

---

EXCERPT 6.5

Example of Research (Alternative) Hypotheses That Are Directional

The purpose of the current study was to determine the effects of fathers' attendance to labor and delivery on the experience of childbirth in a university hospital in Istanbul. The study anticipated that:

1. women whose partners attend labor and delivery view their experience more positively than those who are alone.
2. length of labor and delivery is shortened when fathers attend labor and delivery, and
3. the need for pain-relieving medication is reduced when women are supported by their partners.

Source: Gungor, I, and Beji, NK: Effects of fathers' attendance to labor and delivery on the experience of childbirth in Turkey. Western J Nurs Res 29:213, 2007.

moves to a more general picture. For example, after working many years with people who have type 2 diabetes, you notice that specific observations or patterns emerge every time you talk about blood glucose monitoring. Inductive reasoning is used when these specific observations begin to generate a way to care for this population of people. From these observations, you are able to propose a model or framework for how to incorporate the importance of blood glucose monitoring in working with people who have type 2 diabetes that could possibly be tested through formal research. Certain variables are noted to be related in most situations, which warrants development of a tentative explanation, or hypothesis. Related literature is then reviewed, and a formal hypothesis is formulated.

Deductive reasoning is a process that begins with a general picture and moves to a specific direction or prediction. Deductive hypotheses are derived from theory and contribute to the science of nursing by providing evidence that supports, expands, or contradicts a given theory. A deductive hypothesis that is based on a theoretical framework is illustrated in Excerpt 6.6. Deductive and inductive reasoning are fundamental to the research being conducted. Deductive reasoning is the pattern of "figuring out what's there" whereas inductive reasoning begins with a structure that guides one's search for "what's there."[2]

EXCERPT 6.6

Example of Deductive Hypotheses

According to social cognitive theory, self-efficacy and social support are two key determinants of behavior change and were both successful in explaining physical activity behavior change over 6 months in a large population sample of type 2 diabetes adults. Similarly, Courneya and colleagues' work with cancer patients reported that the constructs of perceived behavioral control (similar to self-efficacy) and subjective norms from the theory of planned behavior were associated with a host of physical activity preferences. Based on social cognitive theory, the theory of planned behavior, and findings from Courneya et al, the exploratory hypotheses were as follows:

1. High self-efficacy (confidence in actions) will be associated with preferring higher intensity activity, engaging in activities alone, engaging in activities at home, and having unsupervised sessions.

2. Social support will be associated with preference for engaging in physical activity with others at a community or diabetes center or having supervised/instructed sessions.

3. Subjective norm (approval of significant others) will be associated with preferring to receive face-to-face counseling from a doctor or an exercise specialist.

Source: Forbes, CC, Plotnikoff, RC, Courneya, KS, and Boule, NG: Physical activity preferences and type 2 diabetes: Exploring demographic, cognitive, and behavioral differences. Diabetes Educ 36:801, 2010.

Testing Hypotheses

Hypothesis testing is what scientific research is all about. To test a hypothesis, the researcher determines the sample, measuring instruments, design, and procedure for collecting data. A testable hypothesis is one that contains variables that are measurable, with a relationship that can be either supported or not supported based on the data collected.

Hypotheses are evaluated by statistical analyses. The choice of an appropriate statistical measure depends not only on the nature of the data, but also on the level of measurement appropriate for those data. Correlational analyses are conducted to determine the existence, type, and strength of the relationship between the variables being studied. Inferential statistics (e.g., t-test, analysis of variance) is used to evaluate hypotheses that examine differences between and among categories or levels of variables. Results obtained from testing a hypothesis are described using certain research terminology. When a study is completed and a significant relationship exists between two variables or there is a difference between groups, the null hypothesis is "rejected." Rejection of the null or statistical hypothesis is similar to acceptance of the research hypothesis. This indicates the possibility that a relationship or difference does exist. Failure to reject the null of a statistical hypothesis implies there is insufficient evidence to support the idea of a real difference.

Research Questions

Research studies do not always contain hypotheses but may instead be organized around research questions. A **research question** is a concise, interrogative statement written in the present tense with one or more variables (or concepts). Research questions focus on describing variable(s), examining relationships among variables, and determining differences between two or more groups regarding the selected variable(s).[3]

Researchers specify the type of research and the purpose of the study by using phrases such as "to identify" and "to describe." Research questions are used when prior knowledge of the phenomenon is limited and the research seeks to identify or describe the phenomenon (as in exploratory or descriptive studies), or in both cases. A general model for writing research questions is as follows:

1. How is X described? (describing variables)
2. What is the perception of X? (describing variables)
3. Is X related to Y? (examining relationships)
4. What is the relationship between X and Y? (examining relationships)
5. Is there a difference between groups 1 and 2 with respect to Y? (determining differences)

The three research questions presented in Excerpt 6.7 focus on describing outcomes of a school nurse referral to a family physician for adolescents identified with elevated cholesterol or blood pressure risk factors. In Excerpt 6.8 the focus of the study is examining relationships—identifying the relationship among metabolic control, self-care behaviors, and parenting in adolescents with type 2 diabetes. Excerpt 6.9 illustrates the third type of research question, determining differences between male and female caregivers.

EXCERPT 6.7

Focus of Research Questions: Describing Variables

Purpose of Study

The purpose of this study was to investigate the outcomes of a grade 9 Health Heart Program nurse referral to a family physician for adolescents identified with elevated cholesterol levels or blood pressure risk factors. The research questions were as follows:

1. Did the adolescents attend a follow-up visit with the family physician after being referred by the nurse?

2. What were the outcomes of the follow-up with the family physician if they did comply with the referral by the nurse (further testing, further referrals, health awareness, and behavioral changes)?

3. If they did not comply with the nurse referral to the physician, why didn't they?

Source: Kilty, HL, and Prentice, D: Adolescent cardiovascular risk factors: A follow-up study. Clin Nurs Res 19:6, 2010.

EXCERPT 6.8

Focus of Research Questions: Examining Relationships

Some studies have explored the effect of diabetes and other chronic diseases on family functioning and relationships. However, less research has documented the relationship among parenting, metabolic control, and self-care behaviors in adolescents, even though parental support is a crucial factor in compliance of young people with diabetes. In addition, no parenting typology or style has been identified as being more conducive to tight glycemic control in adolescents than another. Therefore, this pilot study sought to answer the following research questions:

1. What is the relationship between metabolic control and self-care behaviors in adolescents with type 1 diabetes?

2. What is the relationship between parenting (authoritative, authoritarian, and permissive) and metabolic control in adolescents with type 1 diabetes?

3. What is the relationship between parenting (authoritative, authoritarian, and permissive) and self-care behaviors in adolescents with type 1 diabetes?

Source: Greene, MA, et al: Metabolic control, self-care behaviors, and parenting with adolescents with type 1 diabetes: A correlational study. Diabetes Educ 36:326, 2010.

EXCERPT 6.9

Focus of Research Questions: Determining Differences

The purpose of this study was to examine the psychosocial outcomes in parents caring for children with life-limiting illnesses to determine if there are differences by gender. The specific research questions were the following:

1. Are there differences between male and female parent caregivers on the psychosocial outcomes of (a) meaning in caregiving, (b) self-esteem, (c) optimism, (d) spirituality, (e) depression, (f) burden, and (g) personal growth?

Source: Schnedier, M, Steele, R, Cadell, S, and Hemsworth, D: Differences on psychosocial outcomes between male and female caregivers of children with life-limiting illnesses. J Pediatr Nurs 26:186, 2011.

Research questions are written as interrogative statements. The interrogative form seeks an answer. All research variables and the population to be studied are included in the interrogative statement. In contrast to the problem statement, research questions are more precise and specific. The research question flows naturally from the purpose statement, narrowing the focus of the study.

Qualitative Hypothesis—Generating Research

Quantitative and qualitative approaches to research provide valuable contributions to the development of new knowledge. Quantitative research (traditional approach) describes a phenomenon and tests relationships between and among independent and dependent variables (usually measurable numerically) leading to hypothesis-testing research. Qualitative research provides information regarding individuals' values, beliefs, understandings, and interpretations in order to discover meaningful patterns of a particular phenomenon leading to hypothesis-generating research.

Qualitative research studies are exploratory by nature and use such methods as in-depth interviewing, participant observation, fieldwork, focus groups, and life histories to name a few. A more detailed discussion of qualitative research is presented in Chapter 12. Qualitative research studies are guided by use of research questions rather than hypotheses. Using a qualitative approach to research, data are collected from individuals recruited to participate in a study. The researcher will then use what individuals say (information/data) in order to develop hypotheses. Such an approach does not require a researcher to state hypotheses a priori; rather, the researcher is allowed to discover meaningful patterns related to a particular phenomenon that leads to future hypothesis-generating research.

Classification of Variables

A **variable** is a measurable characteristic that varies among the subjects being studied. As the definition implies, the characteristic or phenomenon under study varies in some way. Research variables are classified as either independent or dependent.

An **independent variable** is a variable that is observed, introduced, or manipulated to determine the effect it has on another variable. Depending on the research approach, the independent variable may be classified as an experimental, treatment, intervention, or predictor variable. The terms "experimental" and "treatment" are not to be confused with experimental treatment that is associated with therapeutic care. "Treatment" means manipulation, not necessarily therapeutic procedures. Consider the following hypothesis:

> Children ages 5 to 10 years old who are provided with prior information about their tonsillectomy will experience less postoperative anxiety than children of the same age who do not receive prior information.

Providing prior information about tonsillectomies, in this case, is the independent variable and is considered the treatment (manipulation) used to discover its effect on postoperative anxiety. "Postoperative anxiety" is the dependent variable, or focus, of the study.

The **dependent variable**, also called the criterion or outcome variable, is the variable that is observed for change or reaction after the treatment is applied. The dependent variable is that which is under investigation; it is this variable that the researcher determines to be a result of conducting the study. The researcher can manipulate conditions that affect the variability in the dependent variable. The researcher intends to understand, explain, or predict the dependent variables; they constitute what the researcher measures about subjects after subjects have experienced or been exposed to the independent variable. Consider the following hypothesis:

> Men ages 25 to 50 years old who experience migraine headaches and perform biofeedback therapy report fewer headaches than do men in the same age range who do not perform biofeedback therapy.

In this hypothesis, the independent variable or intervention (treatment) is biofeedback therapy. This therapy is designed to control the number of migraine headaches among men ages 25 to 50 years old. Another group of men ages 25 to 50 years old does not receive the intervention. The number of headaches is the dependent variable and represents the area of interest under investigation. The number of headaches reflects the effect of and/or the response to the treatment of biofeedback (independent variable). Several independent or dependent variables, or both, can be used in one study.

Extraneous variables are characteristics that are not under investigation but that may, or may not, be relevant to the study. These variables exist in all studies and are primarily of concern in quantitative research. Extraneous variables are classified as controlled or uncontrolled and as recognized or unrecognized. If these extraneous variables are not taken into account, they can confuse the interpretation of the results and confound the effects of the independent variable. Therefore, extraneous variables are sometimes called confounding variables. Attempts should be made to identify and control extraneous variables. Quasi-experimental and experimental designs have been developed to control the influence of extraneous variables.

CRITIQUING HYPOTHESES AND/OR RESEARCH QUESTIONS

Identify a research study to critique. Read the study to see if you recognize any key terms discussed in this chapter. Remember that all studies may not contain all key terms. The following questions[1,4] serve as a guide in critiquing hypotheses and research questions:

1. *Can you identify the hypotheses and/or research questions in the study? Were the hypotheses directional or nondirectional?* Phrases such as "the study tested the following hypotheses" or "it was hypothesized that" help locate hypotheses in a research study. Research questions are easy to identify; they focus on describing variables, examining relationships, and/or determining differences. When research questions are used, the purpose of the study tends to be descriptive or exploratory.

2. *If the study contains hypotheses, are they worded so that there is an expected relationship between two or more variables?* Remember that all hypotheses may not be explicitly stated as described in this chapter.

3. *Is the absence of hypotheses in a research study justifiable?* Consider the research problem and design of the study. Descriptive studies attempt to describe what exists, with no intention to explain relationships, test hypotheses, or make predictions. Results of descriptive studies often lead to the formation of hypotheses that can then be tested.

4. *If the study contains research questions, are they stated clearly and concisely?* Look to see if the research question(s) begin(s) with "why." These research questions are difficult to answer. Such questions may reflect personal values or judgments and are not based on research evidence.

5. *Can you identify how study variables were defined?* Once a problem has been formulated, variables must be defined operationally. Look to see if the study explains how variables are measured, including

the instruments and/or procedures used to obtain those measurements. The operational definitions should be sufficiently detailed so that the procedures can be replicated.

SUMMARY OF KEY IDEAS

1. The hypothesis is the researcher's prediction about the outcome of a study.

2. Hypotheses provide direction for the researcher's efforts and determine the research method and type of data to be collected.

3. A good hypothesis states clearly and concisely the expected relationship (or difference) between two or more variables in measurable terms.

4. Hypotheses can be classified as (1) simple versus complex, (2) nondirectional versus directional, and (3) statistical versus research.

5. A research question is a clear, concise, interrogative statement that is stated in the present tense and includes one or more variables.

6. Research questions are used when prior knowledge of the phenomenon is limited and the research seeks to identify or describe a phenomenon (exploratory or descriptive studies), or both.

7. A variable is a measurable characteristic that varies in a population.

8. Independent variables, sometimes referred to as experimental or treatment variables, are used to explain or predict a result or outcome. Dependent variables reflect the effects of or response to the independent variables; dependent variables are sometimes called outcome variables.

LEARNING ACTIVITIES

1. Identify whether the hypotheses listed here are simple or complex, directional or nondirectional, or statistical (null) or research (alternative).
   a. There is a relationship between self-efficacy and uncertainty among patients with sickle cell disease.
   b. With the use of an imagery protocol for asthmatic children, lower levels of dyspnea and use of fewer pharmacological agents are reported as compared with asthmatic children who do not receive imagery protocol.
   c. Cancer patients receiving chemotherapy who are enrolled in the nursing telephone intervention group have higher hope scores as compared with cancer patients in the control group who receive the standard nursing care.

   d. There is no difference in attitude among junior and senior baccalaureate nursing students toward caring for patients with AIDS.

   e. High levels of perceived stress are significantly related to elevated
blood glucose levels in elderly people with type 2 diabetes.

2. Identify the independent and dependent variables in each of the following hypotheses:

   a. Children with cancer who have a high sense of humor have greater
immune function and less incidence of infections as compared
with children with a low sense of humor.

   b. Attitude and perceived control significantly predict the intention
of newly diagnosed patients with type 1 diabetes to enroll in a
diabetes education program.

   c. Spinal cord–injured patients treated on the kinetic treatment table
have a decreased length of stay in the neurointensive-care unit as
compared with spinal cord–injured patients who are immobilized
on the Stryker frame/wedge turning device.

   d. There is a difference in the intensity, quality, and location of chest
pain in patients who have had internal mammary artery grafting
following coronary artery bypass surgery as compared with patients
who have had only saphenous vein grafting.

   e. There is a relationship between various health-related, physiological, and balloon-related factors and the development of lower-limb
ischemia in patients treated with the intraaortic balloon pump.

3. Read the article cited as the source of Excerpt 6.8. Within the limits
of the information provided in the article, describe how the terms
"metabolic control," "parenting style," and "self-care behaviors"
were operationally defined.

REFERENCES

1. Polit, DF, and Beck, CT: Essentials of
Nursing Research: Methods, Appraisal,
and Utilization, ed. 6. Lippincott
Williams & Wilkins, Philadelphia,
2006, pp 119–124.
2. Haber, J: Developing research questions
and hypotheses. In LoBiondo-Wood,
G, and Haber, J (eds): Nursing Research:
Methods and Critical Appraisal for
Evidence-Based Practice. Mosby

Elsevier, St. Louis, 2006, pp 46–77,
111–114.
3. Burns, N, and Grove, SK: The Practice
of Nursing Research: Conduct, Critique,
and Utilization, ed. 4. WB Saunders,
Philadelphia, 2001, p 171.
4. Langford, RW: Navigating the Maze
of Nursing Research. Mosby, St. Louis,
2001, pp 92–135.

CHAPTER

7

SELECTING THE SAMPLE AND SETTING

JAMES A. FAIN, PHD, RN, BC-ADM, FAAN

LEARNING OBJECTIVES

By the end of this chapter, you will be able to:
1. Define a sample and a population.
2. List the characteristics, uses, and limitations of each kind of probability and non-probability sampling.
3. Distinguish between random selection and random assignment.
4. Discuss the importance of a representative sample.
5. Define external validity.

GLOSSARY OF KEY TERMS

Accessible population. Population that is readily available to the researcher and that represents the target population as closely as possible.

Cluster sampling. Type of sampling in which the researcher selects groups of subjects rather than individual subjects; also called multistage sampling.

Convenience sampling. Type of non-probability sampling in which the researcher selects subjects or elements readily available; also called accidental sampling.

External validity. Extent to which results of a study can be generalized from the study sample to other populations and settings.

Network sampling. Type of nonprobability sampling that takes advantage of social networks.

Nonprobability sampling. Type of sampling in which the sample is not selected using random selection.

Population. Entire set of subjects, objects, events, or elements being studied; also called the target population.

Probability sampling. Type of sampling in which every subject, object, or element in the population has an equal chance or probability of being chosen.

Purposive sampling. Type of nonprobability sampling in which the researcher selects only subjects that satisfy prespecified characteristics; also called judgmental or theoretical sampling.

(Continued)

Quota sampling. Type of nonprobability sampling in which quotas are filled.

Random assignment. Allocation of subjects to either an experimental or a control group.

Random selection. Type of selection in which each subject has an equal, independent chance of being selected.

Sample. A subset of a population.

Sampling. The process of selecting a subset from a larger population.

Sampling frame. A list of all elements in a population.

Simple random sampling. Method of selecting subjects for a sample, in which every subject has an equal chance of being chosen.

Snowball sampling. Type of nonprobability sampling that relies on subjects identifying other subjects with similar characteristics.

Stratified random sampling. Type of random sampling in which the population is divided into subpopulations, or strata, on the basis of one or more variables, and a simple random sample is drawn from each stratum.

Systematic sampling. Type of sampling in which every kth (where "k" is some convenient number) member of the population is selected into the sample.

Target population. Population for which study outcomes are intended. Although the intended (target) population is usually evident, having access to members of this population (accessible) can be difficult.

The purpose of selecting a sample is to gain information from a small group so that findings can be generalized to a larger group. Because generalizations concerning a population are based on characteristics of a sample, the sample must represent the larger population. Matching sampling techniques to the purpose and design of the study determines the meaningfulness of study findings. A clear rationale for sampling techniques helps to ensure correct selection of subjects. This chapter focuses on basic concepts of sampling as they relate to research design, type of sampling, and sample size.

Sampling Concepts

Population and Sample

Regardless of the technique used in selecting a sample, the first step is to define the population. A **population** is an entire set of subjects, objects, events, or elements being studied.[1,2] It is a well-defined group whose members possess specific attributes. Populations may consist of individuals or elements, such as medical records, patient falls, diagnoses, episodes of care, or any other units of interest. For example, researchers may be interested in describing the characteristics of private versus public institutions in different geographic locations. Type of institution and geographic area would be the units that define this population.

Because it is not feasible to study everybody in a particular population, a small subset of the population, called a **sample**, is selected.[1,2] When the sample represents the total population, the researcher may conclude that the study results can be generalized to include the entire population and settings being studied.

The population for a study is often called the **target population** (i.e., the entire set of elements about which the researcher would like to make generalizations). If a researcher studies people with type 2 diabetes, the target population is all people with type 2 diabetes. Finding and contacting all people with type 2 diabetes is impossible. Instead, researchers will identify some portions of the target population that have a chance of being selected. The sample will come from an **accessible population** that is readily available to the researcher and that represents the target population as closely as possible. Perhaps the researcher has access to a large academic health science center, several community hospitals, or home-care services, all of which provide care for people with type 2 diabetes. Individuals with type 2 diabetes from any or all of these institutions constitute an accessible population.

Sampling

Sampling is the process of selecting individuals for a study in such a way that individuals represent the larger group from which they were selected. As mentioned earlier, it is not possible to examine each and every element in a population. When sampling is conducted properly, it allows the researcher to draw inferences and make generalizations about the population without examining every element in the population. Sampling procedures ensure that the characteristics of the phenomena of interest will be, or are likely to be, present in all of the units being studied. With a representative sample, researchers are in a stronger position to draw conclusions from the sample findings that can be generalized to the population.

Types of Sampling

Sampling is classified under two major categories: probability sampling and nonprobability sampling.[1,2] Table 7.1 identifies the most common types of probability and nonprobability sampling. **Probability sampling** occurs when every subject, object, or element in the population has an equal chance, or probability, of being chosen. In **nonprobability sampling**, the sample is not selected randomly. The probability of inclusion and the extent to which the sample represents the population are unknown. Probability and nonprobability sampling strive to represent the population under study, but they employ different methods.

TABLE 7.1	**Types of Sampling**

Probability Sampling

- Simple random sample
- Stratified random sample
- Proportional
- Disproportional
- Cluster (multistage) sample
- Systematic sample

Nonprobability Sampling

- Convenience (accidental)
- Snowball
- Network
- Quota sample
- Purposive sample

Both types of sampling have advantages and disadvantages. In probability sampling, the researcher chooses a random sample considered to be representative of the population from which it is drawn. In nonprobability sampling, the researcher has no way of estimating the probability of each subject's being included in the sample.

There is a misconception about probability versus nonprobability sampling. The assertion that probability sampling is preferred over nonprobability sampling is incorrect. Such a statement can lead to conceptual errors in planning a study. The critical issue in defining a population is the ability to generalize from sample findings back to the population from which the sample was drawn. Probability and nonprobability methods of sampling are both appropriate, based on how the problem is conceptualized and according to the method used to achieve representation.

Probability Sampling

Simple Random Sample

In **simple random sampling**, every subject has an equal and independent chance of being chosen. Selection of one individual in no way affects selection of another. Random samples are only considered to represent the target population; however, it is possible that they do not do so. No sampling technique guarantees a representative sample.

Excerpt 7.1 illustrates simple random sampling. Notice that the word "simple" does not occur in the excerpt. The authors state that a sample of 40 patients experiencing supraventricular tachycardia were randomly selected from a list obtained from the medical records department.

EXCERPT 7.1

Example of Simple Random Sampling

Sample

The target sample included patients aged 20 to 80 years experiencing CABG for the first time. Patients with current valve replacements or valve repairs were not included. A sample of 40 patients experiencing SVT and 40 patients not experiencing SVT was randomly selected from a list obtained from the medical records department with use of the International Classification of Disease code to identify patients undergoing CABG for the first time during the calendar year 1991. The obtained list was not in any systematic chronological or alphabetical order.

Source: Nally, BR, et al: Supraventricular tachycardia after coronary artery bypass grafting surgery and fluid and electrolyte variables. Heart Lung 25:31, 1996.

Whenever researchers use the phrase "randomly selected," the samples being described are simple random samples.

True random sampling involves defining the population and identifying a sampling frame. A **sampling frame** is a list of all subjects, objects, events, or units in the population. After the sampling frame has been identified, there are several ways to conduct random selection. One method is to write each individual's name, or other elements of the population, on separate pieces of paper, put the names into a container, shake the contents, and blindly select names until the desired number of individuals is chosen. This procedure is not always satisfactory or possible. A more appropriate method is to use a table of random numbers, which can be generated by a computer; it contains thousands of digits with no systematic order or relationship. Tables of random numbers, also located in the appendix of most statistics books, usually consist of three or five digits. An example of a five-digit table of random numbers appears as Table 7.2. To select a random sample using a table of random numbers, follow these steps:

1. Identify the population.
2. Determine the desired sample size.
3. List all members of the accessible population.
4. Assign all individuals on the list a consecutive number from one up to the required number.
5. Select an arbitrary number in the table of random numbers (just close your eyes and point to one). From that number, read consecutive numbers in some direction (horizontally or vertically).
6. If you choose a table of random numbers with five digits and your population has 800 members, you need to use only the first three digits of the number. If your population has 75 members, you need to use only the first two digits.

TABLE 7.2	Table of Random Numbers					
23795	97005	43923	81292	39907	67758	10202
57096	70158	36006	25106	92601	54650	27591
52750	69765	42110	38252	80201	21099	70577
90591	58216	04931	78274	10943	27273	28333
20809	23068	84638	99566	41598	25664	02400
57292	76721	75277	37751	79009	75957	22333
02266	97120	05055	34236	42475	80604	02227
61795	15534	45465	68798	02943	90934	63729
18021	45643	82756	50833	16365	87969	78079
52404	24573	72667	17693	04332	43579	24459
53104	80180	30612	24735	63414	67892	37053
78245	43321	64458	95647	57757	82849	15238
96198	06398	76790	63703	85749	07026	46901
64823	65665	43284	84972	92214	97669	62556
65083	67708	58513	18046	88476	13211	11675
30047	05312	47866	90067	41508	44709	70493
27052	80915	10914	62544	01246	59280	95348
84438	29174	15154	97010	53558	58741	53713
09083	21005	15203	76311	39195	62019	29929
96548	06390	56577	99863	58951	08673	26284
68927	37828	17069	73928	26582	08496	19678
07519	29067	53047	49285	05174	86393	19820
15246	16092	88491	46453	01504	61322	55766
97306	47296	94565	29597	34592	67680	33930
72590	71948	34123	04318	55899	96852	90471
89228	75728	32272	24197	71581	14731	42090
35188	64410	86923	25630	91336	05930	16148
79344	21677	43388	36013	37128	48252	36783
92450	37916	46903	53061	38117	65493	06579
42567	05694	82727	39689	77779	53564	49126
88541	53575	41679	00275	42844	21185	56025
48490	44531	58369	05146	29999	49853	70192
48498	60958	77913	74738	27821	56080	46295
66570	93573	73521	99191	90791	94440	83853
14134	59770	58818	47782	14536	08728	26317

7. If the number chosen corresponds to that assigned to any of the individuals in the population, then that individual is in the sample. For example, if a population had 800 members and the number selected was 375, the individual assigned number 375 would be in the sample. If the population had only 300 members, however, in this case individual number 375 would be ignored.

8. Go to the next number in the column and repeat step 7. Continue this process until the desired number of individuals has been selected for the sample.

Simple random sampling is time-consuming. It may also be impossible to obtain an accurate or complete listing (sampling frame) of every element in the accessible population. When random selection is performed appropriately, sample representation in relation to the population is maximized.

Random Selection Versus Random Assignment

Random selection is often confused with random assignment. **Random selection**—the equal, independent chance of being selected—refers to how individuals may be chosen to participate in a study. Random selection is not a prerequisite for random assignment. **Random assignment** is the random allocation of subjects to either an experimental or a control group. Random assignment is often used to provide at least some degree of randomness when random selection is impossible. Figure 7.1 illustrates random selection and random assignment. After researchers choose a target population, the sample is selected to participate.

Stratified Random Sampling

Stratified random sampling is the process of selecting a sample to identify subgroups in the population that are represented in the sample. This process reduces the possibility that the sample might be unrepresentative of the population. Stratified random sampling achieves a greater degree of representativeness with each subgroup, or stratum, of the population. An example of a stratified random sample is seen in Excerpt 7.2. A sampling frame was obtained of 462 female employees in clerical and lower administrative positions at a large public university in southern Brazil. Using stratified random sampling, 60 women were selected. In particular, proportional stratification was used to represent accurately the three clerical categories (strata) of administrative technicians, typists, and clerical staff. Disproportional stratified sampling is sometimes useful if comparisons among strata are needed and strata are very different sizes.

Another example of stratification is seen in Excerpt 7.3. In this study, using purposive nonprobability sampling of 25 Polish immigrants, the sample was stratified according to three historically distinct waves of Polish immigration, yielding three subgroups (strata): post–World War II,

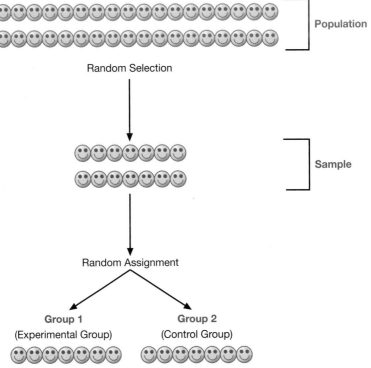

Fig 7•1 Random selection vs. random assignment.

Example of Proportional Stratified Sampling

Sample

This study was part of a larger international research project that incorporated both qualitative and quantitative data analysis in the study design. As a result, the sampling strategy was primarily a function of the quantitative analysis. From a master computer list of the 462 female employees in clerical and lower administrative positions at a large public university in southern Brazil, a stratified random sample of 60 women was obtained. The process of proportional stratification ensured a sample representation of each of the three clerical categories of administrative technician (53%), typist (26%), and clerical staff (21%).

Source: Meleis, AL, et al: Women's work environment and health: Clerical workers in Brazil. Res Nurs Health 19:53, 1996.

---

mid- to late-1970s, and 1980 to 1988. Regardless of the type of sampling reported (purposive sampling), stratification was appropriate to ensure adequate representation. Purposive sampling allows the researcher to select study subjects based on some prespecified characteristic(s). Populations can also be stratified according to age, gender,

EXCERPT 7.3

Stratification: Purposive sample (Nonprobability Sampling)

Sample

A purposive sample of 25 Polish immigrants, who resided in the Seattle area and had been in the United States ranging from 4 months to 39 years, was obtained for this study. Purposive sampling involved stratifying waves of Polish migration (Szulc, 1988), yielding three comparison groups of subsamples. Breakdown of the sample by wave of migration was as follows: subsample 1 (post–World War II era) (n = 6), subsample 2 (mid- to late-1970s) (n=5), and subsample 3 (1980 to 1988) (n=14). The mean length of time in the USA in years was 30.83 (range: 23 to 29), 14.20 (range: 8 to 22), 3.86 (range: 0.4 to 7) for subsamples 1, 2, and 3, respectively. The sample included 15 males and 10 females, and the mean age was 43.92 (range: 26 to 77).

Source: Aroian, KJ: A model of psychological adaptation to migration and resettlement. Nurs Res 39:5, 1990.

ethnicity, socioeconomic status, diagnosis, type of care, type of institution, geographical location, and so on.

Cluster Sampling

In **cluster sampling** (**multistage sampling**), groups, not individuals, are randomly selected. Cluster sampling is used for convenience when the population is very large or spread over a wide geographic area. Sometimes it may be the only feasible method of selecting an adequately large sample. Selection of individuals from within clusters may be performed by random or stratified random sampling. However, it may be impossible to obtain a complete list of all members of the population (sampling frame) to perform a true random selection.

An example of cluster sampling is displayed in Excerpt 7.4. Los Angeles and North Carolina were the identified clusters, representing sites of the Epidemiologic Catchment Area (ECA) study. The ECA was a five-site program initiated by the National Institute of Mental Health, whose primary goals were to estimate the prevalence of specific psychiatric disorders and examine patterns of health and mental health services. Respondents at the Los Angeles and North Carolina sites were selected using multistage probability sampling and were asked questions regarding lifetime sexual assault and current physical functioning.

Systematic Sampling

In **systematic sampling**, individuals or elements of the population are selected from a list by taking every kth individual. The k, which refers to a sampling interval, depends on the size of the list and desired sample size. Systematic sampling is not strictly probability sampling, but pragmatically

EXCERPT 7.4

Example of Cluster (Multisampling) Sampling

Sample

Respondents were selected using multistage area probability sampling from household residents 18 years of age and older at each site. The Los Angeles sample was selected to represent adults in two mental health catchment areas in Los Angeles County, one of which was 83% Latino and the other, 21% Latino. The Latino residents were largely of Mexican cultural or ethnic origin. The interview was translated into Spanish (Karo, Burnman, Escobar, Hough, and Eaton, 1983), and the Spanish version validated before use with ECA respondents (Burnam, Karo, Hough, Escobar, and Forsythe, 1983). The North Carolina sample was selected to represent adults in two mental health areas in North Carolina, one consisting of Durham County, which is primarily urban, and the other of four contiguous rural counties.

Source: Golding, JM: Sexual assault history and limitations in physical functioning in two general population samples. Res Nurs Health 19:33, 1996.

it may be just as good. A major difference between systematic sampling and other types of sampling is the fact that all members of the population do not have an independent chance of being selected for the sample. After the first individual is selected, the rest of the individuals to be included are automatically determined. For example, to select 250 patients from a population list of 1,000 patients, you might divide 1,000 by 250 to determine the size of the sampling interval. Then if $k = 4$, selection involves taking every fourth name. Even though selection is not independent, some researchers consider systematic sampling a type of probability sampling if the population list is randomly ordered. A major advantage of systematic sampling is that data are collected more conveniently and efficiently.

Excerpt 7.5 illustrates the use of systematic sampling without the researchers specifying a sampling interval. Between 1984 and 1986, 4,000 mothers of toddlers who were born full-term and who were delivered vaginally or by cesarean section (sampling frame), were identified. To select 146 mothers from the list of 4,000, every 27th subject was selected.

Nonprobability Sampling

In nonprobability sampling, chance plays no role in determination of the sample. In many studies, the researcher does not begin with a sampling frame in which each member has an independent chance of being included. Many nursing research studies use nonprobability sampling because of the difficulties in obtaining random access to populations. Although these samples are more feasible for the researcher to obtain, the ability to make generalizations about the findings is in jeopardy. The sample chosen may not represent the larger population.

EXCERPT 7.5

Example of Systematic Sampling

Sample

Mothers of toddlers were defined as the biological mothers of children between 12 months and 36 months of postnatal age, inclusive. Full-terms were
defined as infants born at greater than 36 weeks gestation and who weighed
greater than 2,500 grams at birth. The full-term population consisted of
4,000 mothers of toddlers born at a large northeastern metropolitan hospital
between 1984 and 1986, who were full-terms delivered vaginally or by C-
section, and products of single births with no congenital anomalies. Systematic random sampling of hospital chart codes was used to identify a target
population of 146 mothers to contact for participation. The preterm population consisted of 116 mothers of preterm infants born at the same hospital
during the same time period, who had birth weights less than 2,500 grams,
were less than 36 weeks gestation at birth, and who were products of a single birth with no known congenital anomalies.

*Source: Gross, D, et al: Maternal confidence during toddlerhood: Comparing
preterm and full-term groups. Res Nurs Health 12:1, 1989.*

Convenience Sampling

Convenience sampling, sometimes called accidental or nonrandom sampling, is the collection of data from subjects or objects readily available
or easily accessible to the researcher. This type of sample does not use
random selection. Sample subjects are not selected from a larger group
of subjects (population). Instead, the researcher collects data from
whomever is available and meets the study criteria. The advantage of
using a convenience sample is the ease in carrying out the research and
savings in time and money. The disadvantages are the potential for sampling bias, the use of a sample that may not represent the population,
and limited ability for results to be generalized. Excerpts 7.6 and 7.7
illustrate the use of the terms "convenience" and "nonrandom" sampling.
In Excerpt 7.6, a convenience sample was used within a descriptive research design. The study set out to determine if there were differences
between upper arm and forearm blood pressure measurements (BPMs).

Snowball sampling is a useful technique in situations where one cannot get a list of individuals who share a particular characteristic. It is
useful for studies in which the criteria for inclusion specify a certain
trait that is ordinarily difficult to find. Snowball sampling relies on
previously identified members of a group to identify other members of
a population. As newly identified members name others, the sample
"snowballs." This technique is used when limiting a population is not
possible. Excerpt 7.8 illustrates a combination of convenience and
snowball sampling. Women who were at least 18 years of age and who
experienced fatigue as they carried out daily activities at home, school,

EXCERPT 7.6

Example of Convenience Sampling

The purpose of the study was to evaluate the difference between blood pressure measurements (BPMs) obtained at the upper arm and those obtained at the forearm among adults.

Methods

Sample

A convenience sample of adults was recruited by announcements posted in public areas of a 104-unit, low-income apartment building in southwest Missouri and by word of mouth. No incentives were offered for participating other than gaining knowledge about their BPMs. All adults who volunteered were accepted as participants, providing a much higher number of participants (N = 130) than the number recommended by power analysis.

Source: Domiano, KL, et al: Comparison of upper arm and forearm blood pressure. Clin Nurs Res 17:241, 2008.

EXCERPT 7.7

Use of the Phrase Nonrandom Sample

Sample

The sample was a nonrandom convenience sample of 110 parents who called the Children's Careline for advice on managing their child with an uncomplicated febrile illness and whose follow-up care was determined by triage nurses to meet the criteria for home care. All records of calls over a 2-year period about children aged 12–24 months with an uncomplicated febrile illness were reviewed. Excluded were calls about children with other symptoms who required immediate or next-day attention.

Source: Light, PA, Hupcey, JE, and Clark, MB: Nursing telephone triage and its influence on parents' choice of care for febrile children. J Pediatr Nurs 20:424, 2005.

or work were asked to serve as informants to help identify other women who experienced similar fatigue. The researcher had no listing of women who shared similar experiences of fatigue. As one woman was identified, she gave the names of others to contact.

Network sampling is another useful technique in situations where there are limited formal lists or ways of reaching potential subjects. Network sampling procedures also take advantage of social networks and the fact that friends tend to have characteristics in common. When the researcher has found a few subjects with the needed criteria, these individuals are asked to help the researcher get in touch with others having similar characteristics. Obvious biases with network sampling exist because subjects are not independent of each other and because they volunteer to participate. Excerpt 7.9 illustrates use of convenience and

EXCERPT 7.8

Convenience and Snowballing Sampling

Sample and Setting

The study was conducted in a rural setting in the Pacific Northwest area of the United States, with a convenience sample of generally healthy, nonpregnant, premenopausal women who were at least 18 years of age. Regular participation in daily activities at school, work, or home was the first component of the operational definition of "generally healthy." The second component was normal (65%) results on laboratory tests that included a complete blood count (CBC), nonfasting blood sugar, blood urea nitrogen (BUN), serum creatinine, and serum iron. All study participants were premenopausal, as indicated by an established pattern of regular menstrual periods. Forty women participated in the study. Sample size was chosen in anticipation of a large effect size with alpha set at .05. The researchers used "snowball" techniques to recruit women for the study. The process began with women known to the investigators and was extended as participants introduced other women to the investigators for participation.

Source: Dzurec, LC, et al: Acknowledging unexplained fatigue of tired women. J Nurs Schol 34:41, 2002.

EXCERPT 7.9

Convenience and Networking Sampling

The purpose of the study was to explore factors that affect health and social service use among elderly Russian immigrants from the perspectives of the elders, their adult caregiving children, and the health and social service professionals who serve them.

Sample

The sample for this study included 17 elderly immigrants from the former Soviet Union, 8 adult children who were caregivers for elderly parents, and 15 health professionals who served this immigrant group. Elders and adult children were recruited from the primary author's larger study on immigrant adjustment or through network sampling procedures. Providers were identified by key informants and were recruited to include various disciplines and practice areas.

Source: Aroian, KJ, et al: Health and social service utilization among elderly immigrants from the former Soviet Union. J Nurs Schol 33:265, 2001.

network sampling. Elderly parents and adult children caregivers were recruited through network sampling procedures. Networking with other elders and their adult children caregivers was employed to identify other potential elders and caregivers for the sample. Excerpt 7.10 demonstrates the use of a networked sample in the context of a qualitative study without using the word "networked." Adolescents and parents

---

EXCERPT 7.10

Use of a Network Sample: Without Stating the Word "Network"

Sample

Adolescent and parent participants were purposively recruited from the targeted region using key contacts. Key contacts are an essential link to that population of interest and facilitate the recruitment of participants who will provide meaningful data. The four adult key contacts lived in the targeted region, were members of the six-county coalition, and represented local public or private schools (teachers or administrators) or other community organizations. The key contacts recruited participants from their respective schools whom they believed best represented the desired sample in terms of age, gender, and race and who had the ability to meaningfully contribute to a focus group. Both fathers and mothers of adolescents were invited by key contacts to participate in the parent session. The key contacts also used snowball-style recruiting, one participant finding another participant in an effort to recruit an adequate and representative sampling of the region.

Source: Peterson, J: A qualitative comparison of parent and adolescent views regarding substance use. J School Nurs 26:53, 2010.

---

were purposively recruited through use of "key contacts." These key contacts then recruited participants to join the study.

Quota Sampling

Quota sampling is similar to stratified random sampling. A quota sample identifies the strata of the population based on specific characteristics. Quota sampling differs from stratified random sampling in that subjects are not randomly selected for each stratum. The quota is computed proportionally or disproportionally to the population under study. Once the quota for each stratum is determined, subjects are solicited via convenience sampling. Researchers who want to sample proportionally need to know the specific composition of the population. Disproportional quota sampling occurs when the number of elements in each stratum is not proportional to the number in the target population.

Excerpt 7.11 illustrates an example of quota sampling that was used to ensure equal numbers of families expecting a first baby and families expecting a second baby. In this investigation, researchers filled their quota of families expecting a first baby from one site (e.g., public health prenatal clinic) and moved on to another site to find additional subjects (e.g., community Lamaze classes). This process was followed for families expecting a second baby.

Purposive Sampling

Purposive sampling, also known as judgmental or theoretical sampling, is commonly used in qualitative research. It is a type of nonprobability sampling in which the researcher handpicks or selects certain cases to

EXCERPT 7.11

Example of Quota Sampling

Sample

Subjects were 160 women (and their partners when available) selected by a quota sampling technique. This was to ensure equal numbers of families expecting a first baby and families expecting a second baby. Both the woman and her partner were interviewed in 65 of the 160 families. A family was defined as a psychosocial unit composed of two or more adults who have a commitment to each other and who live together. Subjects were drawn from a county public health prenatal clinic (n = 96) and Lamaze classes (n = 64) in a community in the southeastern United States. Families were included in the study if the woman was (1) in the third trimester of pregnancy; (2) anticipating a normal infant; (3) having her first or second child; and (4) living in a family that included at least one other adult (partner, parent, friend, or relative).

Source: Tomlinson, B, et al: Family dynamics during pregnancy. J Adv Nurs 15:683, 1990.

be in the study. Those chosen are thought to best represent the phenomenon being studied and to be typical of the population. In purposive sampling, the researcher makes a judgment regarding the type of subjects needed to provide the most useful information.

An advantage of purposive sampling is that it allows the researcher to handpick the sample, based on his or her knowledge of the phenomenon under study. However, as with any nonprobability sample, sampling bias remains a constant threat. Excerpt 7.12 illustrates purposive sampling and how important it was to sample parents of children with cancer regarding their concerns and issues and to explore what type of support was helpful.

EXCERPT 7.12

Example of Purposive Sample

Participants

Sampling was purposive and targeted parents of children with cancer on active treatment at Princess Margaret Hospital, whose sibling had agreed to participate in the larger study conducted by the researcher. Of the 33 families who met the larger study criteria, 31 families consented to participate, an overall response rate of 94%. Parents were recruited into the focus groups through randomly selecting an initial 8 families from the sample to be approached as participants. Focus groups were held until data saturation was reached. The size of the parent group took into consideration the optimal number of participants, which would facilitate sharing.

Source: Sidhe, R, Passmore, A, and Baker, D: An investigation into parent perceptions of the needs of siblings of children with cancer. J Pediatr Oncol Nurs 22:276, 2005.

Adequacy of the Sample

Sample Size

The most frequently asked question by researchers is "How many subjects do I need?" or "How large a sample should I be worrying about?" The answer is usually, "Large enough!" Although this is not a good answer, there are no hard and fast rules about sample size. In qualitative studies, the purpose is to explore meanings and phenomena; an adequate sample size in these types of studies is one that is large enough to accomplish this goal. Excerpt 7.3 illustrates a qualitative approach to research by using an example of grounded theory methodology (see Chapter 12). In this study, the researcher investigated the implications of migration on emotional status over time among 25 Polish immigrants. The sample was stratified according to the three distinct waves of immigration described earlier. In another study (see Excerpt 7.12), 21 women were interviewed who were at risk for AIDS because of injection drug use or because they were heterosexual partners of injection drug users. In both examples, the exact number of subjects was not determined in advance. The researchers continued sampling subjects until the phenomenon under study was clear.

In quantitative studies, sample size is linked to data collection and the type of analysis. Unfortunately, there is a tendency to believe that results from studies with large sample sizes are more valid than studies with smaller sample sizes. Although this is not true, researchers need to consider the following criteria when evaluating the adequacy of the sample: purpose of the study, research design, sampling method, and data analysis. It is also possible to calculate an exact number of subjects needed by using a statistical procedure called "power analysis." A discussion of power analysis is too complicated to be included in this book. Refer to Burns and Grove,[1] Polit and Beck,[2] or Cohen[3] for specific information on power analysis formulas and tables.

Two critical questions for determining adequacy of a sample include the following:

1. How representative is the sample relative to the target population?
2. To whom does the researcher wish to generalize the results of the study?

The object of sampling is to have a sample as representative as possible with as little sampling error as possible. Every study will contain some error; results will never be 100-percent representative of the population. Samples that are biased or too small, however, threaten the external validity of the design.

External Validity

External validity is the extent to which study results can be generalized from the study sample to other subjects, populations, measuring instruments, and settings. Researchers need to assess how well the sample they studied represents the larger population to which results are to be generalized. Threats to the ability to generalize findings (external validity), in terms of study design, are discussed in the following sections.

Interaction of Selection and Treatment

For subjects who are sampled and selected according to specific characteristics (e.g., diagnosis, age range, race, socioeconomic status), those characteristics define the target population. When samples are confined to certain types of subjects, it is not reasonable to generalize results to those who do not have these characteristics. In addition, selecting subjects who are willing to participate in a study can be difficult and time-consuming. If a large number of subjects approached to participate in a study decline to participate, the sample selected tends to be limited in ways that might not be evident at first glance. The number of subjects who were invited to participate and refused should be reported in order to ascertain threats to external validity.

Interaction of Setting and Treatment

Bias exists when members of different settings agree to participate in studies. For example, if a researcher demonstrates a relationship between the use of an exercise program and functional improvement using patients in a rehabilitation hospital, can these results be generalized to nursing homes? These two types of institutions (rehabilitation hospital and nursing home) may be different in important ways, leading to an interaction of setting and treatment that limits "generalizability." This question can be answered only by replicating effects in different settings.

Interaction of History and Treatment

This threat to external validity concerns the ability to generalize results to different periods in the past or future. For example, researchers examining the results of nutritional studies on reducing cholesterol in the diet would find results today that differ from those obtained 20 years ago. The effects of diet and exercise on cardiovascular fitness were less well known then, as was society's role in promoting health and fitness. This type of generalization is supported when results are replicated in future studies and when previous research corroborates an established relationship. In critiquing a study, researchers need to consider the period of history during which the study was conducted and the effect of the reported findings on nursing practice and societal events during that time.

CRITIQUING THE SAMPLE AND SETTING

Identify a research study to critique. Read the study to see if you recognize any key terms discussed in this chapter. Remember that all studies may not contain all key terms. The following questions[2,4] serve as a guide in critiquing sampling plans:

1. *Can you identify the sample?* Were terms like "target" and "accessible populations" used? Can you determine what the population was? Because populations tend to be inferred rather than directly stated, determining the population to whom results are generalized may be a bit more difficult.

2. *Can you determine whether a probability or nonprobability sampling technique was used?* Look for key words such as "random" for probability samples and "convenience" for nonprobability. If the technique is not specified, chances are great that the sampling technique is nonprobability.

3. *Could you determine any inclusion criteria for study participation?* This is usually discussed under the Methods/Sample section of a research report. In some instances, you might read about reasons why subjects were excluded from the study.

4. *Could you identify the sample size?* Was the sample size adequate enough to yield a representative sample? This may be difficult to answer based on information presented in this chapter. Refer to texts in the reference list for a more detailed discussion of techniques for weighing results to get a better reflection of the population whose characteristics one is trying to estimate. A more appropriate question would have to do with the idea of response rate or impact of refusals.

5. *Can you tell the response rate associated with returned questionnaires or surveys and what percentage of participants elected not to participate in the study and for what reasons?* Response rates are reported as a percentage of returned questionnaires or surveys. However, it is not clear what conclusions can be legitimately drawn if the response rate is 30 percent.

6. *Was the setting described?* There should be an adequate description of the setting in which data were gathered, particularly when aspects of the environment may have been crucial to the study. For example, in nonexperimental research designs, lack of environmental control may be viewed as an uncontrolled extraneous variable. For these reasons, possible ways in which the setting may have influenced the results should be considered.

SUMMARY OF KEY IDEAS

1. Remember, sampling is the process of selecting elements or individuals for a study so as to represent the larger group from which the sample group is selected.

2. There are two major types of sampling procedures: probability and nonprobability.

3. Probability samples (every member of a population has an equal chance of being chosen) are representative samples. Types of probability sampling include simple random, stratified random, cluster, and systematic.

4. Nonprobability samples (members of a population do not have an equal chance of being chosen) are not representative. Types of nonprobability sampling include convenience (snowball and networking), quota, and purposive.

5. Sampling methods must be evaluated to determine if the sample represents the population.

6. Probability and nonprobability sampling are rendered appropriate based on how the study is conceptualized, along with the method used to achieve representation.

7. Sample size, regardless of the type of sampling, affects "generalizability" of study findings.

8. External validity is the extent to which results of a study can be generalized from the study sample to other populations and settings.

9. Power analysis is a statistical method of calculating a needed sample size.

LEARNING ACTIVITIES

1. In each of the studies listed, (1) identify the sample and sample selection procedure used and (2) indicate whether the sample and sample selection procedures are described adequately.
   a. Badr, LK, et al: Determinants of premature infant pain responses to heel sticks. Pediatr Nurs 36:129, 2010.
   b. Hughes, LC, et al: Describing an episode of home nursing care for elderly postsurgical cancer patients. Nurs Res 51:110, 2002.
   c. Moloney, MF: The experience of midlife women with migraines. J Nurs Schol 38:278, 2006.
   d. Peden, AR, et al: Reducing negative thinking and depressive symptoms in college women. Image J Nurs Schol 32:145, 2000.
   e. Knobf, MT: Carrying on: The experience of premature menopause in women with early-stage breast cancer. Nurs Res 51:9, 2002.
   f. Peyrot, M, and Rubin, RR: Access to diabetes self-management education. Diabetes Educ 34:90, 2008.
   g. Yoos, HL: The impact of the parental illness representation on diabetes management in childhood asthma. Nurs Res 56:167, 2007.
   h. Zavala, S, and Shaffer, C: Do patients understand discharge instructions? J Emergency Nurs 37:138, 2011.

REFERENCES

1. Burns, N, and Grove, SK: The Practice of Nursing Research: Conduct, Critique, and Utilization, ed 4. WB Saunders, Philadelphia, 2001, pp 365–384.
2. Polit, DF, and Beck, CT: Essentials of Nursing Research: Methods, Appraisal, and Utilization, ed. 6. Lippincott Williams & Wilkins, Philadelphia, 2006, pp 258–284.
3. Cohen, J: Statistical Power Analysis for the Behavioral Sciences, ed 2. Academic Press, Hillsdale, NJ, 1988.
4. Langford, RW: Navigating the Maze of Nursing Research. Mosby, St. Louis, 2001, p 121.

CHAPTER
8

PRINCIPLES OF MEASUREMENT

JAMES A. FAIN, PhD, RN, BC-ADM, FAAN

LEARNING OBJECTIVES

By the end of this chapter, you will be able to:
1. Compare and contrast the four types of scales of measurement.
2. Discuss the issue of reliability and distinguish among the various types.
3. Discuss the issue of validity and distinguish among the various types.
4. Discuss the relationship between reliability and validity.

GLOSSARY OF KEY TERMS

Construct validity. Extent to which an instrument or test measures an intended hypothetical concept or construct.

Content validity. Extent to which an instrument or test measures an intended content area.

Continuous variable. Variable that takes on an infinite number of different values presented on a continuum.

Criterion-related validity. Extent to which an instrument or test measures a particular concept compared with a criterion.

Cronbach's alpha (coefficient alpha). Widely used index of the extent to which a measuring instrument is internally stable.

Dichotomous variable. A nominal variable that consists of two categories.

Instrument. A device, piece of equipment, or paper-and-pencil test that measures a concept or variable of interest.

Interval level of measurement. Level of measurement characterized by a constant unit of measurement or equal distances between points on a scale.

Measurement. The assignment of numerical values to concepts, according to well-defined rules.

Nominal level of measurement. Lowest level of measurement, which consists of assigning numbers as labels for categories. These numbers have no numerical interpretation.

Operational definition. A definition that assigns meaning to a variable and the terms or procedures by which the variable is to be measured.

(Continued)

Ordinal level of measurement. Level of measurement that yields rank-ordered data.

Psychometric evaluation. Evaluating properties of reliability and validity in relation to instruments being used to measure a particular concept or construct.

Predictive validity. Ability to predict future events, behaviors, or outcomes.

Ratio level of measurement. Highest level of measurement, characterized by equal distances between scores having an absolute zero point.

Reliability. Value that refers to the consistency with which an instrument or test measures a particular concept. Different ways of assessing reliability include test-retest, internal consistency, and interrater.

Test-retest reliability. An approach to reliability examining the extent to which scores are consistent over time.

Validity. Value that refers to the accuracy with which an instrument or test measures what it is supposed to measure. Different types of validity include content, criterion, and construct.

In order to make sense out of data collected, each variable must be defined operationally using a variety of measurement techniques. The specific technique chosen depends on the particular research question and the availability of instruments. One measurement technique is not necessarily better than another. Depending on how each variable is measured, different kinds of data are produced, which represent different scales or levels of measurement. Each level of measurement is classified in relation to certain characteristics. In addition, whether a researcher is testing hypotheses or answering research questions, some characteristics of the instrument are important in terms of determining the accuracy and meaning of results. Two major characteristics that are essential to the meaning and accuracy produced by an instrument are reliability and validity. This chapter focuses on the four levels of measurement and examines the issues of reliability and validity.

Measurement

Measurement is the systemic assignment of numerical values to concepts to reflect properties of those concepts.[1] Whether the data are collected through observation, self-report, or some other method, the researcher must specify under what conditions and according to what criteria the numerical values are to be assigned. Researchers establish the level of measurement for variables under study and decide which statistical analyses are appropriate. The four levels of measurement, in order of increasing sophistication are: nominal, ordinal, interval, and ratio.

Nominal

Nominal level of measurement represents the lowest level of measurement; numbers classify subjects or objects into two or more categories. Questions of "more" or "less" have no meaning in nominal measurement; data simply show the frequency of subjects or objects in each category.

Many variables in nursing research are measured on a nominal scale. Expressions commonly used to denote this level of measurement include nominal scale, nominal data, nominal measurement, and categorical data. Common examples of nominal data include gender (1 for males, 2 for females) and religion (1 for Catholic, 2 for Protestant, and 3 for Jewish). In each case, subjects are put into categories. No one category has "more" gender or "less" religion. The category names are simply labels, arranged in random order, without disturbing their meaning. If there are only two categories associated with nominal data, then the variable of interest is said to be dichotomous in nature.

Numbers are assigned as category names when entering data into a computer. However, these numbers do not represent amounts. Numbers in nominal measurement cannot be manipulated mathematically; the results mean nothing. For example, a person's blood type can be entered into the computer by assigning 1 for type AB, 2 for type A, 3 for type B, and 4 for type O. The numbers have no numerical importance other than to serve as labels for each category. A label of "average blood type," for example, has absolutely no meaning.

Excerpt 8.1 illustrates seven different variables (age, gender, race, marital status, education, employment status, and household income). Each variable is defined as a characteristic that can be measured quantitatively using numbers. An important question in any study is how the variables are measured and defined. When nominal data have just two categories, as in the variable of gender (male or female), they are termed **dichotomous variables**.

Ordinal

Ordinal level of measurement specifies the order of items being measured, without specifying how far apart they are. Ordinal scales classify categories incrementally and rank-order the specific characteristics of each category. Rank-ordered data are measured on an ordinal scale and rank subjects from highest to lowest and from most to least. For example, a researcher interested in patient satisfaction may classify 20 subjects as "1" (very satisfied); another 15 as "2" (somewhat satisfied); and another 25 as "3" (not satisfied). Although ordinal scales show which subjects reported a higher level of patient satisfaction, they do not indicate how much higher. In other words, intervals between ranks are not equal; the difference between "very satisfied" and "somewhat satisfied" is not measurably the same as between "somewhat satisfied" and "not satisfied." Expressions commonly used to denote this level of measurement include "ordinal scale," "ordinal data," "ordinal variables," and "ordinal measurement."

Ordinal data are common in nursing research. Many instruments and scales used to measure psychosocial variables yield ordinal data. Although

EXCERPT 8.1

Illustration of Nominal, Ordinal, and Interval/Ratio Variables

Demographics of the Pretest Sample

Age, y

Mean	51
Range	25–77

Gender

Female	73%
Male	27%

Race

African American	100%

Marital Status

Single, living alone	9%
Single, with children	13%
Married	12%
Widowed	17%
Divorced	4%
Other	4%

Education, y

≤6	24%
8	10%
11–12	52%
13–16	14%

Employment Status

Employed, full-time	43%
Employed, part-time	18%
Unemployed	13%
Disabled	4%
Retired	18%
Other	4%

Household Income

$0–$4999	40%
$5,000–$9,999	20%
$10,000–$19,999	40%
$20,000–$29,999	5%
$30,000–$49,999	5%

Source: Anderson, W, et al: Culturally competent dietary education for southern rural African Americans with diabetes. Diabetes Educ 28:245, 2002.

an ordinal scale results in more precise measurement than a nominal scale, it still does not allow the precision usually warranted in a research study. In addition, ordinal scales do not lend themselves well to other statistical analyses. Knapp[2,3] provides an overview of the ongoing debate among researchers regarding the use of ordinal and interval scales.

In Excerpt 8.1, education and household income are measured and operationally defined by the research on an ordinal scale. An **operational definition** assigns meaning to a variable and the terms or procedures by which it is to be measured. In this example, numbers are assigned to each category and arranged in a natural order (e.g., lowest to highest). Like nominal data, ordinal data are not manipulated mathematically. Ordinal data are simply ranks, specifying which term was first, second, third, and so forth. The variable household income is defined as 1 = $0 to $4,999, 2 = $5,000 to $9,999; 3 = $10,000 to $19,999; 4 = $20,000 to $29,999; and 5 = $30,000 to $49,999.

Interval

Interval level of measurement possesses all characteristics of a nominal and ordinal scale in addition to having an equal interval size based on an actual unit of measurement. Many instruments and scales used in nursing research report "scores" and are usually referred to as "interval data" or "interval variables." When scores have equal intervals, the difference between a score of 20 to 30 is essentially the same as a score of 100 to 110. Because the difference between intervals is the same, it is meaningful to add and subtract these numbers and to compute averages.

Interval scales, however, do not have a true zero point. Temperature is a good example of an interval scale in that a temperature of zero changes, depending on whether the researcher uses a Fahrenheit (F) or Celsius (C) scale. It makes no sense to say that a temperature of 10°F is twice as hot as a temperature of 5°F. Likewise, a temperature of zero is not absolute. Days that are 0°F do not have an absence of temperature.

Many highly reliable psychosocial instruments or scales yield interval data. There are, however, many nurse researchers who interpret ordinal data as if they were interval data and have even shown empirically that it matters little if an ordinal scale is treated as an interval scale. Knapp[2,3] attempts to resolve the controversy by insisting that researchers look to an instrument's "appropriateness" and "meaningfulness"; that is, what descriptive statistics are appropriate for ordinal and interval scales? What meaning does a score associated with each scale have? Does the raw score on a given scale resemble an actual unit of measurement? Does the scale have a true zero point?

Ratio

Ratio level of measurement is the highest level of measurement. The categories in ratio scales are different, ordered, and separated by a constant unit of measurement; ratio scales also have an absolute zero point. A zero point indicates absolutely none of the property. Temperature on the Fahrenheit scale is not a ratio measurement because a temperature of 0°F does not represent absolutely no heat. Ratio data can be manipulated using any arithmetic operation. Ratio levels of measurement include time, weight, and length. From a statistical standpoint, interval and ratio measurements are treated the same. More advanced statistical analyses are used to analyze data collected on an interval and ratio scale. The result of having an increased number of options for data analysis is that the description of what has actually happened in the study is more precise.

Age and education (years) in Excerpt 8.1 were defined operationally by researchers on an interval/ratio scale. Calculating a mean and standard deviation is appropriate for both these variables. Both variables are defined as continuous. A **continuous variable** is one that takes on an infinite number of different values presented on a continuum.

Errors Associated With Measurement

Remember, whenever data are collected, some amount of error is encountered. Researchers attempt to reduce error so data provide a more accurate reflection of the truth. Measurement error refers to how well or how poorly a particular instrument performs in a given population. No instrument is perfect. For a more thorough discussion of measurement error, refer to Burns and Grove.[4]

Measurement Scales

In defining or quantifying concepts or variables within a study, a researcher may use various types of instruments to obtain a score. An **instrument** is a device, piece of equipment, or paper-and-pencil test that measures a concept or variable of interest. Many instruments used in nursing include questionnaires, surveys, and rating scales (Chapter 9). Psychosocial measures are by far the most commonly used data collection methods in nursing research. Some instruments make sense, whereas others may be difficult to follow, irrelevant, or poorly developed. The most important issues to consider when examining the worth of any instrument used to measure variables in a study are *reliability and validity.*

Reliability

Reliability refers to the consistency with which an instrument or test measures whatever it is supposed to measure.[1,4] The more reliable a test or instrument, the more a researcher can rely on the scores obtained to be essentially the same scores that would be obtained if the test were readministered. Reliability can be conceptualized by researchers in three ways.[5] In some studies, researchers ask, *"To what extent does a subject's measured performance remain consistent across repeated testings?"* In other studies, the question of interest takes a slightly different form: "To what extent do individual items that go together to make up an instrument or test consistently measure the same underlying characteristic?" In still other studies, the concern over reliability is expressed in the question, "How much consistency exists among the ratings provided by a group of raters?" Despite the differences among these three questions, the notion of consistency is central.

Reliability is expressed as a reliability coefficient (r). A high reliability coefficient indicates high reliability. Reliability coefficients range from 0.00 to 1.00: A completely reliable test has a reliability coefficient of 1.00, and a completely unreliable test has a reliability coefficient of 0.00.

Reliability testing focuses on three aspects: stability, equivalence, and homogeneity. Within each of these areas, several different types of reliability exist, each dealing with a different kind of consistency. Test-retest reliability (stability), internal consistency (homogeneity), and interrater reliability (equivalence) are measures of reliability and are determined by use of correlations.

Test-Retest Reliability

Stability is concerned with the consistency of repeated measurements. This is usually called **test-retest reliability.** Utilizing this approach to reliability, a researcher measures a group of individuals twice with the same measuring instrument or test, with the two testings separated by a particular period of time. The extent to which scores are consistent over time is frequently referred to as the coefficient of stability. In many studies, a researcher measures a group of subjects twice with the same measuring instrument or test, the two testings being separated by a time interval. A concern with this type of reliability is how to determine the amount of time that should elapse between the two testings. Knapp and Brown[6] argue that there is no methodological justification for greater than a 2-week time interval. However, the time interval may actually be as brief as 1 day or as long as 1 year. Test-retest reliabilities are generally higher when the time lapse between the testing is short, usually no longer than 4 weeks. If the interval is too short, however, memory of the responses given during the first session may influence responses during the second session.

In Excerpt 8.2, the researcher reports several test-retest reliability coefficients, ranging from $r = 0.77$ to $r = 0.86$. However, the researcher does not mention the time interval associated with retesting. Caution is advised when reading research reports regarding how stable the measurement is when researchers do not indicate the length of time between the two testings. In Excerpt 8.3, note how the authors report the coefficient of stability (test-retest reliability) at 2 weeks and 1 month (0.87 and 0.81, respectively).

EXCERPT 8.2

Reporting Test-Retest Reliabilities

Spirituality Index of Well-Being

The Spirituality Index of Well-Being (SIWB) is a 12-item instrument designed to measure two dimensions that the authors considered reflective of the meaningfulness of life and thus of spiritual well-being: self-efficacy and life scheme.

The self-efficacy subscale reliability was demonstrated in previous research (Cronbach's alpha = 0.86; test-retest $r = 0.77$). The life scheme subscale had an alpha of $r = 0.89$ and test-retest of $r = 0.86$. The total scale had an alpha of $r = 0.91$ and test-retest of $r = 0.79$.

Source: Thomas, JC, et al: Self-transcendence, spiritual well-being, and spiritual practices of women with breast cancer. J Holistic Nurs 28:115, 2010.

EXCERPT 8.3

Reporting Test-Retest Reliability With Time Interval

Measurement

The QOL Index (Ferrans and Powers, 1985) was developed to measure the quality of life as perceived by healthy or ill individuals. It consists of 64 items that are rated by using a 6-point Likert-type scale. A total score as well as subscale scores are derived from the instrument. The possible range for each subscale and for overall scores is 0 to 30 (Ferrans, 1990; Ferrans and Powers, 1985; Ferrans and Powers, 1992; Mellors, Riley, and Erlen, 1997; Oleson, 1990). The subscales measure the perception of the individual's health and functioning, socioeconomic, psychological/spiritual, and family-related QOL. Test-retest correlations were performed at 2 weeks and 1 month and were adequate (0.87 and 0.81, respectively). Internal consistency reliability was established through Cronbach's alpha calculations at 0.95 for the total instrument, 0.90 for the health and functioning scale, 0.84 for the socioeconomic scale, 0.93 for the psychological/spiritual scale, and 0.66 for the family scale (Ferrans ane Powers, 1985).

Source: Gerstle, D, et al: Quality of life and chronic nonmalignant pain. Pain Manage Nurs 2:98, 2001.

Internal Consistency Reliability

Researchers sometimes assess the extent to which a measuring instrument possesses internal consistency. From this perspective, reliability is defined as consistency across items of an instrument, with individual items being individual questions. To the extent that certain items "hang together" and measure the same thing, an instrument is said to possess high internal consistency reliability.

To assess internal consistency, a researcher administers a measuring instrument to a group of individuals. After all responses are scored, one of several statistical procedures is applied. The procedure examines the extent to which all the items in the instrument measure the same concept. One of the more popular statistical procedures used to assess internal consistency is **Cronbach's alpha (coefficient alpha)**. This statistical procedure is more versatile than others because it can be used with instruments composed of items that can be scored with three or more possible values. An example is a Likert-type scale (see Chapter 9) in which the response option for each statement is scored from 1 (strongly agree) to 5 (strongly disagree). Another statistical procedure used to assess internal consistency is called Kuder-Richardson 20, or simply KR-20. This procedure is used when the items of an instrument are scored dichotomously (e.g., 1 = yes and 0 = no; or 1 = true and 0 = false).

Use of assessing internal consistencies by Cronbach's alpha is illustrated in Excerpt 8.3, in which the researcher reports the range of internal consistency reliabilities for three subscales associated with the Quality of Life (QOL) Index: 0.90 for the health and functioning scale, 0.84 for the socioeconomic scale, and 0.66 for the family scale. An acceptable level of reliability is an alpha coefficient of 0.80 for a well-developed psychosocial measurement instrument. For newly developed instruments, an alpha coefficient of 0.70 is considered acceptable.[4] Excerpt 8.4 illustrates an example of a researcher reporting the results of KR-20. Participants were asked to fill out the diet-health awareness (DHA) test by answering each question with a "0" for incorrect/do not know or "1" for correct. The KR-20 reliability coefficient reported for the study was 0.81.

EXCERPT 8.4

Use of Kuder-Richardson 20 Reliability

Instruments

Diet-Health Awareness Knowledge

Diet-health association knowledge was defined as awareness of the association between the type of nutrients one consumes and the occurrence of health problems, measured by a diet-health awareness (DHA) test developed by the U.S. Dept. of Agriculture (USDA). The DHA asks participants whether they have heard of any health problems that may be related to the intake of fat, saturated fat, fiber, cholesterol, salt, calcium, sugar, iron, and being overweight. Next to each question, respondents are asked to indicate what health problems are related to the nutrient in question, from a list of 17 diseases. Dichotomous scoring (0 for incorrect or does not know, 1 for correct) was used for the items. A panel of experts from the USDA supported the scale's content validity. Internal consistency testing using Kuder-Richardson Formula 20 (KR-20) showed values of 0.80, 0.77, and 0.76 over 3 years. The KR-20 in the current study was 0.81.

Source: Noureddine, S, and Stein, K: Healthy-eater self-schema and dietary intake. West J Nurs Res 31:201, 2009.

The reliability of instruments can be affected by several factors, including the characteristics of the sample, the number of items or questions, how closely connected the items or questions are, and the response format. Researchers who develop instruments need to understand that these areas potentially affect the reliability of instruments. Gable and Wolf[7] provide a more thorough discussion of developing an instrument and issues of reliability.

Interrater Reliability

In some studies, researchers collect data by having raters evaluate a particular situation. To quantify the amount of consistency among raters, the researcher computes an index of interrater reliability. One popular statistical procedure that quantifies the degree of consistency among raters is called Cohen's kappa. This statistical procedure is used with nominal data and is designed for situations in which raters classify the items being rated according to discreet categories. If all raters agree that a particular item belongs in a given category, and there is total agreement for all items being evaluated, then Cohen's kappa assumes the value of +1. To the extent that raters disagree, Cohen's kappa value becomes smaller. Knapp and Brown[6] report that Cohen's kappa statistic of 0.75 or greater indicates good agreement.

Determining interrater reliability is very common in nursing research and is used in many observational studies. Interrater reliability values should be reported in any study in which observational data are collected or when judgments are made by two or more data collectors. In Excerpt 8.5, several researchers judged patient adjustment by using the

EXCERPT 8.5

Reporting Interrater Reliabilities

Following completion of the interview, the interviewer judged patient adjustment using the Global Adjustment to Illness Scale (GAIS) (Derogatis, 1975), an observational measure of adjustment designed to identify patients' feelings of distress about their current medical condition. Scale values range from 1 to 100 in 10 deciles, with the top decile representing very good adjustment and the bottom decile representing extremely poor adjustment. In four studies examining interrater reliability and validity of brief interview-rated methods of psychosocial adjustment, Morrow et al (1981) reported that the GAIS most accurately reflected clinical impressions by a majority of professional raters. Interrater reliability coefficients reported for experienced interviewers was 0.44, and evidence of construct validity was provided for the four studies with measures such as The Rating of Psychosocial Functioning ($r = 0.68$–0.80). Nurse interviewers collected demographic and illness data from the patient record.

Source: Houdin, AD, Jocobsen, B, and Lowery, BJ: Self-blame and adjustment to breast cancer. Oncol Nurs Forum 23:75, 1996.

Global Adjustment to Illness Scale. The interrater reliability coefficient was 0.44, indicating only a moderate amount of agreement. The use of Cohen's kappa to assess interrater reliability is shown in Excerpt 8.6. In this example, interrater reliability was established between pairs of registered nurses from three visiting nurse services. Each pair of nurses identified patients in their caseload suitable for testing a patient classification instrument. Each nurse separately rated patients in six categories: clinical judgment, teaching needs, physical care, psychosocial needs, multiagency instructions, and number/severity of problems. Percentage of agreement was reported using the kappa statistic.

Validity

Validity is the accuracy with which an instrument or test measures what it is supposed to measure.[1,4] The researcher should not consider whether a test is valid or invalid. Instead, the researcher should simply ask, "*Is it valid for what and for whom?*" For example, an anatomy and physiology test is probably not a valid statistics test. An anatomy and physiology test does not measure any aspects of statistics, regardless of how reliable the test might be. With respect to "for whom," a test in anatomy and physiology would be a valid measure for use by college students, but not for students in grade school.

An instrument may have excellent reliability even though it may not measure what it claims to measure. However, an instrument's data must be reliable if they are to be valid. Thus, high reliability is a necessary, though insufficient, condition for high validity. Because different instruments and

---

EXCERPT 8.6

Use of Cohen's Kappa Statistic

Data Analysis

Percentage agreement and Cohen's kappa statistic were calculated to assess interrater reliability, with percentage agreement of 80% considered acceptable in this early testing. Strength of kappa was assessed using the guidelines proposed by Landis and Koch (1977): less than 0.00 = poor; 0.00 to 0.20 = slight agreement; 0.21 to 0.40 = fair agreement; 0.41 to 0.60 = moderate agreement; 0.61 to 0.80 = substantial agreement; and 0.81 to 1.00 = almost perfect agreement.

Percentage agreement for overall scores in the first investigated charts (Group 1) was 90% (kappa = 0.63) and ranged from 55% to 85% (kappa = –0.04 to 0.55) for category items. For the next 10 charts (Group 2), percentage agreement for overall ratings was 50% (kappa = –0.2) and 80% (kappa = 0.27 to 0.60) for category ratings.

Source: Anderson, KL, and Rokosky, JS: Evaluation of a home health patient classification instrument. West J Nurs Res 23:56, 2001.

tests are designed for a variety of purposes, different types of validity include content validity, criterion-related validity, and construct validity.

Content Validity

Content validity is the extent to which an instrument or test measures an intended content area. Usually this type of validity is used in the development of a questionnaire, interview schedule, interview guide, or instrument. The instrument is constructed using concepts from the literature to reflect the range of dimensions of the variable being measured. Content validity is then determined by a panel of experts. Experts carefully evaluate all items or questions used by the instrument, as well as the instrument's overall appropriateness for use in a proposed study population. Excerpt 8.7 contains the typical sentence seen in most journal articles, indicating that a panel of experts was chosen to evaluate content validity. In this excerpt, individuals with expertise in nutrition were chosen to establish content validity of the Barriers to Healthy Eating Scale (BHES). Excerpt 8.8 provides a more detailed discussion of how (use of literature and members of the Chemical Dependency Issues Task Force) and who (individuals with expertise in substance abuse research, recovering nurses) established content validity.

Criterion-Related Validity

Criterion-related validity is a measure of how well an instrument measuring a particular concept compares with a criterion, providing more quantitative evidence on the accuracy of the instrument. In some instances, a newer instrument is compared with an older, more reputable, instrument. A correlation coefficient is calculated for each set of scores. The two scores are calculated, with the result being referred to as the validity coefficient. A high validity coefficient indicates high

---

EXCERPT 8.7

Content Validity

Results

Content Validity Assessment

Inter-item correlations for the 18-item Barriers to Healthy Eating Scale (BHES) were examined at Time 1 and Time 2. Two items ("I have easy access to a car" and "I like to drink milk") did not meet the criteria for inclusion ($r < 0.30$ with any item within the entire tool or subscale) at either data collection point and were dropped from further analysis, resulting in 16 items. A panel of experts in nutrition reexamined the new 16-item scale and were asked to reassess the relevance of the items to conceptual elements of the subscale and total scale using the aforementioned rankings. The resultant content validity index of the 16-item scale was 0.75.

Source: Fowles, ER, and Feucht, J: Testing the barriers to healthy eating scale. West J Nurs Res 25:429, 2004.

EXCERPT 8.8

Detailed Discussion of Content Validity

Measures

The instruments used in this study were: (a) Demographic and Licensure Information (DLI), administered at Time 1; (b) Lifetime Substance Abuse (LSA), administered at Time 1; (c) Employment History (EH), administered at Time 3; (d) Maintenance of Abstinence (MA), administered monthly; and (e) Current Work Description (CWD), administered at Times 2 and 6. Evidence in support of content validity of all questionnaires was established based on a literature review, review by the National Council of State Boards of Nursing (NCSBN) Chemical Dependency Issues Task Force, and by experts in substance abuse research. In addition, content validity was established by pilot testing the instruments on 10 recovering nurses.

Source: Haack, MR, and Yocum, CJ: State policies and nurses with substance use disorders. Image: J Nurs Schol 34:89, 2002.

criterion-related validity. In addition, an instrument may be selected for comparison that is expected to measure an attribute or concept that is opposite to the dimension of interest. Criterion-related validity can be divided into two types: concurrent and predictive.

Concurrent

When a new instrument is administered at about the same time that data are collected on the criterion, concurrent validity is being assessed. A concern with concurrent validity involves comparing the results obtained from one sample with the results of some criterion measured from a different sample. For example, an instrument measuring stress that has been validated in a healthy normal population will not necessarily provide valid results when used to measure stress in hospitalized patients. Excerpt 8.9

EXCERPT 8.9

Use of Concurrent Validity

Well-being was measured with the Satisfaction with Life Scale (SWLS) (Diener, Emmons, Larsen, and Griffin, 1985) and Purpose in Life Test (PLT) (Crumbaugh and Maholick, 1964). SWLS is a 5-item unidimensional scale that measures subjective global life satisfaction as a cognitive-judgmental process with a 7-point response format ranging from strongly agree to strongly disagree. High scores indicate high satisfaction. Test-retest reliability (0.82), Cronbach's alpha (0.87), concurrent validity with nine measures of well-being, and correlations with self-esteem (0.54) have been reported (Corcoran and Fischer, 1987; Diener et al, 1985). For this sample, the standardized alpha was 0.85 and correlation with self-esteem 0.60.

Source: Anderson, SE: Personality, appraisal, and adaptational outcomes in HIV seropositive men and women. Res Nurs Health 18:303, 1995.

illustrates the use of concurrent validity. In this example, concurrent validity was assessed with nine measures of well-being and self-esteem. Validity coefficients were not reported for the nine well-being measures, and a low-to-moderate validity coefficient was associated with self-esteem ($r = 0.54$).

Predictive

Predictive validity is the ability to predict future events, behaviors, or outcomes. A classic example of predictive validity is the use of Graduate Record Examination (GRE) scores to admit students to graduate school. Many graduate schools require a combined (verbal and quantitative) minimum score of 1,000, in the hope that students who achieve that score will have a higher probability of succeeding in graduate school. This topic has been the subject of many research studies in which various questions are asked, such as, "Are GREs a valid measure, and if so, valid for what, and for whom?"

Construct Validity

Construct validity is the extent to which an instrument measures an intended hypothetical concept or construct. The process of validating a construct is by no means easy. Construct validity is the most valuable, yet the most difficult, way to assess an instrument's validity. Researchers take years to provide evidence of construct validity. To establish the amount of construct validity, researchers can perform a number of tasks, including hypothesis testing, multitrait-multimethod testing, and factor analysis. Refer to Burns and Grove[4] for a more thorough discussion of construct validity. One of the more popular procedures is to produce correlational evidence showing that the construct has a strong relationship with certain measured variables and a weak relationship with other variables. This type of construct validity is referred to as convergent and discriminant validity.

Excerpt 8.10 provides an example of how construct validity was approached. The researchers want to know if their instrument is measuring

---

EXCERPT 8.10

Construct Validity

Sexual Health Practices

Sexual health practices included safe sex behaviors and the new construct, SHRB, as well as rates of sexually transmitted infections (STI) testing and treatment among the respondents. Safe sex behaviors were measured by responses to the Safe Sex Behavior Questionnaire (SSBQ), a self-report instrument containing 27 items with a 4-point Likert response format. Evidence of construct validity was found through significant correlations between the SSBQ and measures of risk-taking and self-expression (Cole and Slocumb, 1995).

Source: Rew, L, Fouladi, RT, and Yockey, RD: Sexual health practices of homeless youth. J Nurs Schol 34:139, 2002.

sexual health practices (construct validity), or if, in fact, it is measuring something else. In order to determine this, several measures (i.e., measures of risk-taking, self-expression) are used to evaluate the construct. The researchers then make predictions about the construct in terms of other related constructs.

Understanding the Importance of Psychometric Properties Associated With Instrumentation

Most research studies use some sort of data collection instrument, often a published, standardized instrument with good reliability and validity. A "good" instrument is essential if research results are to be useful. Assessing the quality of an instrument is done by evaluating the properties of reliability and validity in relation to the instrument being used. This process is called **psychometric evaluation.**

The usefulness of data collection instruments depends on the extent to which researchers can rely on data as accurate and meaningful. Developing instruments or modifying existing instruments requires a certain amount of skill and expertise. Developing psychometrically sound instruments is an important, labor-intensive, and time-consuming task. In the initial search for instruments that might measure a particular concept or construct, one is apt to think about developing one's own instrument. The process of tool development is lengthy and requires considerable research sophistication. Using a newly developed instrument in a study without first evaluating properties of reliability and validity is unacceptable and a waste of time. Identifying whether an instrument used in a study has discussed issues of reliability and validity is important from a researcher's point of view.[4]

At the heart of all measurement is reliability. Reliability is the consistency with which an instrument measures what it is supposed to measure.[1,4] If an instrument is not producing high reliability coefficients ($r = 0.70$ or higher), it is serving no research or evaluation function and jeopardizing the meaningfulness of the data. For example, if a research study reported an alpha coefficient (internal consistency) for the Self-Efficacy Scale (SES) of 0.58, there is concern that the SES measure is not a stable one. Acceptable alpha coefficients vary, depending on the situation and the judgment of the researcher, but normally an alpha coefficient below 0.50 represents poor reliability. A moderate alpha coefficient is considered between 0.50 and 0.70.

Remember, validity is the extent to which an instrument measures what it is supposed to measure.[1,4] Although validity is an important characteristic of an instrument, reliability is necessary before validity can be considered. An instrument that is not reliable cannot be valid.

However, an instrument can be reliable without being valid. For example, an instrument may consistently measure anxiety each time the instrument is administered. However, if the concept to be measured is depression, the instrument is not considered valid.

Appropriateness relates to the fit of the instrument to the intended subjects in order to produce valid data. Many times, researchers will adapt or modify existing instruments that have been developed for other studies with proven reliability and validity with a specific group of subjects. Examine the similarity between subjects in an original study where the development and construction of the instrument began with those subjects in the current study. For example, would an instrument administered to premenopausal women for measuring depression be valid if administered to homeless youth? Other factors such as culture, socioeconomic level, development level, and language must be considered when attempting to administer the same instrument to two different populations. Question the researcher's decision to adapt and/or modify an instrument that has not been tested for reliability and validity with subjects that are different from those involved in the original development of the instrument.

The process of instrument development begins with previous research, which forms the foundation of the new instrument. If there is no relevant previous research, pilot studies are conducted to provide a foundation for the content of the newly developed and/or adapted instrument. Pilot studies help to point out flaws or errors in the construction of the instrument, selection of the sample, and data collection procedures. Pilot testing also gives insight into problems that could be encountered in editing and coding data.

Critiquing Levels of Measurement, Issues of Reliability, and Validity

Identify a research study to critique. Read the study to see if you recognize any key terms discussed in this chapter. Remember that all studies serve as a guide in critiquing levels of measurement and issues of reliability and validity.

1. *Did the study address issues of reliability?* If so, what methods of estimating reliability were used? Look for key terms such as "stability" for test-retest reliability, "Cronbach's alpha" for internal consistency, and "kappa statistic" for interrater reliability. In many studies, information on reliability and validity associated with instrumentation will be reported from earlier studies. Identify if reliability coefficients (Cronbach's alpha) are calculated for both the current study and those reported in previous research. Perhaps both reliability coefficients are compared with one another.

2. *Did the study address issues of validity?* Was there sufficient information available to appraise the instrument's validity? If so, what methods of estimating validity were used? Look for key terms such as "content validity," "criterion-related validity," and "construct validity." The validity of an instrument is critical to the success of any research study. Identify the reason a particular instrument was chosen. If a study is designed to examine parenting skills but the instrument measures coping skills, the results of the study are of little value. Try to understand the usefulness of the instrument given the context in which it is applied.

3. *Can you identify the main study variable(s)?* How were study variables measured: Were nominal, ordinal, and interval/ratio levels of measurement used? Look to see how each variable was measured. Levels of measurement guide the kind of statistical analyses that can be performed.

CRITIQUING INSTRUMENTS

Identify a research study to critique. Read the study to see if you recognize any key terms discussed in this chapter. Remember that all studies may not contain all key terms. The following questions serve as a guide in critiquing instruments.

1. *Does the instrument measure what it claims to measure?* If possible, look over the items in the instrument to see if they make sense. Unfortunately, many research studies will not publish entire instruments. In some instances, a few examples of the items are reported. Look to see if there is mention of where the reader can obtain a copy of the instrument. If the instrument has been adopted from another source, that source should be documented in the reference list. If the instrument is an author-developed instrument, an address may be available at the beginning or end of the research report to indicate where a complete copy can be obtained. All publications related to instrument testing should likewise be referenced. For those instruments that are author-developed with little, if any, information regarding reliability and/or validity, an assessment of the instrument is imperative with respect to validity.

2. *Are there instructions on how to obtain, administer, and score the instrument?* Locating existing instruments is not an easy task. Journal articles sometimes publish a copy of the instrument or examples of items within the instrument. Check the reference list to identify the author of the instrument and some of the early work done on establishing reliability and validity. Many times the author's place of employment, address, and e-mail are listed. The computer database Health Psychological Instruments Online is available and can search

for instruments that measure a particular concept or construct or for information on a particular instrument. Very often, little, if any, information is presented with respect to how and under what conditions instruments are to be administered and scored.

3. *Are scoring procedures explained in sufficient detail?* Refer to the methods section (instrumentation) of the article to find information on scoring procedures.

4. *Does the instrument yield a total score, or are there several subscales associated with the instrument?* Refer to the methods section (instrumentation) of the article, and identify if a total score and subscales are calculated. In many instances, the sentence, "A total score as well as subscale scores are derived from the instrument" is typical. Note that if such a sentence exists, you should be able to identify the names of the various subscale measures.

5. *Has the instrument been pilot tested?* Pilot testing identifies and corrects any problems before the actual study is implemented in its final form. Advantages of a pilot test include an opportunity to evaluate the psychometric properties of instruments, practice in collecting data and uncovering questions and/or instructions that might be ambiguous, assess reliability of subjects, and estimate time associated with data collection. The number of subjects needed for a pilot study varies. If the purpose of the pilot study is to uncover questions and/or instructions that might be ambiguous, 10 to 20 subjects may be sufficient. When the purpose of the pilot test is to evaluate the psychometric properties of an instrument, a much larger sample is necessary. Pilot studies are well worth the time and effort. Problems associated with administering an instrument are costly when they occur after data collection has begun.

SUMMARY OF KEY IDEAS

1. Measurement is the systematic assignment of numerical values to concepts or constructs to reflect properties of those concepts or constructs.

2. The four levels of measurement are nominal, ordinal, interval, and ratio.

3. The lowest level of measurement, nominal, classifies subjects or objects according to different categories.

4. Ordinal levels of measurement specify the order of items being measured, without specifying how far apart they are (interval size).

5. Interval levels of measurement possess all characteristics of nominal and ordinal scales, in addition to having an equal interval size based on an actual unit of measurement.

6. Ratio levels of measurement represent the highest level. In ratio scales, the categories are different, ordered, and separated by a constant unit of measurement, and an absolute zero point exists.

7. Reliability is the consistency with which an instrument measures what it is supposed to measure. Different types of reliability include test-retest, internal consistency, and interrater.

8. Validity is the accuracy with which an instrument measures what it is supposed to measure. Different types of validity include content, criterion-related, and construct.

9. Instruments may have good reliability even if the instrument does not measure what it claims to measure.

LEARNING ACTIVITIES

1. A study was conducted to investigate the effect of dual-earner families on the development of preschool children. Information was collected on the following variables: satisfaction with income (measured as dissatisfied versus satisfied); satisfaction with child care (measured as low, moderate, high); income level (measured as $30,000 to $39,999; $40,000 to $49,999; $50,000 to $59,999; $60,000+); mother's age (measured as mother's actual age); and family stress level (measured as none, very little, moderate, a great deal). Which variable(s) represent(s) an interval/ratio level of measurement?

2. Define the following variables using an ordinal scale of measurement: health status, amount of pain, patient satisfaction, age.

3. Comment on the strength of Cronbach's alpha in the following example:

   Cronbach's alpha was calculated for the Barriers to Cessation Scale in three samples. In study 1 (n = 91), alpha was 0.87; in study 2 (n = 25), alpha was 0.81; and in study 3 (n = 156), alpha was 0.83.

4. What information is missing when evaluating the coefficient of stability in this example?

   State anxiety, the transitory situation-specific response to events, was measured by Spielberger, Gorsuch, Lushene, Vagg, and Jacobs' (1983) 20-item State Anxiety Scale, with items rated from 1 to 4. Internal consistencies ranged from 0.92 to 0.95, with a test-retest reliability of 0.90.

5. What type of validity is discussed in the following sentences?

   Pregnancy risk, intrapartal risk, and infant's health status at birth were measured by revisions of the instruments reported by Hobel,

Hyvarinen, Okada, and Oh (1973) and updated to reflect current diagnostic procedures. A panel of perinatal nurse specialists, a pediatrician, and an obstetrician validated the new scale. The pregnancy risk scale has 80 items, the intrapartal risk scale has 45, and the infant's health status at birth has 69.

REFERENCES

1. Nunnaly, J, and Bernstein, IH: Psychometric Theory, ed. 3. McGraw-Hill, New York, 1994.
2. Knapp, TR: Treating ordinal scales as ordinal scales. Nurs Res 42:184, 1993.
3. Knapp, TR: Treating ordinal scales as interval scales: An attempt to resolve the controversy. Nurs Res 39:121, 1990.
4. Burns, N, and Grove, SK: The Practices of Nursing Research: Conduct, Critique, and Utilization, ed. 4. WB Saunders, Philadelphia, 2001, pp 223–241, 389–406, 441–447.
5. Huck, SW, and Cormier, WH: Reading statistics and research. HarperCollins Publishers, New York, 1996.
6. Knapp, TR, and Brown, JK: Ten measurement commandments that often should be broken. Res Nurs Health 18:465, 1995.
7. Gable, RK, and Wolf, MB: Instrument Development in the Affective Domain, ed. 2. Kluwer Academic Publishers, Boston, 1993.

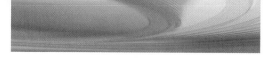

CHAPTER

9

DATA COLLECTION METHODS

JAMES A. FAIN, PhD, RN, BC-ADM, FAAN

LEARNING OBJECTIVES

By the end of this chapter, you will be able to:

1. Identify common instruments and methods used to collect data in quantitative and qualitative research.
2. Distinguish between closed-ended and open-ended questionnaires.
3. List the advantages and disadvantages of using questionnaires.
4. Compare and contrast the different types of scaling techniques.

GLOSSARY OF KEY TERMS

Closed-ended questionnaire. Type of format in which subjects are asked to select an answer from several choices.

Instrument. A device, piece of equipment, or paper-and-pencil test that measures a concept or variable of interest.

Interview schedule. List of topics or an open-ended questionnaire administered to subjects by a skilled interviewer. Sometimes referred to as an interview guide.

Likert scale. Sometimes referred to as a summative scale. Respondents are asked to respond to a series of statements that reflect agreement or disagreement. Most Likert scales consist of five scale points, designated by the words "strongly agree," "agree," "undecided," "disagree," and "strongly disagree."

Open-ended questionnaire. Type of format in which subjects are asked to provide specific answers.

Q methodology. Sorting technique used to characterize opinions, attitudes, or judgments of individuals through comparative rank ordering.

Questionnaire. A structured survey that is self-administered or interviewer administered.

Response set bias. The tendency for subjects to respond to items on a questionnaire in a way that does not reflect the real situation accurately.

Semantic differential scale. Set of scales using pairs of adjectives that reflect opposite feelings.

(Continued)

Scale. A set of numerical values assigned to responses that represent the degree to which respondents possess a particular attitude, value, or characteristic.

Survey. A method of collecting data to describe, compare, or explain knowledge, attitudes, or behaviors.

Visual analogue scale. Type of scale that measures subjective phenomena (e.g., pain, fatigue, shortness of breath, anxiety). The scale is 100 mm long with anchors at each end quantifying intensity. Subjects are asked to mark a point on the line indicating the amount of the phenomenon experienced at that time.

Data collection is a major part of the research process. Methods and instruments for data collection must be chosen according to the nature of the problem, approach to the solution, and variables being studied. Whether the researcher is testing hypotheses or seeking answers to research questions, valid and reliable instruments are essential. The purpose of this chapter is to describe various methods of collecting data for both quantitative and qualitative approaches to research.

Qualitative vs. Quantitative Data

Data are divided into two categories, qualitative and quantitative. Qualitative data can be observed, written, taped, or filmed. Data collection methods include unstructured interviews, direct observation, case studies, field notes, diaries, or historical documents. Qualitative data are useful for preliminary investigation of new areas and for understanding the results of quantitative analyses. The advantages are that collecting the data does not require prior knowledge of the subject and individual variation can be recorded in depth.

Quantitative data are numerical. Numerical data can be used directly (e.g., weight in pounds, height in inches, age in years) or to form categories (e.g., male or female) that can be formulated into counts or tables. The advantages are that data can be analyzed without extreme effort, comparisons can be made, and hypotheses can be tested with well-developed statistical techniques. If data are collected in a standardized, unbiased manner, insights and results may apply to other populations. The distinction between qualitative and quantitative data is not always clear. In qualitative data, each category is assigned a code. These codes are easily entered into a computer and analyzed using statistical techniques based on counts (e.g., chi-square analysis).

Quantitative Data Collection Methods

Quantitative data collection methods include the use of instruments. An **instrument** is a device used to record or gather data on a particular concept.[1] An instrument may be a piece of equipment, structured interview, or paper-and-pencil test. Data-gathering instruments used in research studies include questionnaires, rating scales, checklists, standardized tests, and biophysical measures. Methods for collecting data may be based on a form of self-report that asks individuals to complete a questionnaire, survey, or standardized test.

Surveys and Questionnaires

Surveys are a popular method for collecting data to describe, compare, or explain knowledge, attitudes, and behavior.[2] A **survey** is a series of questions posed to a group of subjects. Questionnaires are structured self-administered surveys. The most common way of distributing questionnaires is through the mail, although many research situations allow for face-to-face administration. Mailed questionnaires are economical and reach a large population in a relatively brief time. One disadvantage of using mailed questionnaires is a low return rate. Responses from 60 percent to 80 percent of a sample are considered excellent. Realistically, researchers can expect return rates from 30 percent to 60 percent for most studies.[3] Excerpt 9.1 illustrates the use of a mailed questionnaire.

EXCERPT 9.1

Use of Mailed Questionnaire

Procedure for Data Collection

The list of potential participants was determined by inserting the inclusion criteria into the cancer registry database and retrieving the names of potential participants for the master list. Thus, this master list contained the names of all women older than 65 years who had been diagnosed with breast cancer during the 5 years prior to the date the list was obtained; it excluded those women diagnosed in the previous 2 months. The master list was locked in a file cabinet in the Cancer Registrar's Office and not made available to the researcher.

The Cancer Registry mailed the prepared packets of information, including a cover letter, the survey—which included the three instruments and a background data questionnaire—a $2.00 bill, and a self-addressed return envelope, to all women on the master list. The women were informed in the cover letter that the money was a token of appreciation for their participation and that they could keep the money whether or not they returned the questionnaire. Follow-up postcards were mailed to all persons on the master list as a reminder to return the survey. This was done by the Cancer Registry 2 weeks after the initial mailing.

Source: Thomas, JC, Burton, M, Griffin, MT, and Fitzpatrick, JJ: Self-transcendence, spiritual well-being, and spiritual practices of women with breast cancer. J Holist Nurs 28:115, 2010.

Closed-ended questionnaires ask subjects to select an answer from among several choices. This technique is often used in large surveys when questionnaires are mailed to subjects. In addition, this type of questionnaire is easily coded. **Open-ended questionnaires** ask subjects to provide specific answers to questions. Open-ended questionnaires are less frequently found in research studies, particularly when quantitative methods for data analysis are planned. The researcher has less control over subjects' answers because there are no fixed choices provided for each question. An example illustrating the difference between open-ended and closed-ended questions is shown in Table 9.1.

Developing a Questionnaire

Designing good questions that are easy to answer, while focusing on the issues and information to be collected, is essential to developing a questionnaire. An example of a questionnaire is illustrated in Figure 9.1. The following are guidelines to consider when designing questions:

1. Ask questions that are specific rather than general.[2,4] For example, if you want to know the level of patient satisfaction, the question

TABLE 9.1	Example of Open-Ended and Close-Ended Questions

Open-Ended Question

Describe some reasons to wear a seat belt when riding in a car driven by someone else.

Closed-Ended Question

1. How often do you wear a seat belt when riding in a car driven by someone else?
   a. Never
   b. Rarely
   c. Sometimes
   d. Most of the time
   e. Always

Open-Ended Question

Explain your beliefs about drinking.

Closed-Ended Question

1. During the past 30 days, how many times did you drive a car when you had been drinking alcohol?
   a. 0 times
   b. 1 time
   c. 2–3 times
   d. 4–5 times
   e. 6 or more times

We are interested in learning more about you. This questionnaire covers a few personal, health, and demographic variables for those in this course. Please answer each question by circling the answer that best describes you. Please return this form to the instructor when requested.

1. What degrees do you currently have?

	Yes	No
BS	1	0
BA	1	0
MS	1	0
MSN	1	0
JD	1	0
MD	1	0
PhD	1	0
Other (specify): _____		

2. Have you taken any of the following exams within the last 5 years?

	Yes	No
GRE	1	0
GMAT	1	0
MCAT	1	0
LSAT	1	0
MAT	1	0
Other (specify): _____		

3. How many semesters of statistics have you taken?

4. Have you ever used a personal computer to analyze data?

Yes   1   No   0

Fig 9•1 In-Class Questionnaire.

Now we would like to know something about your personal habits.

5. How often do you drink coffee?

0   Rarely or never

1   Less than 1 cup per month

2   1–3 cups per month

3   1–6 cups per week

4   1–2 cups per day

5   3–4 cups per day

6   5+ cups per day

6. How many cigarettes do you smoke per day?

0   None, never smoked

1   None now, former smoker

2   Half a pack or less (0–10)

3   Between $\frac{1}{2}$ and 1 pack (11–20)

4   Over 1 pack and up to $1\frac{1}{2}$ packs (21–30)

5   Over $1\frac{1}{2}$ packs and up to 2 packs (31–40)

6   Over 2 packs

7. If you smoke, at what age did you begin smoking?

_____

Please answer if you have ever smoked regularly, even if
you have quit. Leave it blank if you have never smoked.

8. How often do you participate in some sort of physical exercise or sport?

0   Rarely or never

1   Less than once a month

2   1–3 times per month

3   1–3 times per week

4   4–6 times per week

5   Every day

Fig 9•1—cont'd

To help us understand the different groups of people answering these questions, we need to know a little about your background characteristics.

9. How old were you on your last birthday?

_____ Years

10. Gender:

_____Female   _____Male

11. How tall are you?

_____feet   _____inches

12. How much do you weigh?

_____lb

13. Are you currently certified in cardiopulmonary resuscitation (CPR) by either the American Heart Association or the American Red Cross?

Yes   1   No   0

14. Have you ever been told by a doctor that you had any of the following conditions?

	Yes	No
Heart disease	1	0
High blood pressure	1	0
High cholesterol	1	0
Emphysema	1	0
Cancer	1	0

15. Compared with other people your age, how would you rate your health?

Excellent	4
Good	3
Fair	2
Poor	1

Fig 9•1—cont'd

"Are you satisfied or dissatisfied with the care you received?" is too general and might elicit opinions about other aspects of patient satisfaction. The question "How would you rate your level of satisfaction regarding being able to have input into your treatment preferences—excellent, very good, good, fair, or poor?" reflects an answer about respect for values, expressed needs, and input into treatment preferences.

2. Use simple language.[2,4] Make sure the style is appropriate to the education and knowledge of respondents. If you want to know how the respondent thinks lung cancer rates are changing, you could ask a layperson, "Do you think lung cancer is increasing, decreasing, or staying the same?" For an epidemiologist, such basic language would make the question hard to answer. In this case, you should specify period of time, morbidity and mortality rates, race, age, and gender. The question "In the last 5 years, do you think the incidence of respiratory cancer in white males under 65 years of age has increased, decreased, or stayed the same?" assumes a specific respondent.

3. Each question should represent one concept.[2,4] Avoid asking two (or more) questions at the same time. For example, the question "Do you wear seat belts when driving your car?" is really asking several questions: "Can you drive a car?", "Do you own a car?", and "Do you wear seat belts?" If the answer to the original question is "No," it could mean "No, I can't drive or don't have a driver's license" or "Yes, I can drive, but no, I don't wear my seat belt when I drive." The question "When you are in a car, how often do you fasten the seat belt—always, sometimes, or never?" is appropriate.

4. Delimit any reference to time.[2,4] For example, if you ask "Do you exercise often?", it is not clear what "often" means. A more specific question is "In the past week, how often did you exercise— once, twice, or three times; more than three times?"

5. Phrase questions in as neutral a way as possible.[2,4] Try not to let content, structure, or wording favor a certain answer. For example, ask "Do you agree or disagree with the following statement" rather than "Don't you think that . . .?" Make sure there are the same number of positive and negative answers so that respondents will not feel influenced to choose the more heavily weighted point of view.

Designing Good Answers

Asking good questions also involves specifying good answers. Questions can be designed to elicit three main types of answers: open-ended, categorical, and continuous.

Open-Ended Responses. An open-ended question elicits an answer consisting of a free-form statement or essay in which the respondent chooses what to say. Such answers are useful either in the early stages of drafting questions or at the end of a questionnaire in order to enrich or to help interpret shorter responses. Most open-ended responses are not analyzed by using a computer. If such free-form data are to be analyzed by computers, responses need to be coded after the questionnaires have been returned. Coding responses is a tedious and time-consuming task.

Categorical Responses. A categorical response is a type of closed answer that respondents are asked to choose from a limited number of alternatives. When writing categorical responses, answer choices should not leave out any of the most important possibilities. To allow for answers that are rare (occurring less than 5 percent of the time) or that the researcher has not considered, a category such as "Other: Specify" can be placed at the end of the list. Answers should also be mutually exclusive.

Additionally, categories should not overlap. For example, the question, "How old are you: 18 to 21, 21 to 35, 36 to 65, 65 and over?" has two categories that overlap. In this example, if respondents choose more than one answer, the answers may not be mutually exclusive. It is better for the researcher to think of such a question as a series of questions that allow only yes/no answers. For example, the question "Have you had any of the following conditions or illnesses—diabetes, hypertension, high cholesterol, heart attack?" should really be considered as four separate questions.

Continuous Responses. Continuous responses can accommodate a large range of values, representing a continuum. Each value can be entered directly and does not need to be coded. Examples include age, weight, height, blood pressure, and so forth. Researchers should specify the unit of measurement used in each value and the level of precision desired (how many decimal places). For example, a study of nutrition in newborns should ask for weight to the nearest half ounce and age to the nearest month. For a similar study among older adults, weight to the nearest pound and age in years at the last birthday are sufficient.

Ordering the Questions

A **questionnaire** is a collection of questions in which the whole becomes more than the sum of its parts. In addition to wording each question carefully, it is important to plan the order in which questions are asked. Dillman[3] specifies five principles for ordering questions:

1. Start with the topic that the respondent will consider most useful or important.
2. Group questions that are similar in content. Within content area, group questions of the same type. For example, on a given topic, group questions requiring yes/no answers.
3. Take advantage of relationships among groups of questions to build continuity throughout the questionnaire.
4. Questions about sensitive topics should be placed about two-thirds of the way into the questionnaire. Within a topic area, put the questions that are easier to answer first and those that are likely to be more sensitive or objectionable, last.

5. Demographic questions that the respondent might consider boring or personal should be placed at the end of the questionnaire. A respondent might consider demographic questions (e.g., age, sex, marital status, income) intrusive if they are presented at the beginning of a questionnaire. After completing the questionnaire, however, respondents might not consider the demographic questions as offensive.

Scales

A **scale** is a set of numerical values assigned to responses, representing the degree to which subjects possess a particular attitude, value, or characteristic. The purpose of a scale is to distinguish among people who show different intensities of the entity to be measured. Scales are created so that a score can be obtained from a series of items. Several formats are used in creating scales for rating a set of items. Three common types of scaling techniques are Likert, semantic differential, and visual analogue.

Likert Scales

Likert scales, also called summative scales, require subjects to respond to a series of statements to express a viewpoint. Subjects read each statement and select an appropriately ranked response. Response choices commonly address agreement, evaluation, or frequency. Likert's original scale included five agreement categories: "strongly agree (SA)," "agree (A)," "uncertain (U)," "disagree (D)," and "strongly disagree (SD)." The number of categories in the Likert scale can be modified: it can be extended to seven categories (by adding "somewhat disagree" and "somewhat agree") or reduced to four categories (by eliminating "uncertain").

There is no correct number of response categories. Some researchers believe the "uncertain" option should be omitted to force subjects to make a choice. Other researchers believe subjects who do not have strong feelings should be given an option to express that attitude. When the forced-choice method is used, responses that are left blank are generally interpreted as "uncertain." Frequency categories for Likert scales may include terms such as "rarely," "seldom," "sometimes," "occasionally," and "usually." However, these terms are adaptable and should be selected for their appropriateness to the stem question.[5] Table 9.2 displays several 4-, 5-, and 6-point Likert responses for choices addressing agreement, frequency, and evaluation.

Each choice along the scale is assigned a point value, based on the extent to which the item represents a favorable or unfavorable characteristic. Point values could be SA = 5, A = 4, U = 3, D= 2, SD = 1 or SA = 2, A = 1, U = 0, D = –1, SD = –2. The actual values are unimportant as long as the items are consistently scored and follow scoring guidelines. The use of Likert scales is presented in Excerpt 9.2.

| TABLE 9.2 | **Example of Likert Responses** |

Strongly disagree	Strongly disagree	
Disagree	Disagree with reservations	
Agree	Agree with reservations	
Strongly agree	Strongly agree	
Almost never	Never	Always
Occasionally	Rarely	Frequently
Usually	Infrequently	Sometimes
Almost always	Sometimes	Rarely
	Frequently	Never
	Often	
Excellent	Excellent	Excellent
Good	Good	Very good
Fair	Satisfactory	Good
Poor	Unsatisfactory	Fair
	Poor	Poor
Not at all	None	Great deal
A little	Very little	Moderate
Moderately	Moderately	Somewhat
Quite	A great deal	Poor
Extremely		
Almost none	None	A little
Some	A little	Some
Most	Some	Moderate amount
Almost all	A great deal	Great deal
Very satisfactory	Very satisfactory	
Satisfactory	Somewhat satisfactory	
Unsatisfactory	Somewhat unsatisfactory	
Very unsatisfactory	Very unsatisfactory	
Extremely satisfied		
Satisfied		
Dissatisfied		
Extremely dissatisfied		

EXCERPT 9.2

Use of Likert Scales

Operational Definitions

The Herth Hope Scale (HHS) is a 30-item self-report measure of hope as conceptualized by Dufault and Martocchio (1985). The HHS was designed for healthy adults experiencing an acute, chronic, or terminal illness. Participants rate each item on a 4-point Likert scale ranging from 0 (Never Applies to Me) to 3 (Often Applies to Me). Total scores range from 0 to 90, with higher scores suggesting higher levels of hope.

The Mischel Uncertainty in Illness Scale (MUIS) is a self-report scale designed to measure uncertainty in illness as conceptualized by Mishel's uncertainty in illness theory. Measured on a summated 5-point Likert-type scale from 1 (Strongly Disagree) to 5 (Strongly Agree), higher scores indicate higher levels of uncertainty.

The Spiritual Well-Being Scale (SWB) is a 20-item self-report tool designed to measure spiritual well-being as conceptualized by Moberg and Ellison. The scale includes the religious well-being (RWB) and existential well-being (EWB) subscales, each made up of 10 items that are rated on a 6-point Likert-type scale ranging from 6 (Strongly Agree) to 1 (Strongly Disagree). Reverse scoring is required for items that are negatively worded. Possible scores for the total scale range from 20 to 120. A higher score indicates a higher level of spiritual well-being.

Source: Heinrich, CR: Enhancing the perceived health of HIV seropositive men. West J Nurs Res 25:367, 2003.

Some items within an instrument may be worded negatively to avoid creating a response set bias, the tendency for subjects to respond to items based on irrelevant criteria in a way that inaccurately reflects the situation. Instruments dealing with attitudes about psychological or social issues are particularly vulnerable to response sets. For example, subjects who are asked to agree or disagree with a set of statements may tend to respond in a socially acceptable way (social desirability response set). To avoid the possibility of **response set bias**, the researcher may balance the occurrence of positively and negatively worded items on an instrument in order to reduce the tendency for subjects to agree or disagree in a uniform way. A good example is the Personal Resource Questionnaire (PRQ), a two-part measurement of multidimensional characteristics of social support. PRQ-I provides descriptive information about the person's resources and level of satisfaction with these resources. PRQ-II contains 25 items divided into five subscales: intimacy, social integration, nurturance, worth, and assist/guidance. PRQ-II is shown in Table 9.3. The intensity of each item is measured on a 7-point Likert scale, with response choices ranging from "strongly agree" (7) to "strongly disagree" (1). Items are numbered 1 to 25 and scored in a straightforward manner. Mean

TABLE 9.3	Personal Resource Questionnaire (PRQ): Part II

Below are some statements with which some people agree and others disagree. Please read each statement and circle the response most appropriate for you. There is no right or wrong answer.

1 = Strongly Disagree

2 = Disagree

3 = Somewhat Disagree

4 = Neutral

5 = Somewhat Agree

6 = Agree

7 = Strongly Agree

Statements

1. There is someone I feel close to who makes me feel secure.
   1   2   3   4   5   6   7
2. I belong to a group in which I feel important.
   1   2   3   4   5   6   7
3. People let me know that I do well at my work (job, homemaking).
   1   2   3   4   5   6   7
4. I can't count on my relatives and friends to help me with problems.
   1   2   3   4   5   6   7
5. I have enough contact with the person who makes me feel special.
   1   2   3   4   5   6   7
6. I spend time with others who have the same interests that I have.
   1   2   3   4   5   6   7
7. There is little opportunity in my life to be giving and caring to another person.
   1   2   3   4   5   6   7
8. Others let me know that they enjoy working with me (job, committees, projects).
   1   2   3   4   5   6   7
9. There are people who are available if I needed help over an extended period.
   1   2   3   4   5   6   7
10. There is no one to talk to about how I am feeling.
    1   2   3   4   5   6   7
11. Among my group of friends we do favors for each other.
    1   2   3   4   5   6   7
12. I have the opportunity to encourage others to develop their interests and skills.
    1   2   3   4   5   6   7
13. My family lets me know that I am important for keeping the family running.
    1   2   3   4   5   6   7
14. I have relatives or friends that will help me out even if I can't pay them back.
    1   2   3   4   5   6   7

(Continued)

TABLE 9.3	Personal Resource Questionnaire (PRQ): Part II—cont'd

15. When I am upset, there is someone I can be with who lets me be myself.

    1   2   3   4   5   6   7

16. I feel no one has the same problems as I.

    1   2   3   4   5   6   7

17. I enjoy doing little "extra" things that make another person's life more pleasant.

    1   2   3   4   5   6   7

18. I know others appreciate me as a person.

    1   2   3   4   5   6   7

19. There is someone who loves and cares about me.

    1   2   3   4   5   6   7

20. I have people to share social events and fun activities with.

    1   2   3   4   5   6   7

21. I am responsible for helping provide for another person's needs.

    1   2   3   4   5   6   7

22. If I need advice, there is someone who would assist me to work out a plan for dealing with the situation.

    1   2   3   4   5   6   7

23. I have a sense of being needed by another person.

    1   2   3   4   5   6   7

24. People think that I'm not as good a friend as I should be.

    1   2   3   4   5   6   7

25. If I got sick there is someone to give me advice about caring for myself.

    1   2   3   4   5   6   7

Source: Brandt, PA, and Weinert, C: The PRQ: A social support measure. Nurs Res 30:277, 1981.

scores for each subscale are calculated (sum divided by items in subscale); higher scores indicate greater perceived social support in each of the five dimensions. Items 4, 6, 7, 10, and 24 are worded negatively and must be recoded (7 = 1, 6 = 2, 5 = 3, 4 = 4, 3 = 5, 2 = 6, 1 = 7) to reflect the positive direction of the other 20 items. Subscales associated with the PRQ-II are as follows: Intimacy: items 1, 5, 10, 15, 19; Social Integration: items 2, 6, 11, 16, 20; Nurturance: items 7, 12, 17, 21, 23; Worth: items 3, 8, 13, 18, 24; Assistance/Guidance: items 4, 9, 14, 22, 25.

The role questionnaire (RQ) is a 14-item rating scale that has two subscales: role conflict and role ambiguity. Eight items make up the role conflict scale, and six items make up the role ambiguity scale. Excerpt 9.3 discusses how items associated with role ambiguity need to be reverse-scored to reflect the direction of the other eight items. Examples of role ambiguity items include "I know exactly what is expected of me," "I feel certain about how much authority I have," and "Clear, planned goals exist for my job." By reverse-scoring the six role ambiguity items (e.g., 7 = 1, 6 = 2, 5 = 3, 4 = 4, 3 = 5, 2 = 6, 1 = 7), higher scores would indicate higher levels of role ambiguity. The eight role conflict items are already worded positively, so that higher scores indicate higher levels of role conflict. Examples of role conflict items include "I have to do things that should be done differently," "I receive an assignment without the proper support," and "I receive incompatible requests from two or more people." Discussion of reverse scoring is presented in Excerpt 9.3.

Semantic Differential Scales

The **semantic differential scale** is composed of a set of scales using pairs of adjectives that reflect opposite feelings. The technique was developed by Osgood, Suci, and Tannenbaum[6] to measure attitude, beliefs, or both. Subjects are asked to select one point on the scale that best describes

---

EXCERPT 9.3

Reverse Scoring on Items Associated With the Revised Personal Lifestyle Questionnaire (PLQ) for Early Adolescents

Properties of the Personal Lifestyle Questionnaire (PLQ)

Muhlenkamp and Brown (1983) developed the PLQ to assess the extent to which individuals engage in health promotion activities. They labeled these health promotion activities as positive health practices. The PLQ is a 24-item instrument consisting of six subscales: Nutrition (4 items), Relaxation (5 items), Exercise (3 items), Health Promotion (4 items), Safety (4 items), and Substance use (4 items). The items are measured on a 4-point Likert summated rating scale from 1 (Never) to 4 (Always). After reverse scoring of 5 items, higher scores indicate the reporting of more positive health practices; scores range from 24 to 96.

Revision of the PLQ for Early Adolescents

Written permission to revise the instrument was obtained from designated authorities at the College of Nursing, Arizona State University. As stated above, the PLQ has 24 items. Three decisions were made before revising the PLQ. First, maintain 24 items on the revised scale with a similar distribution of items on each subscale. Second, revise the wording of 6 items to make them applicable and readable for early adolescents. Third, eliminate 5 items on the PLQ that were not relevant for early adolescents, such as "Drive after drinking two or more alcoholic beverages" and replace with 5 new items. New items were constructed from the health promotion literature for early adolescents and pertain to the following subscales: Health Promotion, Safety, Nutrition, and Exercise. On the revised PLQ, the number of items per subscale is as follows: Nutrition (4 items), Relaxation (5 items), Exercise (4 items), Health Promotion (4 items), Safety (4 items), and Substance Use (3 items). Five items on the original PLQ are reverse scored, whereas 4 items on the revised PLQ are reverse scored (Items 10, 11, 14, and 17).

Source: Mahon, NE, Yarcheski, TJ, and Yarcheski, A: The Revised Personal Lifestyle Questionnaire for early adolescents. West J Nurs Res 25:533, 2002.

their view of the concept being measured. The scale is different from Likert scales in two ways:

1. Only two extremes are labeled.
2. The continuum is based not on agree/disagree but rather on opposite adjectives that express the respondent's feelings.

The example shown in Figure 9.2 illustrates a 7-point semantic differential scale that explores women's feelings about the labor and delivery experience in childbirth. The middle section represents a neutral position.

The semantic differential scale is scored by assigning values from 1 to 7 to each of the spaces within each adjective pair, with 1 representing the negative extreme and 7 the positive extreme. To avoid biases or a tendency to check the same column in each scale, the order of negative and positive responses is varied randomly. For example, in Figure 9.2, ratings of painful/not painful, slow/fast, lonely/shared, and unprepared/prepared place the negative value on the left. In the other four scales, the positive values are on the left. A total score can be obtained by summing the scores for each rating. Lower total scores usually reflect negative feelings toward the concept being measured; higher scores usually reflect positive feelings. If the researcher decides that higher numbers represent a positive word value, the negative high score items need to be reverse-scored. A score of 7 for the adjective pair "satisfying/unsatisfying" would be scored as a 1 when it was summed, and the adjective pair "unprepared/ prepared" would remain as a score of 7. Excerpt 9.4 describes the use of a semantic differential scale. Women who participated in the study were asked to look at a pair of words and rate their feelings about the 13 different concepts on a 7-point scale. The semantic differential scale is different from the Likert scale in that only two extremes are labeled.

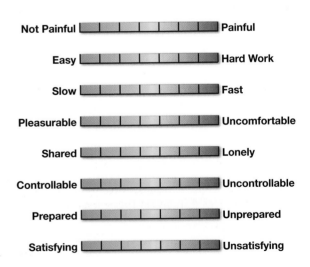

Fig 9•2 Example of Semantic Differential Scale Describing the Labor and Delivery Experience for Women.

EXCERPT 9.4

Use of the Semantic Differential Scale

Power as Knowing Participation in Change Test (PKPCT)

The PKPCT is a semantic differential instrument with four subscales—awareness, choices, freedom to act intentionally, and involvement in creating changes—and a total score. Each subscale is composed of a list of 13 bipolar adjectives. One of the adjective pairs in each list duplicates an earlier item pair, consistent with semantic differential theory. Each subscale item is scored from 1 to 7, with total subscale scores ranging from 13 to 91. Higher scores indicate relatively more power. Women participating in 1997 and 2000 qualitative studies of hypothyroid-like symptoms and fatigue noted that powerlessness was significant in their experiences; thus, the PKPCT was chosen to describe powerlessness.

Source: Dzurec, LC, Hoover, PM, and Fields, J: Acknowledging unexplained fatigue of tired women. Image: J Nurs Schol 34:41, 2002.

Second, the continuum is not based on agree/disagree but on opposite adjectives that express the respondent's feelings.

Visual Analogue Scales

The **visual analogue scale** (VAS) is useful for measuring subjective phenomena (e.g., pain, fatigue, shortness of breath, anxiety). The scale is unidimensional, quantifying intensity only. The VAS is 100 mm long (10 cm), with anchors at each end to indicate the extremes of the phenomenon being assessed. Subjects are asked to mark a point on the line indicating the amount of the phenomenon experienced at that time. The intensity of the phenomenon is scored by measuring the millimeters from the low end of the scale to the subject's mark.[7] The VAS is a reliable and valid measure for assessing subjective patient experiences. An example of a VAS is shown in Figure 9.3. Use of the VAS is illustrated in Excerpt 9.5.

Q Methodology

Q Methodology (or Q sort) is an example of a sorting technique used to characterize opinions, attitudes, or judgments of individuals through comparative rank ordering.[8] The technique involves giving an individual a set of cards containing a series of written items, such as statements or phrases,

Fig 9•3 Example of Visual Analogue Scale (VAS).

Directions: Please place an X at the point on the line that best reflects how much pain you experienced with the venipuncture.

No Pain   Worst Pain Possible

EXCERPT 9.5

Use of the Visual Analogue Scale

Instruments

Two visual analogue scales (VASs) provided ratio-level measures of present pain intensity (I) and pain relief (R). The VAS-I was a horizontal, 10-cm line anchored on the left with *no pain* and on the right with *pain as bad as it could be*. The VAS-R was a horizontal, 10-cm line anchored on the left with *no pain relief* and on the right with *complete pain relief*. The subject placed a red pen mark to show the intensity of present pain or amount of pain relief from all pain therapies. We used a computerized digitizer tablet to measure from the left side of the line to the place marked by the subject and the Dig2 software to automatically enter the score into a database. Validity, reliability, and sensitivity of the VAS as a measure of pain intensity and pain relief have been estimated previously.

Source: Wilkie, D, et al: Effects of coaching patients with lung cancer to report cancer pain. West J Nurs Res 32:23, 2010.

---

each item being placed on a separate card. The individual is asked to sort the cards into piles according to some scaled criterion. The number of cards should range from 40 to 100, depending on the research question.[9] The number of piles is usually 5 to 10, ranging from low priority to high priority. The researcher specifies how many cards are to go into each pile so that the subject is faced with forced choices. Subjects may replace any card or move any card to another pile any time during the sorting process until they are satisfied with the results. Subjects are advised to first select those cards that go into the extreme categories. The method is supposed to yield a normal distribution of responses, with fewer statements in the extreme category.

In Zax's[10] study exploring postpartum concerns of teenage mothers, subjects were asked to sort through cards and place them in five piles, from least to greatest postpartum concerns among teenagers. Each statement was preceded by, "I am worried about. . . ." The Q sort items are shown here. Although considerably fewer than 40 cards were used in this study, it was a beginning attempt to explore self-expressed concerns of first-time teenage mothers during the first 3 postpartum months.

> When my body will look normal again.
> Having my body feel normal again.
> How to take care of my baby.
> How my baby has been acting.
> How I can take care of my baby and do other important things too.
> How things are different with my friends.
> How things are different with my boyfriend.
> Making love.
> School.
> How things are different with my family.

How I'll be able to do household chores.
What it was like being in labor and giving birth.
How my boyfriend feels about my baby.
How I feel emotionally.

Instruments

Phenomena measured by psychosocial instruments (e.g., coping, stress, self-concept, self-esteem, motivation) are studied widely in nursing. Many psychosocial instruments have already been developed, tested, and refined to measure a particular variable or concept. Selecting an appropriate instrument is critical for the researcher. The method of measurement must closely fit the conceptual definition of the variable or concept. Instruments consist of a series of items that may be analyzed either as a total score or independently as separate subscales. Despite the type of instrument sought, certain kinds of information should be available about any standardized instrument.

Psychosocial instruments usually include guidelines for scoring and interpreting scores. Guidelines for scoring include information on criteria for acceptable responses, the number of points to be assigned to various responses, the procedures for computing total scores, and usually, normative data on a wide range of population groups. Journal articles usually do not provide a copy of the questionnaire or instrument(s) used in the study, nor do they give detailed guidelines for scoring and interpreting scores. Excerpt 9.6 provides a discussion of the knowledge, perceived

---

EXCERPT 9.6

Information on How to Score and Interpret Instruments/Scales Associated With the Awareness of HPV and Cervical Cancer Questionnaire

The knowledge portion of the Awareness of HPV and Cervical Cancer Questionnaire consists of 15 multiple-choice items, with each question permitting only one response. The knowledge score for this instrument ranges from 0 to 15 with higher scores indicative of more knowledge of HPV and cervical cancer.

The perceived threat portion of cervical cancer consists of 15 questions, using a 5-point Likert-type scale ranging from 1 (strongly agree) to 5 (strongly disagree). Nine of the 15 questions related to perceived susceptibility and have a possible subtotal score range from 9 to 45. The remaining six questions related to perceived seriousness and have a potential score that ranges from 6 to 30. Higher scores imply greater level of perceived susceptibility and seriousness about HPV and cervical cancer. The last six questions focus on individual sexual behaviors, risk factors, and history of pap smears and are multiple-choice categorical variables.

Source: Montgomery, K, Bloch, JR, Bhattacharya, A, and Montgomery, O: Human papillomavirus and cervical cancer knowledge, health beliefs, and preventative practices in older women. J Obstet Gynecol Neonat Nurs 39:238, 2010.

threat, and seriousness scales associated with the Awareness of HPV and Cervical Cancer Questionnaire.

The construction of an instrument is complex and time-consuming. The development of an effective instrument requires an in-depth knowledge of the phenomena under study and considerable skill in measurement. Beginning researchers should use instruments that have already been developed, ones with established reliability and validity. Standardized instruments are developed by experts in a particular area of study.

Biophysical Measures

Nursing research includes variables measured with physiological instruments. Various monitoring devices have been developed to measure vital signs and other physiological data. These devices yield quantitative data that are easily analyzed. For example, maximal inspiratory pressure is used to indicate inspiratory muscle strength, which provides an index of performance for patients with chronic obstructive lung disease. Excerpt 9.7 provides an example of other types of technology to measure biological measures.

Qualitative Data Collection Methods

Interviews

An **interview schedule**, sometimes called an interview guide, is a list of topics or an open-ended questionnaire administered to subjects by a skilled interviewer. The presence of the interviewer allows for probing of subjects' responses and decreases the possibility of vague answers. Interviewing is often used in qualitative studies to elicit meaningful data; however, open-ended questionnaires may be used with other instruments to generate both qualitative and quantitative data, as shown in Excerpt 9.8

Excerpt 9.7

Use of Technology to Measure Biophysical Variables

Biologic measures included blood glucose, HbA1C, weight, and BMI. Blood glucose was measured using the clinic's glucometer. HbA1C was tested using the Metrika point-of-service monitor. This monitor, certified by the National Glycohemoglobin Standardization Program, requires only one drop of blood and has been found to be as accurate as laboratory testing (Stivers et al., 2000). We used a balance-beam scale with a stadiometer to measure weight and height for calculation of the body mass index (BMI).

Source: Vincent, D, Pasvogel, A, and Barrera, L: A feasibility study of a culturally tailored diabetes intervention for Mexican Americans. Biological Res Nurs 9:130, 2007.

EXCERPT 9.8

Use of Open and Close-Ended Questionnaires to Collect Data

Method

Interview scripts, questions, and probes were used to collect quantitative and qualitative data. Interviews were conducted by research assistants who conducted pilot interviews prior to the study. Multiple sources of information were sought through the use of quantitative and qualitative questions and interviews with parent-teen dyads from the same family. This triangulation research approach supports the idea that no singular method can fully understand problems inherent in complex inquiries. Each method is used to disclose diverse realities, and these can be cross-reviewed and analyzed to increase the validity and results of the study to provide further clarification and verification. Through the use of multiple viewpoints and data sources, triangulation is a tool used for improving the trustworthiness of the data and aids in the interpretation process.

Source: Kilty, HL, and Prentice, D: Adolescent cardiovascular risk factors: A follow-up study. Clin Nurs Res 19:6, 2010.

Audio and video recordings may be used to complement interviews. Researchers must consider the possibility that subjects might be sensitive to the presence of audio and video equipment and should ask for the subject's permission to tape. In Excerpt 9.9, the researcher has indicated each interview will be conducted for 90 minutes and be audiotaped, then later transcribed.

EXCERPT 9.9

Use of Audiotaping During Interviews

Data Collection

In both focus groups, the researcher acted as group moderator, reiterating the purpose of the group conversation and establishing the parameters of confidentiality for the group and study. A quiet and familiar lounge room at the hospital, free from distractions and interruptions, was used as recommended for collecting qualitative data, with parents and researcher seated in a circle.

Probing questions were developed from a review of the literature and clinical experience and were screened by an expert in qualitative research. As parents told their stories and shared similar feelings and experiences, a common bond was formed, and this process facilitated in-depth discussion that was reported as therapeutic by the parents. Each interview was conducted for 90 minutes and audiotaped and later transcribed verbatim.

Source: Sidhu, R, Passmore, A, and Baker, D: An investigation into parent perceptions of the needs of siblings of children with cancer. J Pediar Oncol Nurses 22:276, 2005.

Participant Observation

This type of qualitative data collection is used in ethnographic research. The technique (Chapter 12) involves direct observation through involvement with subjects in their natural setting, participating in their lifestyle activities. Through participation and observation, data are collected in an unstructured manner as field notes written in a journal. The key element in participant observation is involvement with subjects in their environment and development of a trusting relationship.

Focus Group Interviews

Focus groups are acceptable subjects for in-depth interviews. The technique serves a variety of purposes, with the ultimate goal of observing the interactions among focus group members and detecting their attitudes, opinions, and solutions to specific topics posed by the facilitator.[11] Focus groups are designed to be nonthreatening, so participants can express and clarify their views in ways that are less likely to occur one-on-one. There is a sense of "safety in numbers."[12] Focus groups have a value similar to that of an open-ended question; however, with the latter, there is no ability to probe participants for meaning.

Recruiting subjects to participate in a focus group interview is critical. The use of purposive sampling is most often employed when individuals known to have a desired expertise are sought. Recruitment may be sought through the media, posters, or advertisements. Incentives (i.e., money, gifts, certificates, coupons, and so on) may need to be provided to ensure attendance by a sufficient number of participants.[12]

A focus group is typically made up of 6 to 12 individuals who are asked to discuss a particular topic led by a facilitator. Fewer participants may result in an inadequate discussion. Focus group discussions are recorded either manually, by having someone take notes, or by audiotape. If taped, the discussion is transcribed. A transcript of the discussion becomes the data of the focus group interview.

Excerpt 9.10 presents an example of a qualitative approach to research employing focus group methods.

EXCERPT 9.10

Use of Focus Group Interview

Methods

A qualitative design employing focus group methods explored and gathered parental perceptions about the needs and issues of siblings of children with cancer and additionally explored possible supportive interventions. Focus groups were chosen in preference to individual interviews as an efficient means of collecting data from a number of parents. In addition, the dynamics and interplay between the group members were an integral part of this

EXCERPT 9.10

Use of Focus Group Interview—cont'd

process, and the interaction of the "group think" was another key factor in selecting this methodology. The synthesis of information in a group setting was an important component of the research process as it assisted in developing and clarifying the concepts generated.

Source: Sidhu, R, Passmore, A, and Baker, D: An investigation into parent perceptions of the needs of siblings of children with cancer. J Pediar Oncol Nurses 22:276, 2005.

CRITIQUING DATA COLLECTION METHODS

Identify a research study to critique. Read the study to see if you recognize any key terms discussed in this chapter. Remember that all studies may not contain all key terms. The following questions[1,11,12] serve as a guide in critiquing data collection methods:

1. *What types of instruments and/or scales were used to measure the main study variables?* Authors should describe and justify instrumentation used in a study. If you do not know how instruments and/or scales are used, information is lacking that is vital to understanding the data they produce. In quantitative studies, data collected usually take the form of statistical operations when being analyzed. See Chapter 10 for a discussion of the most commonly encountered statistics. In qualitative studies, data are elicited through interviews and participant observation. Refer to Chapter 12 for a more detailed discussion of data collection as it relates to a qualitative approach to research.

2. *Was the data collection process described clearly?* Data collection procedures should be explained in detail. It is not sufficient to read that a questionnaire or survey was used. Readers need to know the details regarding administration of questionnaires, surveys, and scales. It is important to determine if the questionnaires/surveys were administered to individuals or groups, by the researcher or by research assistant(s), with scripted instructions, under conditions that were similar for all subjects, and after administration, if all sections or parts of the questionnaire/survey were to be completed and returned.

SUMMARY OF KEY IDEAS

1. Questionnaires are self-reported forms or interviews designed to collect information.

2. A scale is a set of numerical values assigned to responses, representing the extent to which subjects possess a particular attitude, value, or characteristic.

3. Likert scales consist of a series of statements in which subjects select an appropriately ranked response that reflects their agreement or disagreement.

4. Semantic differential scales measure subjects' feelings about a concept, based on a continuum that extends between two extreme opposites.

5. The visual analogue scale is a 100-mm line used to measure subjective phenomena.

6. Psychosocial instruments for measuring concepts or phenomena in nursing are the most commonly used quantitative method of data collection.

7. Interviews and observation are common methods of data collection in qualitative research.

8. Focus groups present researchers with opportunities to observe the interactions among participants and record their attitudes and opinions.

LEARNING ACTIVITIES

1. Complete the in-class questionnaire in Figure 9.1. As a class, tally the results, and share these with one another. Identify which questions were open-ended, categorical, and continuous responses. Were the questions and answers meaningful and interesting?

2. Design a questionnaire. Write a paragraph that introduces the questionnaire to the respondent and explains how to answer the questions. This paragraph should be encouraging but general. Provide enough specific information. Include a variety of answers to questions that represent open-ended, categorical, and continuous variables.

REFERENCES

1. Polit, DF, and Beck, CT: Essentials of Nursing Research: Methods, Appraisal, and Utilization, ed. 6. Lippincott Williams & Wilkins, Philadelphia, 2006, pp 287–321.
2. Fink, A: The Survey Handbook, ed. 2. Sage Publications, Thousand Oaks, CA, 2003.
3. Dillman, DA: Mail and Telephone Surveys: The Total Design Method, ed. 2. John Wiley & Sons, New York, 2000.
4. Fink, A: How to Conduct Surveys: A Step-by-Step Guide, ed. 4. Sage Publications, Thousand Oaks, CA, 2009.
5. Spector, PE: Summated Rating Scale Construction: An Introduction. Sage Publications, Newbury Park, CA, 1992.
6. Osgood, CE, Suci, GJ, and Tannenbaum, RH: The Measurement Meaning. University of Illinois Press, Urbana, IL, 1957.
7. Gift, AG: Visual analogue scales: Measurement of subjective phenomena. Nurs Res 38:286, 1989.
8. Stephenson, W: The Study of Behavior. Q Technique and its Methodology. University of Chicago Press, Chicago, 1975.
9. Tetting, DW: Q sort update. West J Nurs Res 10:757, 1988.

10. Zax, S: Postpartum concerns of teenage mothers: An exploratory study. Unpublished master's thesis, Yale University School of Nursing, 1985.

11. Burns, N, and Grove, SK: The Practice of Nursing Research: Conduct, Critique, and Utilization, ed. 4. WB Saunders, Philadelphia, 2001, pp 424–426, 671.

12. Gillis A, and Jackson, W: Research for Nurses: Methods and Interpretation. FA Davis, Philadelphia, 2002, pp 234–239, 618.

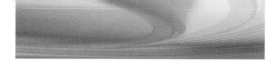

10

ANALYZING DATA

James A. Fain, PhD, RN, BC-ADM, FAAN

LEARNING OBJECTIVES

By the end of this chapter, you will be able to:

1. Differentiate between descriptive and inferential statistics.
2. Compare and contrast the three measures of central tendency.
3. Compare and contrast the three measures of dispersion.
4. Distinguish between parametric and nonparametric procedures.
5. Evaluate a researcher's choice of descriptive and inferential statistics in published research.

GLOSSARY OF KEY TERMS

Analysis of variance (ANOVA). A parametric procedure used to test whether there is a difference among three group means.

Chi-square. A nonparametric procedure used to assess whether a relationship exists between two nominal level variables; symbolized as χ^2.

Correlation. A measure that defines the relationship between two variables.

Descriptive statistics. Statistics that describe and summarize data.

Homogeneity of variance. Situation in which the dependent variables do not differ significantly between or among groups.

Inferential statistics. Statistics that generalize findings from a sample to a population.

Level of confidence. Probability level in which the research hypothesis is accepted with confidence. A 0.05 level of confidence is the standard among researchers.

Mean. A measure of central tendency calculated by summing a set of scores and dividing the sum by the total number of scores; also called the average.

Measures of central tendency. Descriptive statistics that describe the location or approximate center of a distribution of data.

Measures of dispersion. Descriptive statistics that depict the spread or variability among a set of numerical data.

Median. A measure of central tendency that represents the middle score in a distribution.

(Continued)

Mode. The score or value that occurs most frequently in a distribution; a measure of central tendency used most often with nominal-level data.

Negative correlation. Correlation in which high scores for one variable are paired with low scores for the other variable.

Outlier. Data point isolated from other data points; extreme score in a data set.

Parameter. Numerical characteristic of a population (e.g., population mean, population standard deviation).

Positive correlation. Correlation in which high scores for one variable are paired with high scores for the other variable, or low scores for one variable are paired with low scores for the other variable.

Probability. Likelihood that an event will occur, given all possible outcomes.

Range. A measure of variability that is the difference between the lowest and highest values in a distribution.

Robust. Referring to results from statistical analyses that are close to being valid, even though the researcher does not rigidly adhere to assumptions associated with parametric procedures.

Skewed distribution. A distribution of scores with a few outlying observations in either direction.

Standard deviation (SD). The most frequently used measure of variability; the distance a score varies from the mean.

Symmetrical distribution. A distribution of scores in which the mean, median, and mode are all the same.

t-test. A popular parametric procedure for assessing whether two group means are significantly different from one another.

Variance. Measure of variability, which is the average squared deviation from the mean.

The purpose of data analysis is to answer research questions, test hypotheses, or both. The research design and type of data collected determine selection of appropriate statistical procedures. Once data have been collected, statistical procedures describe, analyze, and interpret quantitative data. Application of the appropriate statistics helps the researcher decide if the results and conclusions of the study are justified. Despite how well researchers conduct a study, inappropriate analyses can lead to inappropriate conclusions. Many different statistical procedures are used to analyze data. This chapter provides an overview of the most commonly used statistics that describe and examine relationships and that test for differences.[1] A consumer of nursing research needs to interpret and apply statistical data applicable to nursing practice. This can be accomplished by reading and evaluating data analyses.

Using Statistics to Describe Data

Statistical procedures are classified into two categories, descriptive and inferential statistics. **Descriptive statistics** describe, organize, and summarize data. Inferential statistics make generalizations about populations based on data collected from samples. Descriptive statistics include measures of central tendency and measures of dispersion. **Measures of central tendency** are descriptive statistics that describe the location or approximate the center of a distribution of data. A distribution consists of scores and numerical values and their frequency of occurrence. Measures of central tendency include the mean, median, and mode. **Measures of dispersion** are descriptive statistics that depict the spread or variability among a set of numerical data. Measures of dispersion are described by the range, variance, and standard deviation. Two additional measures of dispersion that are not frequently found in the literature are percentile and interquartile range.

Measures of Central Tendency

Mean

The **mean** is the most commonly used measure of central tendency and is often associated with the term "average." The mean is calculated by adding all the scores in a distribution and dividing the total by the number of scores. One major characteristic of the mean is that the calculation takes into account each score in the distribution.

In defining the mean with a formula, the following notation is used. The symbol that represents the mean is $\bar{X}$, read as "X bar." Σ, the Greek letter Sigma, is used to denote the sum of values.

When data represent either an interval or a ratio scale, the mean is the preferred measure of central tendency. The mean is a stable and reliable measure. If equal-sized samples are randomly selected from the same population, the means of those samples will be similar to each other as compared with either the medians or modes.

Excerpt 10.1 includes a table with results of a study conducted to revise and assess reliability of the revised Personal Lifestyle Questionnaire (PLQ) for use with early adolescents. Descriptive statistics included the mean, standard deviation, and range for the total PLQ and individual subscales. Note that the mean is designated as M and the standard deviation as SD. Within the article, information is provided on how PLQ and various subscales were measured. Scoring methods associated with each scale are not always included in journal articles, because of page limitations. The researcher needs to locate the original publication where major properties and scoring methods associated with the scale are discussed.

The mean is very sensitive to extreme values, or "outliers." An **outlier** is a data point isolated from other data points. In a distribution of scores with outliers, the mean is "pulled" in the direction of those extreme values. For example, in the following distribution of ages in years (e.g., 23, 22, 25, 26, 29, 27, and 23), the mean age is 25. Suppose the 29 becomes 50. The age 50 years is considered an outlier. The mean age is now 28, yet the median and mode remain the same.

EXCERPT 10.1

Use of the Mean, Standard Deviation, and Range as Measures of Central Tendency

Variable	M	SD	Range	Alpha
Total Revised PLQ	67.84	11.26	24–93	0.83
Subscales				
Exercise	10.93	3.10	4–16	0.70
Nutrition	11.25	2.24	4–16	0.37
Relaxation	14.36	3.14	4–20	0.62
Safety	10.92	3.08	5–16	0.60
Substance Use	9.16	1.80	3–12	0.35
Health promotion	10.83	2.85	4–16	0.60

Note: PLQ = Personal Lifestyle Questionnaire.

Source: Mahon, NE, Yarcheski, TJ, and Yarcheski, A: The revised Personal Lifestyle Questionnaire for early adolescents. West J Nurs Res 25:533–547, 2002.

Median

The **median** (Mdn) is the middle score or midpoint of a distribution. Researchers sometimes call it the 50th percentile; 50 percent of the distribution falls below or above the midpoint. The median is calculated by first arranging the scores in rank order. If there is an odd number of scores, the median is the middle score. For example, if a set of scores on a pain scale administered to five patients is 4, 5, 7, 8, and 9, the median is 7. If an even number of scores appears in the distribution, the median is the point halfway between the two middle scores. For example, if the set of scores on the pain scale was 4, 5, 5, 7, 7, and 9, the median is (7 + 5/2) = 6. Thus, the median is not necessarily one of the scores in the distribution.

One major characteristic of the median is that it does not take into account each score in the distribution. The median is not sensitive to extreme scores. For example, if a set of scores on a coping scale administered to five patients is 12, 15, 22, 31, and 35, the median score is 22. The mean for this distribution of scores is 23. However, if one value changes and the set of scores is 12, 15, 22, 31, and 125, the median is still 22, whereas the mean is now 41.

The median is an appropriate measure of central tendency when the data represent a skewed distribution. A distribution that has outlying observations in either direction, above or below the mean, is a **skewed distribution**. A **symmetrical distribution** is one in which the mean, median, and mode are all the same (Fig. 10.1). Skewed distributions have off-centered peaks and longer tails in one direction. The mean, median, and mode do not coincide in skewed distributions; rather, their relative

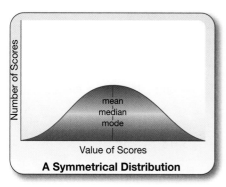

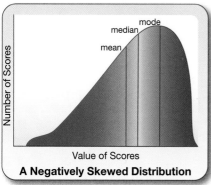
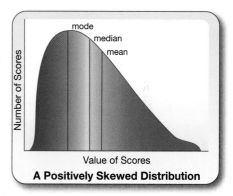

Fig 10•1 Measures of Central Tendency in Normal and Skewed Distribution.

positions remain constant. The mode is closest to the peak of the curve, as this is where the most frequent scores are found. The mean is closest to the tail, where the relatively few extreme scores are located. For this reason, the mean score in positively skewed distributions lies toward the high score values; the mean in the negatively skewed distribution falls close to the low score values (see Fig. 10.1). In a skewed distribution, the median always falls somewhere between the mean and the mode.

The word "median" is abbreviated as "Mdn." Excerpt 10.2 includes a table in which the mean (M) and median (Mdn) are presented for two variables measured on an interval-ratio scale: age and years of education. The mean age of the sample was 56.58 years, with a median of 55. The mean number of years of education was 11.04 years, with a median of 12. In both examples, the mean and median were almost identical, indicating a normal distribution. If the median age was 65, this would represent a negatively skewed distribution.

Mode

The **mode** is the most frequently occurring score in a distribution. It is an appropriate measure of central tendency for nominal data. A distribution

---

EXCERPT 10.2

Use of Mean and Median as Measures of Central Tendency

Demographic and Background Information of Sample

	M	SD	Range	Median	No.	%
N = 65						
Age (yr)	56.58	14.02	29–90	55		
Education (yr)	11.04	3.08	3–18	12		
Race						
Black					27	49
White					28	51
Admission route						
Emergency department				29	53	
Doctor's office					4	7
Transfer					22	40
Annual income (n = 44)						
<$10,000					18	41
$10,000–$24,999					14	24
$25,000–$40,000					7	12
>$40,000					5	9

Source: Warner, CD: Somatic awareness and coronary artery disease in women with chest pain. Heart Lung 24:436, 1995.

---

of scores may have more than one mode. Data with a single mode are called unimodal; data with two modes, bimodal. In Excerpt 10.3, the authors display a frequency distribution for several variables, including marital status and education. In a frequency distribution, the most frequently occurring score (mode) can be identified. Of the 80 subjects who participated in the study, the most frequently occurring category for marital status was married or living with someone (n = 56). Also, the most frequently occurring education category was subjects who had a high school degree (n = 33). Excerpt 10.4 provides sample characteristics about a particular study within the context of the article.

Comparing the Mean, Median, and Mode

Researchers choose a measure of central tendency depending on the level of measurement, shape, or form of the distribution of data and research objective.

Level of Measurement

The use of the mean is appropriate with interval/ratio and sometimes ordinal data (see Chapter 8). The mean is a more precise measure than

---

EXCERPT 10.3

Frequency Distribution

Age–M (SD)	**69 (7 years)**
Gender–Male	**38 (48%)**
Race–White	**79 (99%)**
Marital Status	
Married or living with someone	56 (70%)
Widowed, divorced, or single	24 (30%)
Education	
Less than high school	16 (20%)
High school degree	33 (41%)
Beyond high school	31 (39%)
Annual Income	
<$20,000	26 (35%)
$20,000-$40,000	29 (40%)
>$40,000	18 (25%)
Heart Failure Etiology	
Ischemic	38 (47%)
Nonischemic	42 (53%)
NYHA Class	
Class I	4 (5%)
Class II	28 (35%)
Class III	47 (59%)
Class IV	1 (1%)
Ejection Fraction–M (SD)	**38% (15)**
Cumulative Illness Rating Scale–M (SD)	**15.4 (5.8)**

Source: Klein, DM, Turvey, CL, and Pies, CJ: Relationship of coping styles with quality of life and depressive symptoms in older heart failure patients. J Aging Health 19:22, 2007.

the median or mode because it takes into account every score in a distribution. The mean is also the most stable of the three measures. If a number of samples are randomly drawn from a target population, the mean varies less, compared with the median and mode. The median is an ordinal statistic based on ranks. Applying the mean to ordinal data must yield meaningful results. Likewise, it makes little sense to compute

EXCERPT 10.4

Sample Characteristics Reported Within Text of Article

A total of 20 participants were enrolled and randomly assigned to the usual care control group (N = 10) or to the 8-week intervention (N = 10). The majority of the sample were female (71%) with a mean age of 56 (SD = 9.3, range = 37 to 69). Half (50%) the sample were married. The mean time since diagnosis with type 2 diabetes was 7.9 years (SD = 7.8, range = 1 to 24 years). The majority of participants were in a low socioeconomic bracket with 76% reporting an income of less than $20,000 a year.

Source: Vincent, D, Pasvogel, A, Barrera, L: A feasibility study of a culturally tailored diabetes intervention for Mexican Americans. Biol Res Nurs 9:130–141, 2007.

a median for nominal data (e.g., marital status, religious affiliation). Because the mode requires only a frequency count, it can be applied to any set of data at the nominal, ordinal, or interval/ratio level of measurement.

Shape of the Distribution

The shape or form of the distribution is another factor that influences the researcher's choice of a measure of central tendency. In skewed distributions (see Fig. 10.1), the mean, median, and mode do not coincide, although their relative positions remain constant in moving away from the peak toward the tail. The order is always from mode, to median, to mean. In a skewed distribution, the median always falls somewhere between the mean and mode. It is this characteristic that makes the median the most appropriate measure of central tendency for describing a skewed distribution.

Research Objective

Regardless of the purpose of the study, the researcher uses the mode as a preliminary indicator of central tendency. If a more precise measure of central tendency is warranted, the median or mean is used. To describe a skewed distribution, the researcher chooses the median to give a balanced picture of the extreme scores or outliers. In addition, the median is sometimes used as a point in the distribution at which scores can be divided into two categories containing the same number of respondents. The mean is preferred over the median because the mean is easily used in more advanced statistical analyses.

Measures of Dispersion

Range

The **range** is the simplest measure of dispersion. It is calculated by subtracting the lowest score in the distribution from the highest score.

Excerpt 10.1 illustrates examples of how the range is reported. The researcher reports the range for each subscale associated with the Personal Lifestyle Questionnaire (PLQ). For example, the total PLQ has a potential range of 24 to 93. The subscale exercise has a potential range of 4 to 16, and the subscale relaxation has a potential range of 4 to 20.

The range is considered an unstable measure because it is based on only two values in the distribution. It is extremely sensitive to outliers and does not take into account variations in scores between extremes.

Variance and Standard Deviation

The variance and standard deviation are measures of dispersion. Both measures are based on deviated scores. A deviated score is defined as the difference between a raw score and the mean of that distribution $(x^2 = \overline{X} - X)$. Raw scores below the mean have a negative deviation, whereas raw scores above the mean have a positive deviation. The sum of the deviated scores in a distribution always equals 0. Thus, if researchers use deviated scores in calculating measures of variability, they must find ways to get around the fact that the sum of the deviated scores in a distribution always equals 0. Each deviated score is squared, so that all numbers become positive.

The sum of the squared deviations divided by the number of scores is referred to as the **variance**. Mathematically, the variance is the average squared deviation from the mean. By itself, the variance is not very meaningful. Because each of the deviated scores is squared, the variance is expressed in units that are squares of the original units of measure. For example, if heart rate is measured in beats per minute, the variance is in units of beats^2 per minute^2. To understand what beat^2 per minute^2 means, researchers need to calculate the square root of the variance. This will convert beats^2 per minute^2 back to the original unit of measure (beats/minute).

The square root of the variance is referred to as the **standard deviation** (SD). As an index that summarizes data in the same unit of measurement as the original data, the SD is the most commonly reported measure of dispersion. Like the mean, the standard deviation is the most stable measure of variability and takes into account each score in the distribution. To calculate the SD, two formulas can be used. The first formula involves finding out the deviated scores. Each deviated score is squared, added up, and divided by (N – 1). This is a measure of variability, called variance. In its present form, this measure of variability is not useful.

An example of the calculation is shown in Table 10.1. Suppose a researcher was interested in calculating the variance and standard deviation for the variable age. Age has a variance of 193.33 square years (year^2). Most people would have trouble interpreting a square year. By taking the square root of the variance, the variable is returned to its

TABLE 10.1	Calculation of the Sample Variance and Standard Deviation Using the Deviated Scores	

X	x² (X – X̄)	(X – X̄)²
33	33–38	$(-5)^2 = 25$
68	68–38	$(30)^2 = 900$
28	28–38	$(-10)^2 = 100$
33	33–38	$(-5)^2 = 25$
28	28–38	$(-10)^2 = 100$
56	56–38	$(18)^2 = 324$
42	42–38	$(4)^2 = 16$
29	29–38	$(-9)^2 = 81$
38	38–38	$(0)^2 = 0$
25	25–38	$(-13)^2 = 169$
$\Sigma X = 380$	$\Sigma x^2 = (X - X) = 0$	$\Sigma x^2 = (X - X)^2 = 1{,}740$

$\bar{X} = 38.0$

Variance $(S^2) = 1{,}740\backslash9 = 193.33$ square years

Standard Deviation $(s) = \sqrt{1{,}740\backslash9} = 13.9$ years

original scale of measurement (years). The resulting statistic is an SD of 13.90 years. The SD, like the mean, is sensitive to outliers. It is an appropriate measure of dispersion for distributions that are symmetrical, not skewed.

Comparing the Range, Variance, and Standard Deviation

The range, although quick and simple to obtain, is not very reliable. Although the range is calculated from two scores in a distribution, both the variance and SD take into account every score in a distribution. Despite its relative stability, the variance is not widely used because it cannot be employed in many statistical analyses. In contrast, the SD squares the deviated scores and returns them to their original units of measure. Calculating the SD is the initial step for obtaining other statistical measures, especially in the context of statistical decision making.

Inferential Statistics

Inferential statistics focus on the process of selecting a sample and using the information to make generalizations to a population. Information contained in a sample is used to make inferences concerning a parameter. A **parameter** is a numerical characteristic of a population (e.g., population mean, population standard deviation). Researchers estimate the parameters of a population from a sample. For example, suppose a researcher randomly samples 125 people with type 1 diabetes and measures changes in blood glucose levels. If the mean blood glucose level is 70 mg/dL, this represents the mean sample statistic. If researchers were able to study every individual with type 1 diabetes, an average blood glucose level could be calculated. This would represent the parameter of the population. Researchers are rarely able to study an entire population. The use of inferential statistics allows researchers to make inferences about the larger population (all individuals with type 1 diabetes) from studying the sample (125 randomly selected people with type 1 diabetes).

Inferential statistical procedures are divided into two types. The first involves the estimation of parameters. A parameter estimation is evaluated by a single number or an interval. For example, a researcher might calculate a sample mean and use its value (age of 18) to estimate the mean age of female drivers. Because the estimate consists of a single value, it is called a point estimate. Alternatively, the mean age could be estimated by saying that it is some age between 16 and 22. This is an interval estimate and is associated with some amount of confidence. Confidence associated with an interval estimate is called the confidence interval. A confidence interval is a range of values that has some specified probability (e.g., 0.95 or 0.99) of including a particular population parameter.

The second type of inferential statistical procedure is hypothesis testing, which allows the researcher to formulate a hypothesis concerning the parameter, sample the population of interest, and make objective decisions about the sample results of the study. Central to hypothesis testing is a discussion of probability. Probability helps evaluate the accuracy of a statistic and test a hypothesis. Research findings are often stated and communicated using probability. Two types of hypothesis testing include parametric and nonparametric procedures.

Probability

Probability is an essential concept for understanding inferential statistics. Probability is a means of predicting (e.g., "There is a 50 percent chance of rain for the rest of the week," or "This operation has an 80 percent chance of success."). Probability is a system of rules for analyzing a set of outcomes. **Probability** is the likelihood that an event will occur, given all possible outcomes. The lowercase p signifies probability. For example, the probability of getting heads with the single flip of a coin is 1 out of 2, or 1/2, or 0.5. Therefore, the probability is expressed as 50 percent, or $p = 0.5$. The probability of getting a 4 when a die is thrown is 1 out of 6, 1/6, or $p = 0.17$. Conversely, the probability of not rolling a 4 is 5 out of 6, 5/6, or $p = 0.83$.

To establish whether an outcome is statistically significant, the researcher must set up a confidence level. A **level of confidence** is a probability level in which the null hypothesis can be rejected with confidence and the research hypothesis can be accepted with confidence. Researchers use 0.05 as the standard level of confidence; that is, researchers are willing to accept statistical significance occurring by chance 5 times out of 100. The 0.05 level of confidence is graphically depicted in Figure 10.2. As shown, the 0.05 level of confidence is found in the small areas of the "tails." These are the areas under the curve that represent a distance of ±1.96 SD from a mean difference of 0. A 1.96 SD in either direction represents 2.5 percent of the sample mean differences (50% – 47.5% = 2.5%). In other words, 95 percent of the sample differences falls between –1.96 SD and +1.96 SD from a mean difference of 0.

Confidence levels can be set up for any amount of probability. For example, a more stringent confidence level is 0.01. Using this level of confidence, there is 1 chance out of 100 that the sample difference could occur by chance (1%). The 0.01 level of confidence is represented by the area that lies 2.58 SDs in both directions from a mean difference of zero.

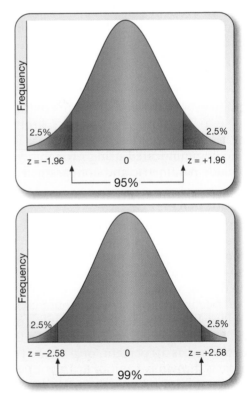

Fig 10·2 Graphic Representation of 0.05 and 0.01 Levels of Confidence.

The magnitude of p does not indicate the amount of validity associated with each research hypothesis. Avoid using terms such as "highly significant" or "more significant." Once the level of significance is chosen, it represents a decision rule. The decision rule is dichotomous: yes or no, significant or not significant. Once the decision is made, the magnitude of p reflects only the relative amount of confidence that can be placed in that decision.

Parametric Versus Nonparametric Statistical Tests

Different statistical tests are appropriate for different sets of data. A decision in choosing an appropriate statistical test depends on whether a researcher selects a parametric or nonparametric procedure. Parametric procedures require assumptions to be met for statistical findings to be valid. General assumptions associated with parametric procedures include the dependent variable being measured on an interval/ratio scale that is normally distributed in the population and groups being mutually exclusive (independent of each other). Random sampling allows every member of the population to have an equal and independent chance of being selected for a sample. If randomization is used, the assumption of independence is met. Specific statistical techniques may have specific assumptions.

Nonparametric tests make no assumptions about the shape of the distribution and are referred to as "distribution-free" tests. Nonparametric tests are usually used when data represent an ordinal or nominal scale. Moreover, nonparametric tests involve simpler and fewer calculations. The major drawback to nonparametric tests is that they are less powerful than parametric tests. Figure 10.3 distinguishes between descriptive and inferential statistics and their various subtypes.

Fig 10·3 Descriptive and Inferential Statistics.

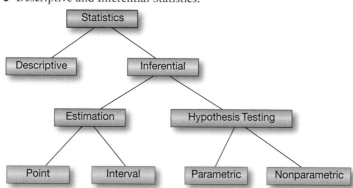

Using Statistics to Examine Relationships

Correlations

A **correlation** is a measure that defines the relationship between two variables. For example, a researcher might be interested in knowing the relationship between smoking and lung capacity. Using correlational techniques, a researcher can determine the nature and size of relationships between variables. The correlation coefficient (r) is an index that describes the relationship between two variables.

The correlation coefficient is a decimal between +1.0 and –1.0. The sign (+ or –) preceding the coefficient shows whether the correlation is positive or negative. A **positive correlation** shows that high scores on one variable are paired with high scores on the other variable. Conversely, low scores on one variable are paired with low scores on the other variable. For negative correlation, low scores on one variable are paired with high scores on the other variable, and high scores on one variable are paired with low scores on the other variable. A **negative correlation** reflects an inverse relationship between two variables.

To judge the strength or size of the correlation, consider the actual number of the correlation coefficient (0.63) and the p value (<0.05). The closer the coefficient is to either +1.0 or –1.0, the higher or stronger the correlation. The closer the coefficient is to zero, the lower or weaker the correlation. The direction of the relationship does not affect the strength of the relationship. A correlation of –0.85 is just as high or strong as +0.85. The following categories show the strength of the correlation coefficients:

0.90 to 0.99: Very high
0.70 to 0.89: High
0.50 to 0.69: Moderate
0.26 to 0.49: Low
0.00 to 0.25: Little, if any

Pearson Product-Moment Correlation

The Pearson product-moment correlation, or simply the Pearson r, is a common correlational technique researchers use to examine the relationship between two variables. The Pearson r is a parametric procedure using interval/ratio data. Refer to Munro[2] for calculation of the correlation coefficient (r).

Correlation Matrix

Researchers can present correlations in a table format or within the text of an article. A specialized form of a correlation table is the correlation matrix. The correlation matrix presents all possible combinations of the study variables. Excerpt 10.5 is an example of a correlation matrix in which the numbers across the top correspond to the study variables listed on the left-hand margin of the table. The number 4 across the top represents the variable social support. Each number in the table represents the correlation coefficient between the variables corresponding to the row and column in which the variable is located. The correlation of 0.56 represents a correlation between perceived health and hope.

A researcher often displays correlation coefficients within the text of an article, as shown in Excerpt 10.6. The Pearson r between self-transcendence (STS) and spiritual well-being (SIWB) was moderately positive ($r = 0.59$). As the level of self-transcendence increased, spiritual well-being increased.

EXCERPT 10.5

Correlation Matrix

Correlations Between Study Variables (n = 125)

Variables	I	2	3	4	5
1. Perceived health	—	0.56**	−0.65***	0.20*	0.31*
2. Hope		—	−0.54***	0.29**	0.63***
3. Uncertainty in illness			—	−0.19*	−0.28**
4. Social support				—	0.29**
5. Spirituality					—

$*p < 0.05$, $**p < 0.01$, $***p < 0.001$

Source: Heinrich, CR: Enhancing the perceived health of HIV seropositive men. West J Nurs Res 25:367–382, 2003.

EXCERPT 10.6

Pearson Correlations Presented Without a Table

Results Related to Spiritual Well-Being

The Spirituality Index of Well-Being (SIWB) had a Cronbach's alpha reliability of 0.90. The SIWB subscale of self-efficacy had a mean score of 25.46 (SD = 3.47); the SIWB subscale of life scheme had a mean score of 25.67 (SD = 3.78), with a minimum of 18 and a maximum of 30. The total SIWB scale had a mean of 51.17 (SD = 6.54) and scores ranging from 31 to 60. Pearson correlation was used to determine the relationship between the SIWB and self-transcendence (STS). The correlation between self-transcendence and spiritual well-being was $r = 0.59$ ($p < 0.000$).

Source: Thomas, JC, Burton, M, Griffin, MT, and Fitzpatrick, JJ: Self-transcendence, spiritual well-being, and spiritual practices of women with breast cancer. J Holist Nurs 28:115–122, 2010.

Using Statistics to Test for Differences

t-test

The *t*-test is an inferential statistical procedure used to determine whether the means of two groups are significantly different. If the sample means are far enough apart, the *t*-test will yield a significant difference, allowing the researcher to conclude that the two groups do not have the same mean. For example, suppose a researcher wanted to know if patients who had open heart surgery using the internal mammary artery as a graft had more chest pain postoperatively than did those using the saphenous vein as a graft. The variable chest pain is measured on a ratio scale using the visual analogue scale (VAS) (see Chapter 9). An example of data from five subjects might look like those seen in Table 10.2.

Based on the group means, it appears that the five patients who had a saphenous vein graft had more intense chest pain postoperatively ($X = 7.2$ versus $X = 5.2$). Both sample means provide the best estimate of the two population means. Some amount of error is inevitable because the means of 7.2 and 5.2 correspond to samples. The statistical question becomes: Is the difference between the two sample means large enough for the researcher to conclude that the population means are different from one another? The *t*-test will answer this question.

Assumptions

Assumptions associated with the *t*-test include those associated with parametric procedures. In addition, both groups must have similar variances with respect to the dependent variable. This is related to the assumption implied by the null hypothesis that the groups are from a single population. This assumption is referred to as **homogeneity of variance**.

TABLE 10.2	
Group 1	**Group 2**
Internal Mammary Artery Graft	**Saphenous Vein Graft**
4	6
3	5
5	8
6	7
8	10
$\Sigma X = 26$	$\Sigma X = 36$
$\overline{X}_1 = 5.2$	$\overline{X}_2 = 7.2$

Forms of the t-Test

Several forms of the *t*-test exist. Researchers use the independent *t*-test when scores in one group have no logical relationship to scores in the other group. Researchers refer to an independent *t*-test as the pooled *t*-test when comparing two independent groups and the four assumptions have been met. If the variances of the groups are significantly different (violation of the assumption of homogeneity of variance), the *t*-test is calculated using the separate *t*-test, which takes into account the fact that the variances are not equal; it is a more conservative measure.

Excerpt 10.7 reports the results of several *t*-tests. Each *t*-test compared men versus women on several variables. The mean age of men (60.22) was compared to the mean age of women (64.51) and found to be significant ($t = -2.03$, $p < 0.05$). The use of the superscripts a and b denote a statistically significant difference between men and women. There was a statistically significant difference between men and women on the following variables: age, weight, waist circumference, total cholesterol, and high-density lipoprotein cholesterol. There was no difference between men and women on the following variables: body mass index, glycosylated hemoglobin, and low-density lipoprotein cholesterol.

The second form of the *t*-test is the dependent *t*-test, also called the "correlated *t*-test," "matched *t*-test," or "*t*-test for paired comparisons." This

---

EXCERPT 10.7

Means, Standard Deviations, and t-Tests of Demographic Characteristics by Gender

	Total Sample (N = 143)	Men (N = 69)	Women (N = 74)	t statistic
Age, years	62.44 (12.76)	60.22 (13.34)	64.51 (11.92)	−2.03[a]
Weight, kg	68.00 (11.54)	75.18 (9.95)	61.31 (8.53)	8.97[b]
BMI, kg/m²	25.77 (3.15)	26.21 (3.24)	25.36 (3.03)	1.61
WC, cm	91.64 (9.25)	96.16 (7.77)	87.43 (8.53)	6.38[b]
TC, mg/dL	189.04 (54.23)	179.49 (49.02)	197.95 (57.58)	−2.06[a]
A1C	7.59 (1.45)	7.67 (1.45)	7.53 (1.46)	0.57
LDL-C, mg/dL	108.52 (39.98)	104.01 (40.28)	112.65 (39.53)	−1.27
HDL-C, mg/dL	44.28 (13.30)	39.14 (11.36)	49.08 (13.25)	−4.80[b]

[a]*p <0.05.*
[b]*p <0.001.*
Abbreviations: A1C, glycosylated hemoglobin; BMI, body mass index; TC, total cholesterol; WC, waist circumference.
  Source: Choi, S: Anthropometric measures and lipid coronary heart disease risk factors in Korean immigrants with type 2 diabetes. J Cardiovasc Nurs 26: 414-422, 2011.

is an appropriate test for situations in which scores in the first group can be paired with a score in the second group. The classic example is a pretest-posttest design, in which a single group of subjects is measured twice. An example of a correlated *t*-test is the two-group study that matches subjects. Excerpt 10.8 displays another situation in which a logical relationship occurs between scores in both groups: husband and wife responses. The purpose of this study was to determine if there were differences in the levels of adjustment, support, symptom distress, hopelessness, and uncertainty

---

EXCERPT 10.8

Display of Six Paired t-Test

Comparison of Women's and Husbands' Scores on the Major Study Variables (n = 74 couples)

Variable	Woman	Husband	Paired t	p
Uncertainty (MUIS)[a]				
M, SD	80.0 (16.9)	84.2 (15.7)	2.08	<0.05
Range	43–148	41–121		
Hopelessness (HS)				
M, SD	3.5 (3.4)	3.8 (3.7)	0.59	0.56
Range	0–16	0–17		
Social Support (SSQ)[b]				
M, SD	98.6 (11.3)	91.9 (10.6)	4.01	<0.001
Range	73–120	69–114		
Symptom Distress (SDS)				
M, SD	25.0 (8.2)	26.0 (7.9)	1.45	.15
Range	13–48	13–46		
Emotional Distress (BSI)				
M, SD	0.50 (0.33)	0.38 (0.36)	2.50	<0.02
Range	0.02–2.3	0–1.5		
Role Adjustment (PAIS)				
M, SD	30.0 (15.8)	27.2 (160)	1.31	0.19
Range	4–73	5–68		

[a]*Scores obtained on a modified version of the MUIS.*
[b]*Scores obtained on a modified version of the SSQ.*

Source: Northouse, LL, Laten, D, and Reddy, P: Adjustment of women and their husbands to recurrent breast cancer. Res Nurs Health 18:515, 1995.

reported by women and their spouses during the recurrent phase of breast cancer. A significant difference was found between levels of uncertainty about the illness, with husbands reporting significantly more uncertainty (M = 84.2 versus 80.0) than their wives. Women also, in contrast to their husbands, reported higher levels of social support (M = 98.6 versus 91.9). On the adjustment measure, significant differences were found between women's and husband's levels of emotional distress, with women reporting more distress (M = 0.50 versus 0.38) than their husbands.

When reading journal articles, the researcher never has to know how to calculate the various forms of the *t*-test or use a *t* table to determine whether a significant difference exists. Refer to Munro[2] to review calculation of the t-test.

Analysis of Variance

Analysis of variance (ANOVA) is an inferential procedure used to determine whether there is a significant difference among three or more group means. The difference between the *t*-test and ANOVA is the number of groups being compared. A simple, or one-way, ANOVA refers to one independent variable with several levels. For example, the variable nursing specialty can be defined as having three levels (i.e., pediatric nursing, community-health nursing, medical-surgical nursing). A two-way ANOVA represents two independent variables with several levels.

Assumptions

Assumptions associated with ANOVA include those associated with parametric procedures, including homogeneity of variance. In ANOVA, the independent variable must be measured on a nominal scale. In some instances, the researcher will recode a continuous variable like age into several categories (i.e., 13 to 19, 20 to 26, and 27 to 33).

Most standard parametric statistical procedures (i.e., *t*-test and ANOVA) list fairly restrictive assumptions that are required to be met if the chosen statistical test is to be valid. A statistical procedure that is appropriate even when its assumptions have been violated is said to be **robust** or thought of as a robust statistic. It is not uncommon for researchers to use parametric procedures for data that are measured on an ordinal scale or data that violate the assumption of normality. The degree of risk depends on how severely the assumptions are broken. It is probably safe to use parametric procedures to analyze ordinal data with roughly equal unit sizes, but these procedures are not reasonable to use for nominal data.

Concept of Variance

In ANOVA, variation is examined to determine whether between-group variance is greater than within-group variance. In conducting ANOVA, both types of variation (between-group and within-group) add up to total variation. Scores within each group vary among one another from the group means and are termed "within-group variance." The distance among group means is called "between-group variance." If the between-group variance is larger than the within-group variance, scores in the different groups are far enough apart for a researcher to conclude that the group means are significantly different. If the between-group variance is smaller than, or about the same as, the within-group variance, the group means are not significantly different. The F-statistic is a three- or four-digit number that indicates the size of the difference between the groups, relative to the size of the variation within each group. The larger the F-statistic (greater between-group variance), the greater the probability of finding a statistically significant difference among the group means.

Results of an ANOVA are presented in an ANOVA summary (see Table 10.3). Table 10.3 has five columns: Source (source of variation), SS (sums of squares), df (degrees of freedom), MS (mean square), and F (F-statistic).[1,3] Refer to Munro[2] for calculation of the ANOVA.

The most important number in the entire ANOVA summary is the single value in the F column. The F value is calculated by dividing the MS associated with between-group variance by the MS associated with within-group variance (27.8 divided by 1.2 = 23.16). As displayed in the table, if a significant difference among the sample means is found, an asterisk next to the calculated F value indicates significance. As in the t-test, the researcher never has to know how to calculate an ANOVA summary. The actual probability of the ANOVA can be evaluated by examining the probability level. If the probability is 0.05 or less ($p < 0.05$), there is a statistically significant difference among the means. In some instances, the researcher reports not the actual probability level but rather that $p < 0.05$.

Nonparametric Statistical Tests

Chi-Square

Chi-square analysis is the most commonly reported nonparametric statistic that compares the frequency of an observed occurrence (actual

TABLE 10.3	ANOVA Summary Table			
Source	**SS**	**df**	**MS**	**F**
Between	55.6	2	27.8	23.16*
Within	14.4	12	1.2	
Total	70.0	14		

*$p < 0.05$.

number in each category) with the frequency of an expected occurrence (based on theory or past experience). The chi-square statistic is the appropriate test when variables are measured on a nominal scale and the researcher counts the number of items in each category.

Assumptions

Assumptions associated with chi-square analyses include the use of frequency data, categories that are mutually exclusive, and a theoretical basis for categorization of variables. Chi-square analyses use nominal (categorical) data. Frequency data represent the actual number of subjects or elements in each category. The chi-square test compares counts, not means. Data that are not normally distributed and that violate the assumptions underlying parametric statistics can be categorized to use the chi-square statistic. Each category is mutually exclusive when subjects are assigned to one category. Theoretical reasons for categorizing variables ensure that the analysis will be meaningful and prevent the researcher from having to recategorize subjects to find relationships between variables. Research questions and methods for analysis are established prior to data collection.

Types of Chi-Square Tests

The two types of chi-square tests are the one-sample and the independent samples tests. The one-sample test is used when a researcher is interested in the number of responses, objects, or subjects that fall into two or more categories. This type of chi-square test compares the set of observed frequencies with the corresponding set of theoretical frequencies that define a specific distribution. This type of test is called a "goodness-of-fit" test. If the two sets of frequencies differ by an amount that can be attributable to sampling error, then there is a "good fit" between the observed data and what would be expected. If sampling error cannot adequately explain the discrepancies between the observed and expected frequencies, then a "bad fit" is said to exist, with a significant difference between the two.[3] For example, a researcher might compare the number of cesarean sections in a local community hospital (observed frequencies) with reported national rates for all community hospitals (theoretical norms). In this example, use of the one-sample chi-square is appropriate.

The independent samples chi-square test is used to determine if two categorical variables are independent of one another. Tests of independence examine the extent of association or relationship between two categorical variables. Researchers frequently compare two or more samples on a categorical response variable. Because the response variable can be composed of two or more categories, there are several options to which the independent samples chi-square test can be applied.

The independent samples chi-square test is calculated with frequency data tabulated in a series of rows and columns called a contingency table. Figure 10.4 illustrates a 2×2 contingency table (two rows and two columns). Each frequency tabulated in the table must be independent and must represent a different individual or unit of observation classified according to two variables. For example, a researcher might want to know if there is a relationship between type of dietary instruction and fasting blood glucose levels. Data from two groups of individuals with diabetes (experimental and control groups) are cross-tabulated with average fasting blood glucose levels. Blood glucose levels can be measured on an interval/ratio scale. Use of chi-square analyses requires that data be tabulated as frequencies. In this example, blood glucose levels are recoded into two categories: less than and greater than the upper limit of normal blood glucose values (Fig. 10.4). The independent samples chi-square test can also be used for a larger number of rows or columns (e.g., 2×3, 3×4, 5×6, 7×7). Refer to Munro[2] for calculation of the chi-square statistic.

As with other statistical procedures, the actual probability associated with the chi-square is evaluated to determine if there is a statistically significant difference. It is often difficult for the reader to know what the actual computed expected cell frequencies are, as these data are not usually reported in tables. Excerpt 10.9 illustrates one format

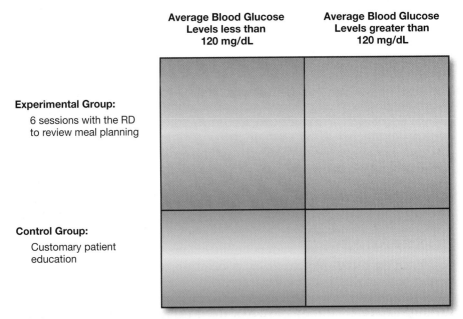

Fig 10•4 2×2 Contingency Table.

EXCERPT 10.9

Reporting Results of Chi-Square Tests in a Table
Sociodemographic Differences Between Men and Women

	Men (n = 77)		Women (n = 50)			
	M	**SD**	**M**	**SD**	**Statistic**	**p**
Age	34.5	7.8	30.5	7.6	$t = -2.89$	< 0.01
Socioeconomic status	38.33	15.25	23.86	12.74	$t = -5.56$	< 0.01
	No. (%)		**No. (%)**			
Race					$\chi^2 = 8.30$	.01
Caucasian	59 (76.6)		26 (52.0)			
African American, Hispanic	18 (23.4)		24 (48.0)			
Education					$\chi^2 = 26.01$	< 0.01
Graduate degree	8 (10.4)		2 (4.0)			
College graduate	14 (18.2)		3 (6.0)			
1–3 yrs college	31 (40.3)		10 (20.0)			
High school graduate	18 (23.4)		14 (28.0)			
7th–11th grade	6 (7.7)		21 (42.0)			
Source of HIV infection					$\chi^2 = 76.15$	<.001
Gay/bisexual contacts	54 (70.1)		0			
Heterosexual contacts	3 (3.9)		31 (62.0)			
Blood transfusions	4 (5.2)		7 (14.0)			
Intravenous drug use	16 (20.8)		12 (24.0)			

Source: Anderson, SE: Personality, appraisal, and adaptational outcomes in HIV seropositive men and women. Res Nurs Health 18:303, 1995.

for presenting the independent samples chi-square test. Researchers actually displayed the observed frequencies for three variables (e.g., race, education, and source of HIV infection). Results of the chi-square analyses indicated that a greater proportion of men had gay/bisexual contacts as their source of infection. In addition, women were younger (note results of *t*-test analysis) and less educated (note results of chi-square analysis).

CRITIQUING DESCRIPTIVE AND INFERENTIAL STATISTICS

Identify a research study to critique. Read the study to see if you recognize any key terms discussed in this chapter. Remember that all studies may not contain all key terms. The following questions[4] serve as a guide in critiquing descriptive and/or inferential statistics:

1. *Were appropriate descriptive statistics used?* Statistics used in descriptive research include measures of central tendency and measures of dispersion. Descriptive statistics summarize important features of numerical data and do not infer anything beyond the data.

2. *Are the reported descriptive statistics appropriate to the level of measurement for each variable?* Remember that nominal and ordinal data can be described by frequency counts; interval/ratio data can be added or subtracted. Tests of statistical inference that require mathematical manipulation should be applied only to variables on the interval/ratio scale. Because ordinal data occur frequently in the behavioral and social sciences, many researchers believe that psychological scales approximate equal intervals fairly well, with results providing satisfactory and useful information.[5,6]

3. *Were appropriate statistics used to answer the research questions or test study hypotheses?* Statistics can be categorized by the purposes for which they are used. As described in this chapter, the function of some statistics is to describe a set of data (using statistics), others are used to examine relationships between or among sets of data (using statistics to examine relationships), and still others are used to detect whether differences exist between groups of data (using statistics to test for differences). Do not get stuck on various statistics reported in research studies. If a particular statistical technique is unfamiliar, look it up in a text, or ask a friend or colleague. If tables are used in the research report, look over the data (i.e., raw scores sometimes reported as totals, averages, ranges, frequencies, or standard deviations), and identify if the author has described the findings within the text.

4. *Is the sample size adequate?* Power analyses are used to identify appropriate sample sizes based on the type of statistical analyses performed. Other nursing research textbooks describe power analysis in more detail, but several pieces of information need to be available to readers of research reports. First, a clear explanation of how the sample size was derived needs to be provided. If the number of subjects imposes limitations on the study, these need to be stated.

5. *If tables were used in the research report, were results clearly and completely stated?* Look over the entire table before trying to absorb specific information contained in the table. All tables should be adequately referenced within the research report, with author(s) directing the reader's attention to particular sections of the table. Is the title of the table adequate in describing the content of the table? Have any of the numerical pieces of data within the table been subjected to statistical tests of significance? If so, are the results

adequately marked and is appropriate information provided concerning how to interpret the results?

SUMMARY OF KEY IDEAS

1. Descriptive statistics are used to summarize measures of central tendency (mean, median, mode) and dispersion (range, variance, standard deviation).

2. Inferential statistics focus on determining how likely it is that results based on a sample are the same as those which would be obtained for the population.

3. Researchers need to establish the level of measurement for data collected in order to select appropriate statistical procedures.

4. Parametric and nonparametric procedures are two types of statistical tests. Parametric procedures require assumptions to be met in order for statistical findings to be valid. Nonparametric procedures make no assumptions about the shape of the distribution and are often described as "distribution free."

5. Parametric statistical tests include Pearson correlations, the *t*-test, and ANOVA.

6. The Pearson *r* (Pearson product-moment correlation) is a measure that defines the relationship or association between two variables. The *t*-test is a parametric procedure that determines if there is a significant difference between two group means.

7. ANOVA is a parametric procedure that determines if there is a significant difference among three or more means.

8. Chi-square analysis is a nonparametric procedure used to assess whether a relationship exists between two categorical variables.

9. A statistical procedure that is appropriate even when the assumptions are violated is said to be robust.

LEARNING ACTIVITIES

1. Using the data in Excerpt 10.2, write three or four sentences describing the sample characteristics using measures of central tendency (mean, median, mode) and measures of dispersion (range, variance, standard deviation).

2. As a researcher, collect data on marital status (measured as married or not married); family stress level (measured as low, moderate, and high); height (measured as inches); and satisfaction with care (measured as very satisfied, somewhat satisfied, somewhat dissatisfied, and very dissatisfied). Identify the appropriate measures of central tendency and dispersion for each of these variables.

TABLE 10.4	t-Test for Length of Second Stage of Labor in Minutes by Weight Group				
Groups	**n**	**M (in minutes)**	**SD**	**t value**
≤25%	50	72.42	46.69	
−2.05	0.02*			
≥25%	46	93.28	52.87	

p < 0.05.

3. Interpret the results of the following *t*-test. "Groups" refer to primigravidas who increased their prepregnancy weight by 25 percent or less and those who increased their weight by 25 percent or greater.

4. Use the results in the table and write two or three sentences describing the findings.

REFERENCES

1. Burns, N, and Grove, SK: The Practice of Nursing Research: Conduct, Critique, and Utilization, ed. 4. WB Saunders, Philadelphia, 2001, pp 499–567.
2. Munro, BH: Statistical Methods for Health Care Research, ed. 5. Lippincott Williams & Wilkins, Philadelphia, 2005.
3. Huck, SW, and Cormier, WH: Reading Statistics and Research, ed. 2. Harper-Collins Publishers, New York, 1996.
4. LoBiondo-Wood, G, and Haber, J: Nursing Research: Methods, Critical Appraisal, and Utilization, ed. 4. Mosby-Year Book, St. Louis, 1998, pp 365, 383.
5. Knapp, TR: Treating ordinal scales as interval scales: An attempt to resolve the controversy. Nurs Res 39:121, 1990.
6. Knapp, TR: Treating ordinal scales as ordinal scales. Nurs Res 42:184, 1993.

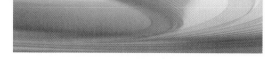

11

SELECTING A QUANTITATIVE RESEARCH DESIGN

James A. Fain, PhD, RN, BC-ADM, FAAN

LEARNING OBJECTIVES

By the end of this chapter, you will be able to:
1. Define and explain the purpose of a research design.
2. Describe characteristics of a good research design.
3. Compare and contrast differences between experimental and quasi-experimental research designs.
4. Understand a selected group of quantitative research designs.
5. Appreciate the process that underlies research design selection.

GLOSSARY OF KEY TERMS

Analytic epidemiological studies. Studies concerned with testing hypotheses to determine if specific exposures are related to the presence or absence of specific diseases.

Control. Elements built into a design to reduce or eliminate interpretations of the cause of the results. These elements include the use of randomization, manipulation of experimental conditions, and use of comparison groups.

Control group. The group that does not receive the experimental treatment in an experiment or intervention.

Descriptive study. A study designed to describe the meaning of existing phenomena.

Descriptive correlational study. A study used to describe and explain the nature and magnitude of existing relationships.

Descriptive epidemiological studies. Studies concerned with the distribution and patterns of disease or disability in a population.

Double-blinded study. Treatment assignment (to either experimental or control group) is unknown to patients and health-care providers. Sometimes referred to as patient-provider masking.

Experimental group. The group that receives the "new" treatment in an experiment.

External validity. The extent to which the results of a study can be generalized from the study sample to the target population.

(Continued)

Extraneous variable. Any variable that is not directly related to the purpose of the study but that may affect the dependent variable; sometimes termed "intervening" or "confounding variables."

Internal validity. Refers to whether the independent variable made a difference.

Paradigm. Organizing framework that contains a set of assumptions or values that underlie how scientists view reality, truth, and research.

Qualitative research. Research directed at the discovery of meaning and underlying philosophical inquiry or psychological and sociological underpinnings.

Quantitative research. Research directed at the discovery of relationships and cause and effect. Methods used are based on the scientific method of inquiry.

Randomized clinical trial (RCT). A prospective study evaluating the effectiveness of an intervention/treatment in a large sample of patients. Essential features of a clinical trial include use of an experimental and control group, randomization, masking of patients and health-care providers, and sufficient sample sizes.

Research design. Set of guidelines by which a researcher obtains answers to questions.

Single-blinded study. Treatment assignment (to either experimental or control group) is unknown to patients.

A research design is a guide chosen by the researcher to answer questions or test hypotheses. Selection of an appropriate design compels the researcher to address critical issues to ensure that data produced are credible and interpretable. The design is the crucial link connecting the researcher's framework and research questions with resultant data. The topic of interest under investigation, the amount of knowledge on the topic, and the individual's philosophy may guide the choice of research design.[1]

Several factors guide the selection of a research design. Most often the purpose of the study, along with level of knowledge about the topic, determines what research design is most appropriate.[2] If little is known about a particular topic, a descriptive or exploratory research design is used. In this instance, the focus is on describing and understanding a phenomenon. If the particular phenomenon is well defined and measured, a more structured design, such as an experimental or quasi-experimental research design, may be appropriate to answer research questions or test hypotheses. This chapter focuses on assisting the researcher in selecting a quantitative research design.

Quantitative Versus Qualitative Research

The terms "quantitative" and "qualitative" are defined in a variety of ways. Researchers often define quantitative research as that which uses numbers to represent reality. **Quantitative research** is directed at the discovery of relationships and cause and effect. Methods used are based on the scientific method of inquiry (see Chapter 1). Quantitative refers to measurement and analysis of relationships between and among variables at a particular point in time.

Qualitative research is directed at the discovery of meaning rather than cause and effect. Qualitative research involves the use of language, concepts, and words rather than numbers to represent evidence from research. The word "qualitative" also implies an emphasis on process and meanings in context. The focus is on the creation of social experience and emergent meanings, the relationship between participant and researcher, and the environmental issues that may shape inquiry. Quantitative and qualitative research also refer to a researcher's worldview, or paradigm. Although defined in several ways, a **paradigm** is an organizing framework that contains a set of assumptions or values that underlie how scientists view reality, truth, and research.[3] Within the quantitative-qualitative perspectives, these views are profoundly different.

Quantitative and Qualitative Approaches to Design Selection

Assumptions underlying quantitative and qualitative paradigms reveal different views of reality. Table 11.1 presents major quantitative and qualitative contrasts emerging from the nature of reality, view of humans, source of knowledge, and research orientation. Review this table and classify your own beliefs.

Researchers often believe in the predominance of one paradigm over another. Depending on whether they emerge from a quantitative or a qualitative perspective, researchers ask questions in different ways. Belief in the elements of a quantitative perspective direct a researcher to ask questions focused on relationships among variables, with an outcome orientation. Belief in characteristics that compose a qualitative paradigm guides a researcher toward process-oriented exploratory questions with use of more flexible research designs.

For example, nurses might ask different questions to research management of postoperative pain, depending on their perspective. From a quantitative perspective, pain is viewed as a single reality, one that can be captured objectively. The nurse might ask questions focused on the pain as well as its relationship to other variables such as preoperative teaching and amount of pain medication given. Measurement of pain and related variables at specified times might be the focus of these questions. The nurse might ask, "*What is the relationship among timing of pain medication, amount of medication, and*

TABLE 11.1	**Nature of Reality and the Conduct of Research**

Quantitative	Qualitative
Nature of Reality	
Reality obtainable in objective terms	Social construction of reality
Single reality	Multiple realities
Parts separate and manipulable	Parts interrelated
Variables independent of each other	Variables dependent on each other
Context free and objective	Context interrelated and subjective
Narrow in scope	Broad, inclusive in scope
View of Humans	
Human data collected are objective	Subjective data
Human is made of parts	Holistic view
Source of Knowledge	
Logical positivism and empiricism	Research traditions:
	Anthropology, social psychology, philosophy
Use of observation	Intuition, gestalt
Psychological and biophysical facts	Social interventions, values, culture
Orientation of Research	
Outcome, product-oriented	Process, phenomena; person-oriented

pain relief (as measured by a visual analogue scale) in a postoperative population?"

Quantitative design is structured so that measurement and testing are prominent characteristics. Research emerging from this perspective centers on explanation, verification of facts, testing of theoretical relationships, and prediction of events.

From a qualitative perspective, the nurse would consider the patient an active participant in a socially constructed context. Many realities might exist for this patient regarding the pain experience. The nurse would be interested in discovering how the patient is encountering the pain experience. Research is process-oriented, with a focus on the patient's perspective of the pain experience in a social context. The nurse might ask, *"What is the pain experience like for the patient postoperatively?"* The design is flexible, to capture social and thinking processes. Research emerging from this perspective would center on understanding from the patient's viewpoint, discovery of social processes, and description of happenings.

What Is a Research Design?

A **research design** is an overall plan or blueprint that outlines aspects of sample collection and analyses based on specific research questions and/or hypotheses.

Research designs may be defined from a broad or narrow perspective. From a broad perspective, the design suggests approaches for observation and analysis but does not specifically tell the researcher what to do. Researchers regard design as the total strategy for the investigation, connecting theoretical perspective and problem identification with data collection and analysis. From a limited perspective, researchers consider design as a precisely conceived blueprint that brings empirical evidence to bear on the research problem. It provides methodological direction, such as sampling and random assignment. How one selects or arrives at sample selection is probably the single most important aspect of a good research design.

A research design is a general, nonspecific approach to a particular study or precise question. Specifics constitute the specific plan. Just as a soccer player must link general rules of the game to a specific strategy of play, the research design guides the researcher's specific plan. The researcher's plan includes specification of procedures or strategies, such as site selection, selection of essential instruments, timing and types of observations, sampling techniques, and data analysis.

Classification of Research Designs

Research designs are classified from various perspectives and include elements that reflect quantitative or qualitative viewpoints (see Table 11.2). This classification is neither mutually exclusive nor exhaustive.

For example, quantitative designs develop from a strong theoretical base, emerge from questions regarding explanation and relationships between and among variables, and generally derive from evolving

TABLE 11.2	**Design Structure as a Function of Quantitative-Qualitative Dimensions**
Quantitative Dimension	**Qualitative Dimension**
Strong theoretical base	Strong philosophical perspective
Explanation among variables	Understanding of human action
Objective approach to phenomena	Subjective approach
Measurement of variables	Meaning of concepts
Precision in measurement	Description of phenomena
Control of error: internal validity	Trustworthiness of findings

knowledge in the area of inquiry. Qualitative designs emerge from a strong research tradition and perhaps theoretical base, evolve from questions about understanding and description of phenomena, and generally emerge from evolving knowledge.

Consequently, quantitative designs focus on approaches that emphasize explanations of variables, verification of data, measuring variables, use of instruments for data collection, statistical significance, and internal validity. Qualitative designs emphasize understanding social action, discovery of information, meaning of concepts, participatory involvement of researcher as a means of data collection, and trustworthiness of findings as corroborated by the participants in the research.

Quantitative Research Designs

Design of an experiment can take a variety of forms and be classified as experimental or quasi-experimental.[4] Classifying a research design as experimental versus quasi-experimental refers to the amount of control (little or no control) a researcher has over independent variables. Research designs that offer the greatest amount of control are referred to as experimental designs.

Characteristics Associated With Experimental Designs

Three important characteristics associated with conducting experimental designs include control, random assignment, and manipulation,

Control Control is the essence of an experimental design. The researcher must be able to control the experimental situation by eliminating actions of other possible variables beyond the independent variable. Control is achieved through use of control groups.

Random Assignment The researcher must be able to select subjects randomly from the population and then randomly assign them to the control and experimental group. Random assignment is similar, but not identical, to random selection (See Chapter 7).

Manipulation In an experiment, the researcher must be able to manipulate the action of the independent variable. In essence, the researcher directly determines what form an independent variable will take. Some independent variables can be manipulated (e.g., type of intervention; teaching methods; educational programs) while other independent variables cannot be manipulated (e.g., gender, religious preference, ethnicity). As a researcher, you can manipulate the type of educational program subjects are exposed to. However, you cannot manipulate a variable such as religion. That is, subjects cannot be made into Catholics or Protestants.

Extraneous Variables

The essence of an experiment is the ability of the researcher to manipulate and control variables so that rival hypotheses are ruled out as possible explanations for the observed response. An **extraneous variable** (sometimes called intervening or confounding variable) is any variable that is not directly related to the purpose of the study but that may affect the dependent variable. Extraneous variables can be external factors emerging from the environment and the experiment or internal factors that represent personal characteristics of the subjects of the study. When extraneous variables are not controlled, they exert a confounding influence on the independent variable in such a way that their separate effects are obscured.

For example, a researcher concerned about patients' pain relief after surgery wonders if there is a better way to treat postoperative pain. Theory-based research suggests that patients have better pain control if they receive 2 to 4 mg of morphine sulfate intravenously (IV) every 1 to 2 hours. Patients in a particular unit have traditionally been given 5 to 8 mg of morphine sulfate intramuscularly (IM) every 3 to 4 hours, as needed. The question is raised, *"Will there be a difference in patients' pain relief if some patients receive the traditional method (5 to 8 mg of morphine IM every 3 to 4 hours) and others receive the research-based approach of 2 to 4 mg of morphine IV every 1 to 2 hours?"*

An experimental design is set up where patients are randomly assigned to a control group (the group receiving the traditional medication regimen) or an experimental group (the group receiving the new or experimental intervention). The only difference between the two groups is the difference in the administration of pain medication. Pain is measured by use of a visual analogue scale.

In this example, control over extraneous influences has been achieved by creating control and experimental groups and randomly assigning patients to each group. The independent variable was manipulated through use of an experimental intervention. The hypothesis in this research predicts (based on theory and research) which of the two types of pain interventions will give "better" pain relief.

Types of Experimental Designs

Campbell and Stanley[4] identify three basic experimental designs, including randomized pretest-posttest control group design, randomized posttest-only control group, and one-group pretest-posttest design.

The randomized pretest-posttest control group design is one of the most commonly seen designs in the literature. The design is shown diagrammatically in Figure 11.1. Pretesting provides the researcher with information about the similarity of experimental and control groups on measures of the dependent variable before the independent variable is introduced.

The pretest-posttest control group design is sometimes referred to as a "before-and-after" design. Vincent, Pasvogel, and Barrera[5] used this type of design to test the feasibility of and examine the effects of a culturally tailored intervention for Mexican Americans with type 2 diabetes.

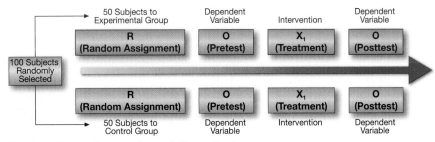

Fig 11•1 Pretest-Posttest Control Group Design.

Twenty participants were randomly assigned to an intervention (8-week 2-hour group session based on cultural modifications associated with a diabetes education program) or control group (usual care and diabetes education two to four times a year for 15 minutes) using a list of random numbers from the Microsoft Excel random-number generator function. Outcome measures (e.g., diabetes knowledge, self-efficacy, glucose control) were evaluated before, after, and 4 weeks postintervention.

A second commonly seen experimental design in the literature is the randomized posttest-only control group. Some researchers argue that pretesting is not always necessary, especially when randomization is used. In many nursing studies, it may be inappropriate or impossible to pretest before the independent variable is manipulated. The posttest-only control group is shown in Figure 11.2.

Excerpt 11.1 illustrates the use of a randomized posttest-only control group to determine which of two groups (those receiving a monograph on growth disorders among children with an individualized health care plan [IHP] versus those not receiving the monograph and IHP) had greater knowledge of growth assessment.

A third experimental design is the one-group pretest-posttest design. In this type of research design, a group of participants are pretested on a dependent variable and then tested after the treatment condition has been administered. The one-group pretest-posttest design is a weak experimental design in that this type of design does not control for potentially

Fig 11•2 Posttest-Only Control Group Design.

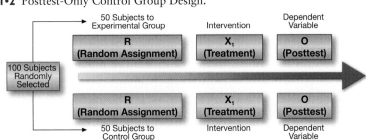

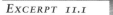

Use of Posttest-Only Control Group

Methods

A questionnaire was developed to obtain information on school nurses' experiences, concerns, and knowledge related to caring for children with growth disorders in schools. A descriptive survey design was used to identify school nurses' experiences and concerns with children with growth disorders. To assess knowledge and the impact of the use of a monograph, a posttest-only, two-group survey design was used. This design was chosen to avoid potential sensitization to the study topic that might occur with a pretest-posttest design. School nurses' baseline knowledge of growth disorders and their management was evaluated by having one group of school nurses (n = 112) complete a questionnaire on growth disorders before receiving the monograph. To assess the impact of the monograph on school nurses' knowledge, the other group (n = 224) was provided the monograph and the questionnaire at the same time.

Source: Williams, JK, et al: School nurses' experiences, concerns, and knowledge of growth disorders in children: Development of a monograph. J Sch Nurs 18:25, 2002.

confounding extraneous variables such as history, maturation, testing, and instrumentation; thus, it is difficult to identify the effect of the treatment. The design is shown diagrammatically in Figure 11.3.

Rossen and Knafl[6] employed the use of a one-group pretest-posttest design to investigate the impact of older women moving from a private residence to an age-specific congregate independent living community (ILC). A convenience sample of older women were recruited from 12 ILCs. Data were collected in participant's homes at two points in time; a month prior to the move and between the third and fourth month after the move. Outcome measures (dependent variables) collected prior to and after the move included physical well-being, emotional well-being, and person-environment interaction.

For other variations of experimental designs (e.g., Solomon four-group design, factorial designs), refer to Campbell and Stanley.[4]

Quasi-Experimental Designs

Like experimental designs, quasi-experimental designs dictate manipulation of the independent variable. The outcome is "predicted" by theory

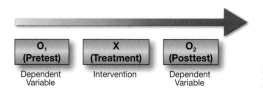

Fig 11•3 One-Group Pretest-Posttest Design.

and research. However, random assignment and/or control groups are absent.

Often, researchers are obliged to use a quasi-experimental design because of the nature of the study or clinical setting. Additionally, a researcher may find it impossible to develop a control group or to randomly assign patients to groups owing to the nature of the clinical setting. Although the researcher may use control and experimental groups in quasi-experimental designs, these designs may use convenience (no random assignment) sampling or matched groups.

Several different quasi-experimental designs are outlined in the research literature. Campbell and Stanley[4] illustrate more than 10 different quasi-experimental designs. The most common and basic type seen in nursing research is the nonequivalent control group design, also called a comparison group. When reading a research report, do not confuse this with the experimental randomized pretest-posttest control group design (see Fig. 11.1). With nonequivalent groups, there is no randomization of subjects into groups. The researcher selects two samples from two similar available groups. The nonequivalent control group is shown in Figure 11.4.

Refer to the previous example of the researcher interested in patients' pain relief after surgery. Suppose that two surgical floors (6-East and 7-West) decide to change their approach to pain medication intervention. Nurses on 6-East decide to use 2 to 4 mg of morphine IV every 1 to 2 hours for the postoperative population; 7-West still wants to continue using 5 to 8 mg of morphine intramuscularly (IM) every 3 to 4 hours. Both floors have similar numbers of surgical patients. Unfortunately, the researcher cannot create control and experimental groups because of the nature of the clinical setting. It is decided to group all patients and compare the pain relief received from the different interventions. In this example, the researcher must assign patients to groups randomly. Patients are assigned as a function of the floor location (or by convenience); consequently, the groups are nonequivalent. The research question focuses on which of the two medication interventions might be "best" for pain relief.

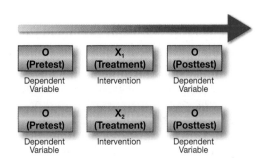

Fig 11•4 Nonequivalent Control Group Design.

A more elaborate quasi-experimental design might test each group before and after the intervention. Similar to the before-and-after experimental design, this approach allows the researcher to compare the before-and-after scores within each group (within-group comparison). Additionally, the researcher may compare scores of one group against those of another (across-group comparison). This design is called "quasi-experimental before-and-after." For other variations of quasi-experimental designs, refer to Campbell and Stanley[4] and Cook and Campbell.[7]

Randomized Clinical Trials

A **randomized clinical trial** (RCT) is the most widely accepted approach to evaluating the effectiveness of an intervention/treatment in a sample of patients. RCTs require the researcher to adhere strictly to principles of experimental design. Clinical trials typically use a pretest-posttest control group design, follow subjects in time (prospective), collect outcome data after an extended period, and frequently sample from multiple sites. Essential features of clinical trials include use of an experimental and control group, randomization, blinding of patients and health-care providers, and sufficient sample sizes.

Experimental designs typically involve two groups, experimental and control. Sometimes there may be three groups, where more than one intervention/treatment is presented. The **experimental group** receives the intervention/treatment, and the **control group** usually receives the standard, customary care. Use of a control group enables the researcher to compare the performance of the treatment group(s) to that of a group that did not receive the intervention/treatment but was exposed to the same passage of time.

A major feature of the clinical trial is that patients are assigned to the treatment group(s) by a method that maximizes the probability that the two groups will be similar in demographic characteristics that may influence either the response to the intervention/treatment or various outcome measures. With randomization, treatment group assignment is based on probability alone and not on the health-care provider's preference.

Blinding of patients and health-care providers is important because it reduces biasing of perceptions or ways of acting on everyone's part. Blinding means that the treatment assignment is not known to certain individuals. Patients who know they have been assigned to receive a particular treatment/intervention, might anticipate or look forward to favorable outcomes. On the other hand, those patients not assigned to receive a particular treatment/intervention might feel deprived or even relieved. In either case, knowledge of being assigned to a particular group could possibly affect outcomes. In a **single-blinded study**, the treatment assignment is unknown to patients; in a double-blinded study, the treatment assignment is unknown to the patients and to the health-care providers. In **double-blinded studies**, the treatment assignment is revealed only if there are serious or unexpected side effects from the intervention/treatment. Blinding is sometimes referred to as masking.

Sufficient sample sizes are required in clinical trials to ensure that the effectiveness of the intervention/treatment can be detected by statistics used to compare the groups' outcomes. With small samples, the study is said to lack statistical power, meaning the study has a low chance of confirming a difference between groups that really does exist. If the study has adequate statistical power, it is important to conduct a power analysis to determine the appropriate number of subjects needed to have a certain chance (usually 80 percent) of detecting a significant difference if one actually does exist. Refer to other research textbooks for a detailed discussion of power analysis.

Excerpt 11.2 displays part of the methods section of a randomized clinical trial. The purpose of the study was to evaluate the effect of music on pain and anxiety in children undergoing lumbar punctures. Twenty children were randomly assigned to a music group (intervention group, n = 20) and 20 children were assigned to a control group receiving no music. Children in the music group chose songs they liked to play into earphones from an iPod (portable music player with earphones). Children in the control group used earphones without music being played. All children were given identical preprocedural information about the procedure and study. Data collection started immediately before the procedure and included measuring the following variables: heart rate (HR), blood pressure (BP), oxygen saturation (O_2SAT), respiratory rate (RR), and self-reported pain and anxiety scores. The HR, BP, O_2SAT, and RR were monitored during the procedure with children listening or not listening to music according to their group assignment. Directly after the procedure, the self-reported pain and anxiety scores were repeated.

EXCERPT 11.2

Example of Methods Section From a Randomized Clinical Trial

Design and Procedure

The study design was a randomized clinical trial followed by interviews with open-ended questions. After informed consent, the children were randomized to two groups: use of earphones with music (music group) or earphones without music (control group). Randomization was carried out using opaque envelopes, half of which contained a paper that said "music" and half that said "no music." The children in the music group chose songs they liked to be played into the earphone from an iPod, that is, a portable music player with earphones. In the control group, earphones without music were used. All the children were given identical preprocedural information about the procedures and study.

Source: Nguyen, TN, et al: Music therapy to reduce pain and anxiety in children with cancer undergoing lumbar puncture: A randomized clinical trial. J Pediatr Oncol Nurs 27:146, 2010.

Evaluating the effectiveness of an intervention/treatment utilizing an RCT is considered the "best" form of evidence, or "gold standard," for clinical research. However, it is important to realize that not all clinical researchable questions can be answered with RCTs. Other research designs can also generate very useful and valid scientific information.

Validity in Relation to Research Design

Two kinds of validity related to research design are internal validity and external validity. **Internal validity** refers to whether the independent variable actually made a difference: Did the intervention or treatment lead to the results, or were the results a response to extraneous variables? Extraneous variables present threats to internal validity because they offer competing explanations for the relationship between independent and dependent variables. True experiments have a great amount of internal validity because of the use of control groups and randomization. Campbell and Stanley[4] have identified several types of threats to internal validity that can be experienced in clinical studies. **External validity** refers to the extent to which the results of a study can be generalized from the study sample to the larger population (see Chapter 7).

The term "internal validity" poses to a researcher two important questions: Did the treatment (intervention) actually bring about a change in the dependent variable? and Did the independent variable really make a difference? Both questions cannot be answered by researchers unless the design provides adequate control of extraneous variables. That is, if the design provides control of variables, then the researcher is able to eliminate alternative explanations of the observed outcome and interpret it as showing some kind of relationship between variables.

Campbell and Stanley[4] have identified six "threats" to internal validity that may produce an effect that could be mistaken for the effect of the experimental treatment/intervention.

History

History refers to the confounding effects of specific events, other than the experimental treatment that occurs after the introduction of the independent variable or between the pretest and posttest.[4] For example, if a researcher studies the effect of an educational intervention to increase compliance with the American Diabetes Association (ADA) diet regimen, history may be more influential to compliance than is the educational intervention. History can also refer to more global events. For example, a researcher interested in health promotion among adolescents studies the effect of an educational program for increasing the use of seat belts. If, during the course of the study, the state passes a law mandating seat belt use, that also represents a history effect.

The history effect is more of a threat for one-group research designs compared to multigroup research designs. This is because in two or more group designs, researchers are comparing a treatment group(s) to a comparison group. As long as the history effect occurs for both groups the difference between groups will not be due to a history effect.

Maturation

A second threat to internal validity is maturation: biological or psychological processes that occur with the passage of time and are independent of any external events.[4] Maturation is a concern in many areas of clinical research, especially in studies involving long periods between measurements (longitudinal studies). For example, a researcher studying children might encounter physical and developmental changes, unrelated to an intervention, that may influence performance.

The maturation effect is more of a threat in one-group designs. Maturation is not a threat in two-group designs because participants in both groups mature at the same rate. The difference between the two groups is not due to maturation.

Testing

The third threat to internal validity is the potential effect of pretesting or repeated testing on the dependent variable. Individuals usually score higher when they retake an achievement or intelligence test. Testing effects refer to improved performance or increased skill occurring because of familiarity with measurements.[4] For example, subjects may actually learn information by taking a pretest, thereby changing their responses on a posttest, independent of any instructional intervention. Again, testing is not a threat in the two-group design. As long as participants are equally affected by the use of a pretest, the difference between the two groups will not be due to testing.

Instrumentation

Instrumentation effects involve the reliability of measurement (see Chapter 8). The effect of any change in the observational technique or measurement instrument might account for observational differences. In particular, the problem of instrumentation becomes crucial when human beings are used as judges, observers, raters, coders, or interviewers. Observers can become more experienced at measurement between the pretest and the posttest.[4] This threat to internal validity can be addressed by documenting test-retest and interrater reliabilities. In addition, instrumentation is not a threat in the two-group design. As long as participants are equally affected by the instrumentation effect, the difference between the two groups will not be due to instrumentation.

Statistical Regression

Statistical regression is also associated with reliability of a test. When measures are not reliable, there is a tendency for extreme scores on the pretest to regress toward the mean on the posttest.[4] This effect occurs in the absence of intervention. Extremely low scores tend to increase; extremely high scores, to decrease. Statistical regression is of concern when groups are selected on the basis of extreme scores. For example, a researcher wanting to examine the effect of self-efficacy on subjects who comply and on those who do not comply with their diet regimen might assign subjects to two groups based on their pretest scores (e.g., extent of compliance). The effect of the regression will be to move both groups toward their combined average in posttests. The amount of statistical regression is directly related to the extent of measurement error in the dependent variable. Like several other threats to internal validity, use of a control or comparison group (two-group design) handles statistical regression to the mean.

Mortality

Researchers are often faced with the fact that subjects drop out of a study before it is completed. Mortality, or attrition, refers to the loss of subjects from both experimental and control groups for various reasons.[4] Researchers should determine whether attrition occurs for random or biased reasons and if one particular group is affected more than others.

Nonexperimental Designs

Nonexperimental research is clearly distinguishable from experimental and quasi-experimental research in that it does not manipulate the independent variable. In nonexperimental designs, the researcher observes the actions of variables as they occur in the natural state. The major purpose of nonexperimental research is to uncover new knowledge and describe relationships among variables. This type of research is also a rich source of data that helps the researcher to formulate questions to use in an experimental or quasi-experimental design. Two basic categories of nonexperimental designs are descriptive and correlational.

Descriptive Designs

Descriptive studies gather information about conditions, attitudes, or characteristics of individuals or groups of individuals. The purpose of descriptive research is to describe the meaning of existing phenomena. Enumeration and brief description of characteristics are the key elements in this design. For example, a researcher decides to survey the religious affiliations of patients because there has been little pastoral care at a particular institution. A brief description and enumeration of affiliations will help support the need for further religious support within the institution.

Domiano et al[8] presents an example of a descriptive study. The purpose of the study was to evaluate the difference between blood pressure measures (BPMs) obtained at the upper arm and those obtained at the forearm among adults. Measurements were taken according to the American Heart Association (AHA) guidelines. Two BPMs at the upper arm and two BPMs at the forearm were obtained for each participant. A 1-minute rest period between each BPM was provided to allow for normal blood flow in the extremity. Such a study was considered descriptive in that there was no consensus in the literature about what numerical value of difference between upper arm and forearm BPMs should be considered clinically significant.

Excerpt 11.3 illustrates the use of an exploratory descriptive design whose purpose was to investigate the outcomes of a grade nine Healthy Heart Program nurse referral to a family physician for adolescents identified with elevated cholesterol levels or blood pressure risk factors. Note that both quantitative and qualitative data were collected (referred to as triangulation or mixed-methods).

Correlational Designs

A correlational design arises from a level of knowledge needing further refinement of variable measurement or clarification of relationships among variables. Unlike the experimental and quasi-experimental designs, the independent variable is not manipulated. However, this design gives support to later work, using more sophisticated designs that explicate causal relationships. Correlational research investigates the relationship among two or more variables. The researcher can use this approach to describe relationships, predict relationships, or test relationships supported

---

EXCERPT 11.3

Example of a Descriptive Research Design

Design

This exploratory descriptive research study used a telephone survey that had both quantitative and qualitative questions. Data were collected using a semi-structured telephone interview developed for the study. Quantitative questions were used to query if adolescents attended the follow-up referral appointment with the family physician and whether they were prescribed medications, referred to specialists, or made lifestyle changes as a result. Additional qualitative questions were designed to explore further perception and opinions related to their experience.

Source: Kitty, HL, and Prentice, D: Adolescent cardiovascular risk factors: A follow-up study. Clin Nurs Res 19:6, 2010.

by clinical theory. In correlational studies, no attempt is made to control or manipulate the variables under study.

Correlational research can be conducted retrospectively or prospectively. Retrospective research involves examination of data collected in the past, often obtained from medical records or survey. Many epidemiological studies use retrospective data. Prospective research involves the examination of variables through direct recording in the present. Prospective studies are more reliable than retrospective ones because of the potential for greater control of data collection methods.

Descriptive Correlational Design

The purpose of a **descriptive correlational design** is to describe and explain the nature and magnitude of existing relationships, without necessarily clarifying the underlying causal factors in the relationship. The nature of a relationship explains the type of relationship that exists, that is, whether the relationship is positive or negative. The relationship between the number of cigarettes smoked and lung function has been shown to be negative and is referred to as an inverse relationship. People who smoke more cigarettes have a lower lung function and people who smoke a lower number of cigarettes have a higher lung function. Descriptive correlational designs are essentially exploratory and often target the generation of hypotheses.

Thomas et al[9] used a descriptive correlational design to describe the relationship between self-transcendence and spiritual well-being and identify spiritual practices among older women recovering from breast cancer. A sample of older women diagnosed with breast cancer not currently undergoing chemotherapy or radiation treatment were recruited.

Excerpt 11.4 reports the results of the above-mentioned descriptive correlational study whose purpose was to examine relationships among variables and provide additional information about women recovering from breast cancer.

EXCERPT 11.4

Reporting Results of a Descriptive Correlational Study

Results

A total of 203 surveys were mailed to women older than 65 years who lived in the community and who had a diagnosis of breast cancer. Of the 203 survey packets mailed, 103 surveys were returned. Of the 103 packets returned, one was eliminated because of incomplete information and 15 surveys were eliminated as it was noted that participants had recorded recurrence of breast cancer and did not meet study criteria.

Current age ranges were 65 to 74 years (82.8%), 75 to 84 years (13.8%), and 85 to 94 years (3.4%). Most of the women were married (n = 61; 70.1%) and not employed outside the home (n = 51; 58.6%).

(Continued)

Reporting Results of a Descriptive Correlational Study—cont'd

Results Related to Self-Transcendence

Reliability of the Self-Transcendence Scale (STS) was demonstrated with a Cronbach's alpha of 0.86. Cronbach's alpha is in the range of previous studies using the STS (range 0.73 to 0.95). The STS mean average score was 3.52 (SD = 0.18) and the range was 2.53 to 4.0.

Results Related to Spiritual Well-Being

The Spirituality Index of Well-Being (SIWB) had a Cronbach's alpha of 0.90. The SIWB subscale of self-efficacy had a mean score of 25.46 (SD = 3.47); the SIWB subscale of life scheme had a mean score of 25.67 (SD = 3.78), with a minimum of 18 and a maximum of 30. The total SIWB scale had a mean of 51.17 (SD = 6.54), and scores ranged from 31 to 60. Pearson correlation was used to determine the relationship between SIWB and STS. The correlation between STS and SIWB was $r = 0.59$ ($p < 0.0000$).

Source: Thomas, JC, Burton, M, Griffin, MT, and Fitzpatrick, JJ: Self-transcendence, spiritual well-being, and spiritual practice of women with breast cancer. J Holist Nurs 28:115, 2010.

Other Types of Research Designs

Numerous other designs exist that do not fit into the aforementioned classification system. Usually these designs originate from specific questions arising from unique purposes.

Historical Research

Historical research systematically investigates and critically evaluates information related to past events. Its purpose is not to review literature about past events but to shed light on present events through analysis of cause, effects, and trends of historical events. The goal is to create new insights, not to rehash historical information. Qualitative and quantitative approaches and data collection techniques are used. Fairman[10] presents a historiographical analysis of the social, political, and culture context of nursing scholarship in the postwar period, with an understanding of how this context shaped nursing scholarship. Fairman[10] speaks of the development of nursing scholarship being influenced by three contextual strands: nurses' use of experiential clinical knowledge, development of an intellectual genealogy, and the creation of a growing cadre of nurse scholars.

Secondary Analysis

Secondary analysis uses previously gathered data to test new hypotheses, explore new relationships among variables, or create new insights. Because the process of data collection is time-consuming and expensive, use of these data is an efficient way to create new insights and new knowledge.

However, data may be deficient or problematic in areas of variables or populations studied. Despite this caveat, a number of groups are attempting to organize and make available databases for secondary analysis. Melkus, Whittemore, and Mitchell[11] offer a comprehensive article discussing data collected from two independent study samples, using different instruments to measure some variables and answer new study questions as to what differences, if any, exist between rural white and urban black women with type 2 diabetes. One data set contained information on women recruited from an outpatient diabetes education center in rural Connecticut, and a second data set consisted of information from a large urban center in Southern Connecticut. Common variables collected at each site were extracted from each study's original database on demographic, physiological, psychosocial, and self-management outcomes.

Excerpt 11.5 illustrates a write-up from the methods section of a secondary analysis conducted to explore the relationship between the symptoms of schizophrenia experienced by older adults with diabetes and their response to a health-promoting intervention. Note that authors have created a subheading within the article titled "Original Study," where some details of the original study were discussed.

Meta-Analysis

Meta-analysis is a technique that uses the findings from several studies to create a data set that may be analyzed as a single piece of datum. By

---

EXCERPT 11.5

Illustration of Methods Section From a Secondary Analysis

Original Study

A study conducted by McKibbin et al investigated the efficacy of a 24-week lifestyle intervention to reduce obesity in middle-aged and older adults with schizophrenia and type 2 diabetes. Details about the study design and results can be found in the original publication of the study. Briefly, the hypothesis was that the intervention group receiving the diabetes awareness and rehabilitation training (DART) would demonstrate greater reductions in body mass index (BMI) in comparison to the usual care plus information (UCI) group.

Methods

The primary article describing the study specifically addressed the outcome between pre- and postintervention across variables. The authors of the primary article, however, did not examine moderators of treatment outcome. Therefore, the current study explored the role of schizophrenia symptoms experienced by older adults with schizophrenia and comorbid type 2 diabetes in response to the diabetes education program.

Source: Leutwyler, HC, Wallhagen, M, and McKibbin, C: The impact of symptomatology on response to a health promoting intervention among older adults with schizophrenia. Diabetes Educ 36:945, 2010.

applying statistical procedures to these findings, this technique can be a unique approach to integrate knowledge. Meta-analyses are common in nursing literature. Cochran and Conn[12] conducted a secondary meta-analysis to describe the influence of diabetes self-management on quality of life (QOL) among adult patients with diabetes. The study used data from a larger meta-analysis that examined effects of interventions designed to increase physical activity in adults with chronic illnesses. A subset of the larger study that examined diabetes self-management training in adults with diabetes with reported QOL outcomes were analyzed.

Epidemiological Research

Epidemiology studies the distribution and determinants of disease and injury frequency in human populations.[13] Epidemiological questions often arise out of clinical experience and public health concerns about the relationship between social practices and disease outcomes.

Epidemiology began as the study of "epidemics," concerned primarily with mortality and morbidity from acute infectious disease. As medical cures and treatments developed to control many of these problems, and as patterns of disease have changed, chronic diseases and disabilities have gained increased prominence in epidemiology. Today, epidemiology encompasses a broader context of "epidemic" and "disease," including studies of AIDS, outbreaks of controlled diseases such as measles, and more chronic conditions such as cardiac disease, arthritis, diabetes, traumatic injuries, and birth defects.

Epidemiology includes the basics of experimental, descriptive, and correlational research designs. It is distinguished as a research approach because of its unique concern with the identification of risk factors associated with disease and disability.[13] Risk factors are exposures that increase or decrease the likelihood of developing certain diseases or disorders. Examples of risk factors include lifestyle practices such as smoking, substance abuse, drinking alcohol, eating foods high in cholesterol or salt, occupational hazards (repetitive task of using computers), and environmental influences (second-hand smoke).

Epidemiological studies are generally classified as descriptive or analytic.[13] **Descriptive epidemiological studies** are concerned with the distribution and patterns of disease or disability in a population. These studies provide valuable information that can be used to generate hypotheses and set priorities for health-care planning. Descriptive epidemiological studies usually take the form of case reports, correlational studies, or cross-sectional surveys.

Analytic epidemiological studies involve testing hypotheses to determine if specific exposures are related to the presence or absence of specific diseases or disabilities. Analytic epidemiological studies allow the researcher to determine if the disease rate is different among those exposed or unexposed to the factor of interest and, thus, establish that certain exposures either increase or decrease one's risk of developing that disease. Analytic studies are broadly categorized as observational or interventional. Observational studies use surveys, interviews, or review of medical records, whereas the researcher documents the natural course of events, noting who is and who is not exposed and who does and does not develop the disease. There is no direct intervention and no control over who receives the exposure. These observational studies take the form of case-control and cohort studies.

Research Design Selection

How does one select a research design? There are several questions you may want to ask yourself as you move toward understanding design selection. Each question lays a foundation for the next question so that choice of design emerges from your philosophical approach, theory, and research questions:

1. How do you approach reality? What are your beliefs about the world, nursing, and patient care? Are your thoughts aligned with a quantitative or qualitative paradigm?
2. With what research tradition are you allied? Do you think holistically, or do you think in terms of a medical, sociological, or psychological viewpoint?
3. Is there an existing theoretical framework to guide inquiry of your chosen phenomena of interest? How much research exists in your area of inquiry? Are the concepts labeled, defined, and/or measured?
4. What question are you asking? Is your question more outcome-oriented or process-oriented? Does your question lend itself to a quantitative or qualitative design?
5. What type of research design emerges from this sequence of questions? Does your design fit with your worldview, theory, and research question?

QUESTIONS TO CONSIDER WHEN CRITIQUING RESEARCH DESIGNS

Identify a research study to critique. Read the study to see if you recognize any key terms discussed in this chapter. Remember that all studies may not contain all key terms. The following questions serve as a guide in critiquing research designs:

1. *Was the research design of the study described along with a rationale for the selection?* In the methods section of a research report, the word "design" should appear as a subheading followed by the particular type: experimental, quasi-experimental, or nonexperimental.

The author(s) should have clearly described their choice of design. In some research reports, there is no mention of what type of research design was employed. Based on the specific stated purpose of the study, you should be able to judge the type of design.

2. *Is the research design appropriate for answering the research questions and/or testing the hypotheses of the study?* Although research studies have a number of common components (i.e., problem statement, research questions and/or hypotheses, findings/results, conclusions/discussion), procedures specific to a study are to a great extent determined by the particular research design involved. Read over the research study, and evaluate if the type of research question and/or hypothesis posed is suitable to the research design employed in the study.

3. *If the study utilizes an experimental design, was randomization used to assign subjects to the experimental and control groups?* The validity of an experimental design depends on how subjects are assigned to groups and whether a control group was included in the design. Look to see if random assignment has occurred and if the process is described. Random assignment to groups is important because it distributes known and unknown extraneous (confounding) variables equally across groups, ensuring that the composition of groups is unbiased.

SUMMARY OF KEY IDEAS

1. A research design is a set of guidelines by which researchers obtain answers to inquiries.

2. Quantitative and qualitative approaches to research constitute an organizing framework that contains a set of assumptions or values that underlie how scientists view reality, truth, and research.

3. Quantitative research, which is directed at the verification of relationships, involves measurement and analysis of relationships. Qualitative research is concerned with the discovery of meaning and the use of language, concepts, and words rather than numbers to represent evidence from research.

4. All research designs are classified as experimental or nonexperimental.

5. Experimental designs are classified as true experimental or quasi-experimental. A true experimental design is actually an experiment in which the researcher tries to assess whether an intervention or treatment (independent variable) makes a difference in a measured outcome. Subjects are randomly assigned to an experimental or control group.

6. Three basic types of true experimental designs include the randomized pretest-posttest control group design, randomized posttest-only control group, and the one-group pretest-posttest design.

7. A quasi-experimental design dictates manipulation of the independent variable. In this type of design, random assignment, control groups, or both, are absent.

8. The basic type of quasi-experimental design is the nonequivalent control group design.

9. In nonexperimental designs, the researcher observes the actions of variables as they occur. The major purpose of nonexperimental designs is to uncover new knowledge and describe relationships. Two basic categories of nonexperimental research are descriptive and correlational research.

10. Randomized clinical trials (RCTs) are prospective studies that evaluate the effectiveness of an intervention/treatment in a large sample of patients. Some researchers consider RCTs to be the "best" form of evidence, or the "gold standard" for clinical research.

11. Quantitative designs focus on internal validity. Internal validity refers to whether the independent variable made a difference or whether the results were a response to some extraneous variable(s).

12. Threats to internal validity include history, maturation, testing, instrumentation, statistical regression, and mortality.

LEARNING ACTIVITIES

1. Identify several articles from research-oriented journals published within the last 5 years that describe experimental and quasi-experimental designs.
   a. Describe the type of research design used in each article. Did it follow the definition of an experimental design, quasi-experimental design, or both, as defined by this chapter? Describe the characteristics that make each study an experiment or quasi-experiment.
   b. In studies describing an experimental design, what two or three groups were being compared? Was there equivalence between or among the groups?
   c. In studies describing an experimental design, were the extraneous variables controlled to the greatest possible extent? Describe how each variable was controlled.
   d. In studies describing a quasi-experimental design, what characteristics of the study make it quasi-experimental rather than experimental?

REFERENCES

1. Brockopp, DY, and Hastings-Tolsma, MT: Fundamentals of Nursing Research, ed. 3. Jones and Bartlett, Boston, MA, 2003, pp 221–222.
2. Gillis, A, and Jackson, W: Research for Nurses: Methods and Interpretation. FA Davis, Philadelphia, 2002, p 94.
3. Guba, E: The Paradigm Dialogue. Sage, Newbury Park, CA, 1990.
4. Campbell, D, and Stanley, J: Experimental and Quasiexperimental Designs for Research. Rand McNally College Publishing, Chicago, 1966.
5. Vincent, D, Pasvogel, A, and Barrera, L: A feasibility study of a culturally tailored diabetes intervention for Mexican Americans. Biol Res Nurs 9:130, 2007.
6. Rossen, EK, and Knafl, K: Women's well-being after relocation to independent living communities. West J Nurs Res 29:183, 2007.
7. Cook, T, and Campbell, D: Quasi-experimentation: Design and Analysis Issues for Field Settings. Rand McNally College Publishing, Chicago, 1979.
8. Domiano, KL, Hinck, SM, Savinske, DL, and Hope, KL: Comparison of upper arm and forearm blood pressure. Clin Nurs Res 17:241, 2008.
9. Thomas, JC, Burton, M, Griffin, MT, and Fitzpatrick, JJ: Self-transcendence, spiritual well-being, and spiritual practices of women with breast cancer. J Holist Nurs 28:115, 2010.
10. Fairman, J: Context and contingency in the history of post World War II nursing scholarship in the United States. J Nurs Schol 40:4, 2008.
11. Melkus, G, Whittemore, R, and Mitchell, J: Type 2 diabetes in urban black and rural white women. Diabetes Educ 35:293, 2009.
12. Cochran J, and Conn, VS: Meta-analysis of quality of life outcomes following diabetes self-management training. Diabetes Educ 34:815, 2008.
13. Greenberg RS, et al: Medical Epidemiology, ed. 2. Appleton & Lange, Norwalk, CT, 1996, pp 1–15.

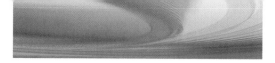

CHAPTER

12

SELECTING A QUALITATIVE RESEARCH DESIGN

James A. Fain, PhD, RN, BC-ADM, FAAN

LEARNING OBJECTIVES

By the end of this chapter, you will be able to:
1. Define phenomenology.
2. Describe phenomenological research methods.
3. Describe the relevance of phenomenology to nursing research and practice.
4. Review and critique phenomenological research in nursing.
5. Define major characteristics of ethnographic research.
6. Outline three states of an ethnographic research study.
7. Identify potential applications of ethnographic research for nursing practice.
8. Define grounded theory.
9. Discuss the steps in the research process for grounded theory.
10. Explain the constant comparative method of data analysis.
11. Discuss criteria for judging grounded theory.
12. Define descriptive qualitative research.

GLOSSARY OF KEY TERMS

Bracketing. Identification of any previous knowledge, ideas, or beliefs about the phenomenon under investigation.

Category. Type of concept that is usually used for a higher level of abstraction.

Coding. Process by which data are conceptualized.

Confirmability. Method used to establish the scientific rigor of phenomenological research. It has three elements: auditability, credibility, and fittingness. Auditability requires the reader to be able to follow the researcher's decision path and reach a similar conclusion. Credibility requires that the phenomenological description of the lived experience be recognized by people in the situation as an accurate description of their own experience. Fittingness requires that the phenomenological description is grounded in the lived experience and reflects typical and atypical elements of the experience.

(Continued)

Constant comparative method. Form of qualitative data analysis that categorizes units of meaning through a process of comparing incident to incident until concepts emerge.

Essences. Elements or structured units that give an understanding of the lived experience.

Ethnography. A qualitative research approach developed by anthropologists, involving the study and description of a culture in the natural setting. The researcher is intimately involved in the data collection process and seeks to understand fully how life unfolds for the particular culture under study.

Fieldwork. An anthropological research approach that involves prolonged residence with members of the culture that is being studied. Field notes are written as detailed descriptions of researchers' observations, experiences, and conversations in the "field" (research setting).

Grounded theory. Discovery of a theory from data that have been systematically obtained through research.

Lived experience. The focus of phenomenology. It consists of everyday experiences of an individual in the context of normal pursuits. It is what is real and true to the individual.

Memos. Write-up of ideas about codes and their relationships as they occur to the researcher while coding.

Participant observer. A technique in anthropological fieldwork. It involves direct observation of everyday life in study participants' natural settings and participation in their lifestyle and activities to the greatest extent possible.

Phenomenology. A philosophy and research method that explores and describes everyday experience as it appears to human consciousness in order to generate and enhance the understanding of what it means to be human. Phenomenology limits philosophical inquiry to acts of consciousness.

Purposive sampling. Selecting and interviewing participants who have actually lived and experienced the phenomena of interest.

Saturation. Point when data collection is terminated because no new description and interpretations of the lived experience are coming from the study participants.

Symbolic interaction. Theoretical orientation to qualitative research; focus is on the nature of social interaction among individuals.

Theoretical sampling. Process used in data collection that is controlled by the emerging theory; researcher collects, codes, and analyzes the data.

Qualitative research is a way to gain insight through discovering meanings. The qualitative approach emphasizes an understanding of human experience, exploring the nature of people's transactions with themselves, others, and their surroundings. Research questions that lend themselves to qualitative inquiry are generally broad, seeking to understand why something occurs, what certain experiences mean to individuals, or how the dynamics of an experience influence subsequent behaviors or decisions. The purpose of qualitative research is to examine such experiences using a holistic approach that is concerned with the nature of "reality" as the participants understand it.

Qualitative designs are approaches used to discover knowledge and understand rich descriptions of meanings from social experiences. Methods associated with qualitative designs are conducted within a framework guided by a particular philosophical approach. Table 12.1 displays common types of qualitative designs based on philosophy, theory/research tradition, and research questions.

The tradition known as *phenomenology* seeks to draw meaning from complex realities through careful analysis of narrative subjective material. This perspective is based on the belief that experience can be interpreted *only* by the individual who has lived it and that the meaning of that experience to the individual is relevant and important.

A second common perspective, called "ethnography," is the study of a specific cultural group of people. Ethnographic research examines the attitudes, beliefs, and behaviors of sociological units. In ethnographic research, the researcher becomes immersed in the subject's way of life to understand cultural forces that shape behavior and feelings.

One of the unique features of qualitative research methodologies is that it allows the researcher to develop research hypotheses as the data unfold. Because it is an exploratory technique, qualitative research will not always begin with predetermined expectations. Instead, the researcher can use the data to develop a theory that will explain what is observed. For this approach, called "grounded theory research," the researcher collects, codes, and analyzes data simultaneously and identifies relevant

TABLE 12.1	Comparison of Selected Types of Qualitative Designs		
Design	**Philosophy**	**Theory/ Research Tradition**	**Type of Research Question**
Phenomenological	Phenomenology	Philosophy	Meaningful questions eliciting the essence of experiences
Ethnography; participant observation	Historical/ cultural	Anthropology; sociology	Descriptive questions of values, beliefs, practices of cultural groups; meaning from social encounters
Grounded theory	Symbolic interaction	Sociology	Process and core concept questions; experiences over time or change with stages and phases

variables, leading to the development of theoretical concepts that are "grounded" in observations.

In this chapter, a brief introduction to phenomenological, ethnographic, and grounded theory research is presented to help researchers gain an appreciation for these approaches and develop familiarity with techniques and terminology associated with qualitative methodology.

Phenomenological Research

Phenomenology is a qualitative research approach that provides the researcher with an opportunity to gain a deep understanding of the nature or meaning of everyday experiences. In phenomenological terms, these experiences are called the **lived experience**. Phenomenology systematically uncovers and describes the meaning or essences of an experience. **Essences** are elements or structural units that give an understanding to the phenomenon under study. When using a phenomenological approach to research, there is less interest in the facts of an experience and more interest in the meaning facts hold for the person experiencing them. Phenomenology uncovers the meaning of everyday experiences and brings these experiences to the reader through language.

Phenomenology is both a philosophy and a research method that explores and describes everyday experiences in order to generate and enhance an understanding of what the experience is like. Phenomenology is a way of viewing ourselves, others, and everything else that comes in contact with our lives. In this sense, phenomenology is a system of interpreting and studying the world of everyday life.[1] It is the instant when experience, reflection, and ideas come together and make sense to the individual.

Phenomenology as a Philosophy and Research Method

Philosophy assesses and systematically relates human knowledge and experience from an integrating perspective.[2] Phenomenology is a reflective philosophy focusing on exploration of the inner world of human beings, with phenomenological interpretations deriving content immediately and continuously from the human experience.

Phenomenology, as a research method, is a rigorous, critical, and systematic investigation of phenomena (human experience). The approach is a descriptive, retrospective, in-depth analysis of a conscious lived experience. Phenomenology has appeal as a research approach because it views human beings as subjects, rather than objects, who can make choices based on meaning and values. The purpose of phenomenology is to describe the intrinsic traits or essences of the lived experience. A content outline associated with a phenomenological research report is displayed in Table 12.2.

TABLE 12.2	Content Outline for a Phenomenological Research Report

Introduction

Lived Experience Under Study

- What is the lived experience?
- What is the aim/purpose of the study?
- Why is it important to study this lived experience?

Bracketing

- What is the researcher's interest in the lived experience?
- What is the specific context of the lived experience?

Historical/Experiential

- What are the researcher's assumptions and preexisting knowledge?
- Define concepts and terms.

Methods

Research Design Sample

- Criteria for inclusion.
- How access to the sample was obtained.

Human Subjects' Considerations

- IRB review and approval.
- Process of obtaining and maintaining informed consent described.

Data Collection

- How were data collected?
- Researcher's log as source of data.

Data Analysis

- Description of procedures used to analyze and interpret data.
  Content Outline for a Phenomenological Research Report

Confirmability

- How was scientific rigor ensured?

Findings

- Description of themes or essences uncovered.
- Themes and essences substantiated with direct quotes from study participants.

Discussion

- Discussion of meanings and understandings explicated.
- Related meanings and understandings to scientific literature and researcher's bracketed preknowledge and assumptions.

Source: Adapted from Boyd, C, and Munhall, P: Qualitative research proposals and reports. In Munhall, P, and Boyd, C (eds): Nursing Research: A Qualitative Perspective, ed. 2. National League for Nursing, New York, 1993, pp 424–453.

Characteristics of Phenomenological Research

Research Problem/Question

The research question in phenomenological research focuses on the meaning of the lived experience. The goal of phenomenological research is to develop rich, full, insightful descriptions of the lived experience. Any experience that presents itself to one's consciousness is a potential topic for phenomenological research. To be conscious is to be aware of some aspect of a lived experience. Because the focus of phenomenological research is consciousness, phenomenology is always a retrospective reflection on experience.

Conducting Phenomenological Research

The first step is to identify a lived experience appropriate for phenomenological study. Phenomenology is the appropriate research method in the following circumstances:[3]

1. The goal is to understand the meaning of a lived experience.
2. The lived experience of interest is not well described or understood; there is little, if any, published research; and/or what is published about the lived experience demonstrates the need for greater depth of description.
3. People who are living or have lived the experience are accessible and are a source of rich and descriptive data; literary or artistic portrayals of the lived experience are available/accessible.
4. There is an audience for the research.
5. The resources and time, along with researcher's style and strengths, must be compatible with this mode of inquiry.

Nursing practice offers a rich source of human experience suitable for investigation using the phenomenological method. Excerpt 12.1 is an example of how the authors made it explicit to readers why a phenomenological approach to research was chosen to study the meaning of family members' experiences of living with an individual with moderate or severe traumatic brain injury (TBI).

Sample

It is common to use a small, **purposive sample** selected from persons who have actually lived the experience under study and who are able and willing to describe the experience. Participants are solicited until there is redundancy in the data, or saturation. **Saturation** refers to the participants' descriptions becoming repetitive, with no new or different ideas or interpretations emerging. Excerpt 12.2 describes a purposive sample in a phenomenological study with discussion of how data collection continued until saturation.

EXCERPT 12.1

Rationale for Using a Phenomenological Approach to Research

In summary, previous research using both quantitative and qualitative methods confirms that traumatic brain injury (TBI) has far-reaching consequences for close relatives. The research also shows that they experience various burdens and have a great need for different kinds of support; however, these needs are not always met. To meet the needs of these families, more knowledge is required about the experience of daily life with a person with TBI. The understanding gained from quantitative research is useful for predicting and enabling interventions to reduce harmful consequences of illness. However, to provide holistic care, more understanding is needed about the meaning of living with a person with TBI from close relatives' perspective.

Source: Jumisko, E, Lexell, J, and Soderberg, S: Living with moderate or severe traumatic brain injury: The meaning of family members' experiences. J Fam Nurs 13:353, 2007.

EXCERPT 12.2

Description of Purposive Sample With Discussion of Data Saturation

Sample

The purposive sample included 20 dyads of a spinal cord injured person and a family member who had lived with the injury for 5 to 10 years. All participants were English speaking. All of the spinal cord injured participants had a complete spinal cord injury. The time frame of 5 to 10 years was selected based on a review of literature. Woodbury and Redd (1987) determined that psychological distress occurred approximately 3 to 5 years following the injury, when spinal cord injured patients felt the total impact of the injury on their lives. Most recent research has revealed that adapting to spinal cord injury is an evolving process. Djkers (1996) suggested that adjustment may take anywhere from 2 to 7 years. The meaning of living with spinal cord injury, therefore, would emerge and best be reflected in the years following this psychological adjustment period.

Data Collection

Interviews continued until data saturation occurred—that is, when new themes or patterns about the major construct under study no longer emerged from the data and when concepts and relationships were validated with a variety of participants. Although data saturation had been achieved after the completion of 12 interviews, interviews continued rather than close the study to those who already had volunteered to participate.

Source: DeSanto-Madeya, S: The meaning of living with spinal cord injury 5 to 10 years after the injury. West J Nurs Res 28:265, 2006.

Ethical Considerations

Munhall[4] describes several ethical considerations unique to phenomenological research that relates to the researcher as well as participant. There is concern for the nurse as researcher and the potential conflict of professional practice ethics and the ethics of research.

Informed consent is the knowledgeable and expressed choice of an individual to participate in a research project without coercion, deceit, or duress. The consent document explains the research and procedures to be used, a description of risks and benefits to the participant, specific permission to tape and record interviews (if appropriate), and a discussion of how the researcher will ensure confidentiality and privacy to the participant. The participant's freedom to withdraw from the project without penalty and to ask questions is also stated. Munhall[4] advocates that the consent be renegotiated as the research project proceeds and circumstances change.

The institutional review board (IRB) is used by most academic and health service institutions to oversee research activities. IRBs deal regularly with quantitative research proposals. However, the phenomenologist may have to educate the IRB about the philosophical underpinnings and design of phenomenological research. Some IRBs have an expedited review process for qualitative research proposals because restricting access to treatment and manipulation of the interventions are not part of these study designs. Providing readers with evidence that research studies/projects have been brought forth to IRBs is usually found in the Methods section of a research report; sometimes under a subheading entitled "Ethical Consideration" (see Excerpt 12.3).

EXCERPT 12.3

Discussion of Institutional Review Boards in Phenomenological Research

Ethical Considerations

All participants gave their informed consent and were provided a guarantee of confidentiality. The Ethical Committee at Lulea University of Technology in Sweden gave permission for the study.

Settings and Participants

The study took place in an inpatient and outpatient pediatric cancer unit located in a city in west Canada. Permission to carry out the study was first secured from the Research Ethics Board of the University of Manitoba.

Source: Jumisko, E, Lexell, J, and Soderberg, S: *Living with moderate or severe traumatic brain injury: The meaning of family members' experiences. J Fam Nurs* 13:353, 2007.

Source: Woodgate, R: *The importance of being there: Perspectives of social support by adolescents with cancer. J Pediatr Oncol Nurs* 23:122, 2006.

Data Collection

The phenomenological method embraces a unique approach to data collection. Before data are collected, the researcher should conduct an exercise called bracketing. **Bracketing** is a reflective self-assessment whereby the researcher articulates assumptions, knowledge, and ideas that are brought to the research project about the particular phenomenon. Some phenomenological methods require that these be bracketed, or suspended, during the study so that the lived experience can be approached from a fresh perspective.

Primary data collection techniques in phenomenological research elicit descriptions of lived experience from study participants by means of interviews or written descriptions. Participants are asked, "What is the experience like?" Interviews are usually unstructured. Interaction between the researcher and the participant is focused on achieving a full description of the lived experience. The researcher must be an empathetic and skilled listener and encourage fuller description by rephrasing the participant's statements. Sometimes a second or third interview is needed to elicit full description. The researcher is encouraged to log his or her reflections on the process of the interviews as a source of valuable data for analysis. Some phenomenologists use literary and artistic expressions of the lived experience under study as another source of data. Interviews are recorded and transcribed verbatim. Information presented in Excerpt 12.4 describes

---

EXCERPT 12.4

Use of Interviews: Phenomenological Research Report

Data Collection

Data were collected using audio-tape recorded, semistructured, in-depth interviews, all of which were conducted by the author. In the interview process of phenomenological inquiry, the participant is encouraged to give details of the lived experience so that the researcher can discover and interpret meaning. The injured person and family member were asked to participate in two interviews. The spinal cord injured person and family member were interviewed together to gain insight into the experience of living with spinal cord injury for both spinal cord injured persons and their family members. This allows the researcher to look at interactions and contexts from the combined perspective rather than each individual.

The first interview was conducted in the spinal cord injured person's home. The person's home was the ideal location because it provides a comfortable interview atmosphere with no distractions and because data were not limited to interviews, but also included participant observation, field notes, and unobtrusive samples of behavior and interaction in natural settings.

The purpose of the first interview was to gain insight into the experience of living with spinal cord injury. An interview guide was used to help the spinal cord injured person and family member describe the experience of

(Continued)

EXCERPT 12.4

Use of Interviews: Phenomenological Research Report—cont'd

living with spinal cord injury without leading the discussion. The initial statement asked, "Please describe your experience, including circumstances, situations, thoughts, and feelings that you think reflect your experience of living with spinal cord injury." The interview lasted 1 to 2 hours.

The second interview took place 4 to 6 weeks later via telephone. Prior to the second interview, the transcripts from the first interview were returned to the spinal cord injured persons and their family members for reflection. The purpose of the second interview was to provide the injured person and family member the opportunity to reflect and further elaborate on personal and family issues uncovered during the first interview or disclose feelings that emerged after hearing the spinal cord injured person's and family member's response. The second interview, which lasted from 20 to 60 minutes, was conducted and audio-taped, having the spinal cord injured person and family member on two phone lines simultaneously.

Source: DeSanto-Madeya, S: The meaning of living with spinal cord injury 5 to 10 years after the injury. West J Nurs Res 28:265, 2006.

---

a typical write-up on data collection (interviewing) in a phenomenological study. Note the detail in which the researcher describes the first and second set of interviews.

Data Analysis

Several methods for data analysis exist in phenomenological research. All methods require the researcher to engage in a dialogue with the data and use inductive reasoning and synthesis. Tables 12.3 through 12.5 present the most commonly used methods. Regardless of method selected, the researcher must read and listen to the data many times. The researcher must not rush and describe the lived experience prematurely. The researcher needs to take his/or her time and become immersed in the participant's descriptions to identify themes and essences related to the lived experience.

A real difficulty researchers might experience is managing large amounts of narrative data. A system for filing, coding, and retrieving data is a necessary first step in the analysis of data. Early transcription and analysis of recorded interviews help the researcher maintain the essence of the interview. Some computer programs are now available to assist in data management (e.g., Atlas/ti, Ethnograph v5.07, Nudist, NVivo8, XSight).

Question of Scientific Rigor

In quantitative research, the researcher is expected to address the validity and reliability of the measurement instruments as a sign of scientific rigor. Although the phenomenologist is also concerned with reliability, validity is not relevant. Because phenomenology is the study of lived

| TABLE 12.3 | Giorgi's Method of Data Analysis |

Participants: 2 to 10 persons who have lived the experience under study

Data generation: Interview or written description

Data Analysis

1. Read the entire disclosure of the lived experience straight through to obtain a sense of the whole.
2. Reread the disclosure to discover the essences of the lived experience under study. Look for each time a transition in meaning occurs. Abstract these meaning units or themes.
3. Examine meaning units for redundancies, clarification, or elaboration. Relate meaning units to each other and to a sense of the whole.
4. Reflect on the meaning units, and extrapolate the essence of the experience for each participant. Transform each meaning unit into the language of science when relevant.
5. Formulate a consistent description of the meaning structures of the lived experience for all participants.

Source: Adapted from Giorgi, A: Psychology as a Human Science: A Phenomenologically Based Approach. Harper and Row, New York, 1970.

| TABLE 12.4 | Colaizzi's Method of Data Analysis |

Participants: 2 to 10 persons who have lived the experience under study

Data generation: Lengthy and repeated interviews to facilitate full description

Data Analysis

1. Describe the lived experience under study.
2. Collect participant descriptions of the lived experience.
3. Read all participants' descriptions of the lived experience.
4. Extract significant statements.
5. Articulate the meaning of each significant statement.
6. Aggregate the meanings into clusters of themes.
7. Write an exhaustive description.
8. Return to participants for validation of the exhaustive description.
9. Incorporate any new data revealed during validations into a final exhaustive description.

Source: Adapted from Colaizzi, P: Psychological research as a phenomenologist views it. In Vaille, R, and King, M (eds): Existential Phenomenological Alternatives for Psychology. Oxford University Press, New York, 1978.

TABLE 12.5	Van Manen's Method of Data Analysis

Participants: Persons who have lived the experience under study

Data generation: See following

Data Collection and Analysis

Turn to the Nature of Lived Experience

1. Orient to the lived experience.
2. Formulate the phenomenological research question.
3. Explicate assumptions and preunderstandings.

Experiential Investigation

4. Generate data.
   a. Use personal experience.
   b. Trace etymological sources.
   c. Search idiomatic phrases.
   d. Obtain experiential descriptions from participants.
   e. Locate experiential descriptions in the arts.
5. Consult phenomenological literature.

Phenomenological Reflection

6. Conduct thematic analysis.
   a. Uncover themes.
   b. Isolate thematic statements.
   c. Compose linguistic transformations.
   d. Glean thematic descriptions from artistic sources.
7. Determine essential themes.

Phenomenological Writing

8. Attend to spoken language.
9. Vary examples.
10. Write.
11. Rewrite often.

Source: Adapted from Van Manen, M: Researching the Lived Experience. State University of New York Press, Buffalo, NY, 1990.

experience, it is contextual; no generalizations can be made. It is the nature of the research rather than a limitation of the method. Guba and Lincoln[5] suggest confirmability as a measure of scientific rigor. **Confirmability** has three elements: auditability, credibility, and fittingness.

Auditability Auditability requires readers to be able to follow the decision path of the researcher and arrive at the same or comparable (but not contradictory) findings, given the researcher's data, perspective, and situation. Bracketing, the identification of knowledge, presuppositions, and ideas, helps to fulfill this element.

Credibility Credibility requires that findings are faithful descriptions or interpretations of the lived experience. The findings are recognized by people in the situation as an accurate description of their own experience. Through multiple interviews with participants and by giving the participants the opportunity to review and amend the descriptions and themes that emerge from the data analysis, this requirement is met. To enhance credibility, the researcher's experiences in collecting and analyzing data, often recorded as a diary or log, are included in the discussion of the findings.

Fittingness Fittingness is the extent to which study findings fit the data; that is, findings should be truly grounded in the lived experience under study and reflect the typical and atypical elements of that experience. Using direct quotes from the study, participants help the researcher to meet this element of confirmability. The ultimate test of fittingness is the affirmation of the existence and meaning of the lived experience by the reader. Information provided in Excerpt 12.5 addresses how methodological rigor was evaluated in one particular phenomenological research report.

Writing Phenomenological Findings

The final step in any research study is the dissemination of findings. In phenomenology, this means to let the essential structures of the lived experience "be seen" through language.[6] There are several conventions for the write-up of phenomenological research. Bracketing requires the researcher to identify and suspend foreknowledge, preconceived ideas, and assumptions—to approach the lived experience under study from a fresh perspective. Therefore, extensive literature review and synthesis does not precede the study. Literature and experience that are part of the researcher's knowledge base and natural attitude are discussed early in the report under the topic of bracketing. A more comprehensive literature review on the themes, essences, and meaning structures of the lived experience uncovered during data analysis is integrated into the discussion of the study findings.

EXCERPT 12.5

Methodological Rigor

Credibility was demonstrated when the study participants recognized the transcribed data as their own experience. Auditability was ensured by providing a written decision trail of the abstraction process from raw data to significant statements, formulated meanings, supportive data, themes, and thematic categories. An expert in phenomenological research audited the study process and confirmed that the data and findings were internally consistent. Transferability was accomplished by providing thick, rich descriptions of data to demonstrate that research findings have meaning to others in similar situations.

Source: DeSanto-Madeya, S: The meaning of living with spinal cord injury 5 to 10 years after the injury. West J Nurs Res 28:265, 2006.

The phenomenologist is not concerned with the frequency or prevalence of a theme but rather descriptions and understandings of the experience uncovered. Numbers, percentages, and statistical measures are not usually used in the analysis and discussion of the findings. Instead, the phenomenologist develops an accurate, integrated, literary description of an experience and its meaning. The use of direct quotes from the participants illustrates the researcher's analysis and affirms the accuracy of the analysis by providing the reader access to the original data.

Finally, writing, editing, rewriting, and returning to the original data is a repeated cycle. It is helpful to have faculty, informed colleagues, or coresearchers in this process. It requires concentration, attention to detail, and time to do it well. A rich description of the essence or meaning of a lived experience is the product of a well-done phenomenological study. This description is powerful in itself. It enables the reader of phenomenology to gain greater insight into what it means to be human and to engage in the experience under study. This insight can guide future nursing activities and personal actions.

Ethnographic Research

Ethnographic research is a qualitative approach that provides an opportunity for researchers to conduct studies that attend to the need for intimacy with members of a culture. Researchers play a significant role in identifying, interpreting, and analyzing the culture under study. More than just observing, the researcher often becomes a participant in the culture.

Ethnography means "study and description of a culture of a particular group of people." It is the oldest qualitative research method in use today, having originated in the mid-1800s. The case study method in sociology (later called participant observation) represents another qualitative research method with a long and distinctive tradition.[7] It is used to describe and understand social life, mainly in urban settings of Western societies. Over the last 15 years, numerous qualitative research methods have emerged from this tradition, some of which have been called ethnography.[8,9]

Anthropologists developed ethnography as a way to study cultures at a time when they were frustrated with existing research methods. Having relied on data gathered by travelers and explorers, it was often superficial, haphazard, and ethnocentric (i.e., interpreting behaviors in light of one's own culture). Even when anthropologists were able to provide direction on what and how to observe thoughts, feelings, and behaviors of another group of people, accounts were often misleading. It was hard for the outsider not to reinterpret strange behavior in familiar terms because it is easier to understand something familiar.[10] The notion of anthropologists going to the field to collect their own data was a highly innovative, almost revolutionary idea in 1885. Today,

fieldwork is the essence of conducting an ethnography. Fieldwork is an approach that involves prolonged residence with members of the culture being studied.

Ethnography became a way of "getting the whole configuration of culture down correctly before it disappeared" and dealing with cultural problems, such as deciphering what are the most stable and enduring cultural traits (e.g., the kind of tools a people used and the techniques for making them, the form of the family, or a people's beliefs about healing and the supernatural world).[11] Currently, ethnography remains central to the study of culture within anthropology, although it has been refined and explicated more fully over time, and a variety of other types of cultural research have emerged.

Ethnographic Research and Nursing

Nurses first became interested in ethnography as a source of information and research method for better understanding patients from diverse cultures in the mid-1950s. Madeline Leininger,[12] one of the first nurse anthropologists, wrote that her interest in culture began to emerge when she was working as a child psychiatric mental health nurse.

Over the years, several new questions emerged about how cultures influence people's experiences with health and illness. The interest in culture was further augmented by the general movement of nurses into doctoral education, some of whom pursued their doctorates in anthropology under the nurse scientist program. Graduates of these programs began writing about how ethnography and its findings could enhance nursing practice and be a useful method for nursing research.[12-14]

In the 1980s, ethnographic research and nursing studies gained momentum. By 1995, ethnographic research began to emerge everywhere in nursing, although not always conveying much meaning and adding considerably to the cross-disciplinary confusion of the term. Initially, the term "ethnography" was used more often to refer to a particular type of computer software ("ethnograph"); a specific style of interview ("ethnographic interview"); or other types of field research (e.g., participant observation unrelated to culture) than to depict fieldwork aimed at the study of a particular culture.

Characteristics of Ethnographic Research

Research Problem/Question

The research problem in ethnographic research focuses on describing and understanding a specific culture. The researcher lives for an extended time among a given group of people who share a common culture. As a **participant observer**, the researcher enters into the everyday life and activities of the people of the culture being studied. By watching what goes on, talking with individuals, and participating in activities, the researcher comes to know the culture shared by this group of people. Researchers may supplement their observations (which are recorded as field notes) with a wide variety of additional data collection tools (e.g., key informant interviewing, collections of life histories, structured interviewing, questionnaires, documents, photographs).

In ethnographic research, "entering the field" means entering as a stranger into an unfamiliar setting. The researcher uses this position of stranger to learn how it is to think, feel, and act like the people around him or her. It is the difference between the researcher's own culture and that of the people being studied that helps in identifying distinctive behaviors, thoughts, and emotions, as well as the rules influencing these in the culture under study.

Researchers tend to reside in the field for about a year, although the exact time can vary from as little as 5 months to as long as 5 years. Generally, 1 year has been considered a reasonable time to be accepted by persons in the culture and to learn the subculture's manifest and latent aspects, to attend to a wide variety of the subculture's activities, to see members in various contexts, and to follow certain events to their conclusions. More time or less time in the field may be required, depending on the research question(s) and complexity of the culture. The goal is in-depth knowledge of the culture rather than surface familiarity.

Conducting Ethnographic Research

The planning and implementing of an ethnographic research study takes place in three stages: pre-fieldwork, fieldwork, and post-fieldwork (Table 12.6).

Pre-Fieldwork

The researcher usually starts by choosing a group of people, a field, and/or a problem. Once a particular group of people or culture is chosen, the researcher seeks more specific and detailed knowledge about the people and culture under study as well as the problem to be examined.

In Excerpt 12.6, the author talks about the group of people and culture she decided to study and the purpose of the ethnographic study.

Work done in the pre-fieldwork stage enhances the researcher's ability to understand the context and orientation of the people in the culture being studied. It alerts the researcher to the kinds of beliefs and practices that might be encountered later. It also helps the researcher in formulating a more specific and systematic plan of investigation for the fieldwork stage. This plan is looser than "research designs" you see in more quantitative research. It usually includes three phases. In the first phase, the researcher focuses on gaining entry, establishing relationships, and beginning to describe the culture (or some major aspect of it). In the second phase, the researcher usually concentrates more directly on the specific problem.

TABLE 12.6	Stages of Implementing an Ethnographic Research Study

Pre-Fieldwork

- Choosing a people, field, problem
- Searching the literature and gathering information on the people and the problem
- Formulating a systematic plan of investigation
- Making preparations

Fieldwork Phase I

- Making contacts and gaining experience
- Settling in and establishing a role
- Beginning to gather information and mapping out visible features of culture

Phase II

- Working with informants
- Identifying major themes
- Focusing on gathering information on selected problem
- Doing some sampling
- Selecting additional techniques for further data collection

Phase III

- Continuing with participant observation—now raising more sensitive questions
- Double-checking data
- Obtaining large volumes of information

Post-Fieldwork

- Finalizing the analysis and findings
- Writing up the study (selecting an audience, a voice, and data for presentation)

EXCERPT 12.6	

Purpose of Ethnographic Studies

The purpose of this ethnographic study was to describe experiences of hospice residents who received complementary therapies and to describe hospice culture patterns where complementary therapies were delivered. Specifically, the research question was "What are the experiences of hospice residents who use complementary therapies?" In the current study, experience is defined as the participant's inner beliefs and thoughts, and pattern is defined as abstracted cultural beliefs and practices that describe behaviors or group rules.

Source: Nelson, J: Being in tune with life: Complementary therapy use and well-being in residential hospice residents. J Holist Nurs 24:152, 2006.

In the third phase, the researcher often spends considerable time double-checking and validating analyses and interpretations emerging from the first two phases. The amount of time devoted to any of these phases, but particularly the first two, varies widely across researchers. In the past, when the primary focus was on describing an unrecorded culture, the greatest amount of time was spent in the first phase. More recently, researchers have focused more attention and time on a specific problem under study (phase two) and used the initial phase only to gain entry, establish contacts, and obtain an overall sense of the culture, more as a backdrop than as the central focus of investigation.

As final preparation for the field, the researcher also has to give thought to a host of practical considerations (e.g., training in the language; arranging for funding; locating a specific site and planning for residence in a new location, one in which there may be potential political, social, or other deterrents to overcome). Even with all this preparation and preplanning, the researcher needs to remain open-minded and ready to "shift gears," as it is often the unexpected that leads to the most important discoveries in the field.

Fieldwork: Phase I

The researcher's main overall approach in the field is participant observation. Participant observation and taking field notes begin immediately as the researcher enters the field and settles in. During this phase, the researcher focuses on making contacts, developing trust, and gaining acceptance as well as establishing a consistent role and becoming familiar with daily routines. For most researchers, this is a period of considerable personal adjustment. Excerpt 12.7 provides an example of ethnographic data collection.

EXCERPT 12.7

Ethnographic Data Collection

Data collection began by observing the staff in routine care and delivering complementary therapies, attending weekly interdisciplinary team meetings, and interacting with the interdisciplinary staff and families. During participant observation, the investigator continually informed staff, residents, and families of her role in the hospice setting as a researcher and wore a hospice photo name tag identifying her as a researcher.

Informal interviews occurred with residents, staff, and family about responses and behaviors immediately before and after the administration of complementary therapies. Formal interviews were conducted with participants who were purposively selected by the researcher, based on their complementary therapy experiences and their willingness to participate. Residents who agreed to study participation were asked to sign a consent form.

Source: Nelson, J: *Being in tune with life: Complementary therapy use and well-being in residential hospice residents. J Holist Nurs* 24:152, 2006.

Researchers give much thought to what role to take and how to introduce themselves. Whatever role is chosen, it enhances the researcher's exposure to certain people, activities, and events and decreases the chances of seeing or participating in others. Because every role has a particular vantage point, the researcher tries to find one that allows maximum exposure to the culture as a whole and the specific problem of interest.

Also during this initial period of adjustment, the researcher develops a daily set of activities to provide some sense of order and begins to collect data on those features of the new environment that can be recorded without much assistance. These tend to include the less personal and socially intense elements of the setting and culture.

Fieldwork: Phase II

During the middle phase of the fieldwork, the researcher augments his or her continuing participant observation by working closely with a small number of informants: individuals who are willing and able to express cultural information verbally. Also during phase II, researchers begin to identify emerging themes and categorize and analyze general features of the culture.

During this second phase, researchers often use additional techniques for collecting data, although some methods (e.g., mapping and census taking) are frequently begun in phase I. Researchers usually do not decide on what additional techniques to use until they have been in the field for quite awhile. They like to closely fit and refine selected techniques to the particular language and practices of the people being studied and the specific problem of interest. Table 12.7 lists some of the more frequently used data collection techniques in ethnographic research.

TABLE 12.7	Data Collection Techniques in Ethnographic Research

1. Census taking: Collection of basic demographic data about people being studied (e.g., age, occupation, marital status).
2. Mapping: Identifying the location of people, culture, environmental features in order to understand how people interact.
3. Document analysis: Examination of data such as vital statistics records, newspapers, personal diaries to supplement information collected through interviewing and participant observation.
4. Life histories: Comprehensive biography of an informant's life, which also provides an example of the way in which cultural patterns are integrated in a person's life.
5. Event analysis: Detailed written and photographic documentation of such events as weddings, funerals, and festivals in the culture under investigation.

Fieldwork: Phase III

In the final fieldwork phase, the researcher can raise more sensitive questions and obtain an increasingly large volume of information. Phase III is when researchers concentrate on double-checking and monitoring field information to support and further refine themes, evaluate data gathered, and broaden understanding of how representative the research findings are of members of the culture.

Post-Fieldwork

The researcher reviews the findings and begins to write up the findings of the field research, although this will have already been started in the field. In writing up the findings, the researcher makes several major choices related to what audience to address, which voice to use, what data to present, and how to organize the findings. These choices are reflected in the various formats you might see in published ethnographies.

Writing Phenomenological Findings

Most researchers choose to write for a scholarly audience, take an authoritative voice (as though they were neutral observers), and begin with the findings. This is followed by a presentation of selected data to support those findings. The "classic" ethnography usually begins with a brief overview of the setting and the people being studied, followed by a review of the specific problem being addressed and a discussion of the fieldwork phase. The description of the researcher and his or her relationship to the subjects is usually provided in this section of the write-up. The bulk of the text follows, consisting of impersonally written, monologic descriptions of the culture that analyze the specific problem. The presentation of data is usually rich in detail and well ordered, first with regard to the culture as a whole and second with regard to the specific cultural problem being addressed. In this classic format, the researcher is intent on capturing the culture as a whole and tries to avoid depicting any one individual in too much detail for fear of confusing individual personality characteristics with attributes of the culture as a whole. At the same time, these presentations vary somewhat according to the specific theories, interpretations, or styles of analysis used by the researcher.

Grounded Theory

Grounded theory is a qualitative research method developed in the 1960s by two sociologists, Barney Glaser and Anselm Strauss, based on the symbolic interactionist perspective of human behavior. Grounded theory is the discovery of theory from data that have been systematically obtained through research.[15] Grounded theory combines both inductive and deductive research methods. With the use of inductive processes, theory emerges from the data. Deduction is then used to test the theory empirically.

Grounded theory differs from quantitative research. In quantitative research, the investigator identifies a research problem, selects a theory or conceptual framework, and deduces hypotheses to test. Grounded theory does not start with an existing theory; it generates a theory to explain a substantive area. The research product ends with a theoretical formulation or integrated set of conceptual hypotheses.[15]

Symbolic Interaction

Symbolic interaction provides the theoretical underpinnings of grounded theory. **Symbolic interaction** focuses on the nature of social interaction among individuals. Basic principles central to symbolic interaction include the fact that human beings act in relation to one another, take each other's acts into account as they themselves act, and provide meaning to specific symbols in their lives.[16]

To understand human behavior, one must examine the nature of social interaction. Within natural settings, social behavior is examined from an individual and group perspective. The researcher examines the world from an individual's perspective and discovers how to interpret himself or herself in the context of others. As an observer, the researcher translates the meaning obtained from interactions into a language understood by others.

Characteristics of Grounded Theory Research

Research Problem/Questions

Grounded theory is especially suited to knowledge development in nursing because nursing is a practice discipline whose essence lies in processes.[15] Through grounded theory, the processes that underlie social experience are discovered and become the basis for nursing interventions. As emphasized by Glaser,[17] one of the best arguments for use of grounded theory is that it frees the researcher to discover what *is* going on rather than assume what *should* be going on. Because grounded theory involves an emerging theory from data, the main problem or concern for people in a social setting also must emerge from the data. The researcher remains sensitive to how participants in the social setting interpret and give meaning to their situation. Discovering the problem or focus of the study and what processes account for its solution helps ensure the clinical relevance of the emerging theory.

In grounded theory, the research problem is discovered, as is the process that resolves it.[15] The grounded theorist moves into an area of interest with no specific problem in mind. Researchers should be careful not to force the data to fit with the grounded theorist's own preconceived problem, keeping an open mind to allow the emergence of the participant's problem.

The research question asked is *"What is the chief concern or problem of the people in a substantive area, and what accounts for variation in processing the problem?"* Excerpt 12.8 displays the introductory paragraphs that guided a grounded theory study on decision-making about mammography screening among African American women.

Conducting Grounded Theory Research

Data Collection

Grounded theorists must view the environment as informants do and focus on the interaction under study. Participant observation, informal interviewing, and formal interviewing are the three main sources of data generation. Unstructured observational data are gathered by participant observation. While participating in the functioning of a social group, the researcher is observing and recording data. Participant observation is combined with informal interviewing. Like everyday conversations, informal interviewing can last from a few minutes to more than an hour. The grounded theorist writes field notes to record data obtained through participant observation and interviewing.

Formal interviewing is also used, when the researcher wishes more in-depth information. Unstructured formal interviews are used most frequently to obtain detailed information in the participant's own words. Formal interviews are audio-taped to capture the participant's interview

---

EXCERPT 12.8

Rationale for Grounded Theory Study

Despite improvements in mammography screening in women during the past two decades, African American (AA) women of diverse socioeconomic status continue to experience later discovery and premature deaths attributed to breast cancer. Although health disparities of serious magnitude exist, little is known about the social processes characteristics of AA women when making decisions about mammography screening. This gap in the literature has been partly acknowledged by some researchers who have encouraged studies by listening closely to what women themselves have to say about their decisions regarding mammography screening. Additionally, published reports have not included information about the social processes used by AA women in making decisions about mammography screening. The important new approach from a grounded perspective allows one to consider the social processes that are implicit in the words or perspectives of AA women to describe their decisions associated with mammography screening.

Source: Fowler, BA: Social processes used by African American women in making decisions about mammography screening. J Nurs Schol 38:247, 2006.

word-for-word. A researcher may use an interview guide consisting of several questions related to the topic. A time and place for conducting the interview are agreed to by the researcher and participant. Informed consent must be obtained before starting the interview.

At the beginning of a grounded theory study, the researcher asks general research questions. As theory begins to emerge, the researcher asks more specific questions to elicit information needed to saturate developing codes and categories. Based on the evolving theory, the grounded theorist asks different participants different questions. Excerpt 12.9 addresses the data-gathering techniques used in the study on decision making about mammography screening among African American women.

Theoretical Sampling

Theoretical sampling is the process of data collection for generating theory, whereby the researcher jointly collects, codes, and analyzes data and then decides what data to collect next in order to develop the grounded theory. This process of data collection is controlled by the emerging theory.[18] The grounded theorist uses theoretical sampling for emergence to fill in thin areas and extend the substantive theory. This is the process by which data collection is continually guided.

Theoretical sampling is done to discover categories and their properties. Unlike statistical sampling used in quantitative research, a predetermined sample size is not calculated. In theoretical sampling, sample size is determined by generated data and analyses. Theoretical sampling is continued until the categories are saturated. Saturation indicates repetition of data when nothing new is found. Information presented in Excerpt 12.10 discusses and illustrates the process of theoretical sampling.

EXCERPT 12.9

Data Collection Techniques Used in a Grounded Theory Study

Interview data were obtained using a researcher-designed, semistructured interview guide (IG) that was pilot tested on a similar group of women. The IG provided structure to potentially sensitive interview questions about mammography screening. Interview questions were read to each participant with ample time for response. Repeated questions included: "What are your thoughts and feelings when you hear the words mammography screening?" "What else comes to mind when you hear the words mammography screening?" "What sort of things do you consider when making decisions about mammography screening?" "Are others involved when making decisions about mammography screening?"

Source: Fowler, BA: Social processes used by African American women in making decisions about mammography screening. J Nurs Schol 38:247, 2006.

EXCERPT 12.10

Discussion of Theoretical Sampling

Consistent with grounded theory methodology, data collection continued until theoretically with a sample of an additional 14 women who were recruited through contacts with influential women in the AA community at professional or social organizations. The theoretical sample was chosen specifically to include women who were of interest in light of the analysis. Data collection and qualitative analysis occurred simultaneously from the beginning of the study.

Source: Fowler, BA: Social processes used by African American women in making decisions about mammography screening. J Nurs Schol 38:247, 2006.

Coding

From the first day of fieldwork, the grounded theorist is simultaneously collecting, coding, and analyzing data. **Coding** is a process to organize data into patterns called concepts. The **constant comparative method** of data analysis is a form of qualitative data analysis that makes sense of data by constantly comparing incidents until categories and concepts emerge.

The goal of grounded theory is to generate a theory around a core category. A **category** is a type of concept identified in a higher level of abstraction. A core category represents a pattern of behavior that is relevant and/or problematic for persons involved in a study. Discussion of coding in a grounded theory study is presented in Excerpt 12.11.

EXCERPT 12.11

Example of Data Analysis Section in a Grounded Theory Research Report

Analysis

Data were analyzed using constant comparative analysis beginning with the first audio-taped interview. Interviews were compared with written field notes by this researcher and were transcribed verbatim by an experienced transcriptionist. Pseudonyms were used to ensure confidentiality. Approximately 60 codes were identified, such as valuing the church ministry, relying on the Bible and other religious supports, and acknowledging prior negative experiences with health-care professionals and systems. Data were compared with each other to ensure that they were mutually exclusive and covered the behavioral variations. Caution was used in selecting the most descriptive and explicit codes that were reported by the majority of women. Codes were linked to subcategories by noting the interrelationships. For example, reading the Bible scriptures and seeking health-related information were linked to the category of relying on religious beliefs and supports.

Source: Fowler, BA: Social processes used by African American women in making decisions about mammography screening. J Nurs Schol 38:247, 2006.

Review of the Literature

In a grounded theory study, the review of literature does not occur at the start. The grounded theorist begins by collecting data in the field and generating a theory. When the theory appears to be sufficiently grounded and developed, the literature is reviewed and related to the developing theory.[17] By waiting to complete a literature review, the researcher avoids contaminating the data with preconceived concepts that may or may not be relevant. Grounded theory discovers concepts and hypotheses rather than tests or replicates hypotheses.

Memos

Memos are the write-up of ideas as they emerge while the grounded theorist is coding for categories, properties, and their relationships. Memos are written up as ideas occur to the grounded theorist while he or she is comparing, coding, and analyzing the data. The length of a memo can be a sentence, a paragraph, or even several pages. The researcher is not constrained by having to "write correctly" at all times. The purpose of memos is to record the researcher's ideas and get them on paper. Sorting memos in a theoretical outline is an essential step in grounded theory research.

Criteria for Judging Grounded Theory

Glaser[17] identified four criteria for judging grounded theory: fit, work, relevance, and modifiability. Fit refers to categories identified by the emerging theory corresponding to the data collected. Data should not be forced to fit preconceived categories or be discarded in favor of keeping an existing theory intact. Work involves indicating that the grounded theory explains what happens, predicts what will occur, and interprets an area of substantive or formal inquiry. An area of study must be relevant and comprehensible to individuals in the setting. The final criteria for judging grounded theory is modifiability. Theory is always being modified. A grounded theory can never be more correct than its ability to work the data. As new data reveal themselves in research, the theory is modified.

CRITIQUING PHENOMENOLOGICAL RESEARCH

Identify a phenomenological research study to critique. Read the study to see if you recognize any key terms discussed in this chapter. Remember that all studies may not contain all key terms. The following questions serve as a guide in critiquing phenomenological research:

1. *Is the research phenomenon of interest clearly stated?* A description of the phenomenon along with a statement why the phenomenon requires a qualitative approach should be provided within the opening paragraphs of the research report.

2. *Does the description help you understand the lived experience of study participants?* It is the lived experience that gives meaning to an individual's perception of a particular phenomenon. Look to see if the authors have captured a perception of the lived experience while emphasizing the richness, breadth, and depth of those experiences.

3. *Is the method used to collect data compatible with the purpose of the research?* Phenomenology is a type of qualitative research approach whose purpose is to describe particular phenomena as lived experience. There should be congruency between the methodology and purpose statement.

4. *Is purposive sampling used?* Purposive sampling is used most commonly in phenomenological research. Identify if the method of sampling selects individuals for participation based on their particular knowledge of a phenomenon.

5. *Have the researchers described the procedures for collecting data?* Look to see if the researchers conducted interviews. Data collection involves open-ended, clarifying questions to facilitate the process of participants describing the lived experience.

6. *Have strategies for analyzing the data been described?* Data analysis requires the researcher becoming immersed in the data. A variety of methods, each reflecting a different way to analyze data, are presented in Tables 12.2 through 12.7. Look to see if the researchers have identified one of these methods and followed the procedures for analyzing data.

7. *Do the themes maintain the integrity of the original data? Have the researchers used examples to support the interpretation?* In preserving the uniqueness of each person's description of the lived experience, verbatim responses from the interviews are used to identify themes and categories.

8. *What evidence is provided that the conduct of the research meets the criteria of rigor?* Participants acknowledge that the findings of the study are understood and viewed as credible and true. The researcher sends a copy of the transcribed interview to the participants, asking them if the description reflects their experiences. Content may then be added or deleted as appropriate.

CRITIQUING ETHNOGRAPHIC RESEARCH

Identify an ethnographic research study to critique. Read the study to see if you recognize any key terms discussed in this chapter. Remember that all studies may not contain all key terms. The following questions serve as a guide in critiquing ethnographic research:

1. *Has the researcher clearly identified the culture to be studied?* Ethnography as a qualitative approach provides an opportunity for

intimacy with members of a culture. Identify if the researcher has focused on a particular culture and described the culture in detail.

2. *Was the study conducted in the field? Was fieldwork performed?* A characteristic of ethnographic research is the participant's cultural immersion. This requires researchers "living" among the people being studied, making contacts, and establishing a role. Has the researcher provided evidence that cultural immersion occurred?

3. *Does the researcher clearly describe his or her role in the study?* Researchers must understand the role they play in the discovery of cultural knowledge. Because the researcher becomes the "instrument," he or she is required to participate in the culture, observe the participants, document observations, interview members of the cultural group, examine documents, possibly collect artifacts, and report the findings. Is there evidence that the researcher has participated in various activities to discover the cultural knowledge needed to organize and interpret a variety of experiences?

4. *Were multiple sources of data (i.e., participant observations, document analysis, life histories, analysis) used?* After identifying the type of culture being studied, identify if data sources were appropriate.

5. *Was time in the field adequate to meet the purpose of the study?* The length of time spent in the field varies among studies and depends on the research question, complexity of the culture, time required to build relationships, and access to data. Fieldwork requires complete commitment through constant observation and participation in various cultural activities. Look to see if the researcher has identified time spent in cultural immersion and if it makes sense.

CRITIQUING GROUNDED THEORY RESEARCH

Identify a grounded theory research study to critique. Read the study to see if you recognize any key terms discussed in this chapter. Remember that all studies may not contain all key terms. The following questions serve as a guide in critiquing grounded theory research:

1. *Does the question lend itself to be researched in a social setting?* Grounded theory research is an interactionist perspective and is appropriately used when the phenomena of interest can be examined through social interaction. The research question should lead to data collection from multiple sources as well as from a range of people in the social setting, focusing on how they perceive themselves and others.

2. *Were multiple data sources used to collect data?* When evaluating grounded theory research, it is important to pay particular attention to data collection techniques. Identify data collection strategies used in the study (i.e., observation, interview, document analysis, participant observation). Interview data should be backed up with

observational data whenever possible. Likewise, a wide range of subjects should be contacted to ensure that the researcher is seeing as much diversity as possible in responses.

3. *What is the nature and scope of the literature review?* One of the most important functions of the literature review is to allow the reader to "see" the phenomenon of interest as the researcher did at the beginning of the study. The literature review does not dictate the focus of the research. Thus, there is usually no conceptual or theoretical framework presented in a grounded theory research report. The purpose of grounded theory is to generate theory, not test it. However, the literature may suggest directions for early fieldwork and add depth to the theoretical scheme once it is developed.

4. *Does the theory make sense?* Evaluating the theory is the most important step. Does the integration of categories and constructs make sense? Do the concepts hang together logically? Is there sufficient evidence (data) to support the concepts? One of the most time-consuming aspects of conducting grounded theory research is coding and the ability to coin terms that are meaningful to others. Researchers are constantly coming up with drafts and asking colleagues to review their coding structures to be sure the terms and jargon used are understandable as the theoretical scheme is presented.

SUMMARY OF KEY IDEAS

1. Phenomenology is both a philosophy and a research method.

2. The purpose of phenomenological research is to describe the meaning of life through the interpretation of the "lived experience."

3. Understanding behavior or experiences requires that the individual interpret the experience for the researcher.

4. Data are collected through interviews, videotapes, or written descriptions by individuals.

5. Data are analyzed through interpretive analysis or hermeneutics.

6. Ethnographic research includes both anthropological and historical research strategies.

7. In ethnographic studies, the researcher becomes immersed in the subjects and their way of life in order to understand the cultural forces that shape behavior.

8. The aim of the ethnographer is to learn from (rather than to study) members of cultural groups to understand their worldview as they define it.

9. The planning and implementing of an ethnographic study takes place in three stages: pre-fieldwork, fieldwork, and post-fieldwork.

10. The goal of grounded theory is to generate a theory around a core variable that accounts for a pattern of behavior that is relevant and problematic for those persons involved.

11. Symbolic interaction is the theoretical underpinning of grounded theory.

12. In grounded theory the research problem is as much discovered as the process that resolves it.

13. Literature review is delayed until the theory is grounded in the data to avoid contaminating the researcher's efforts to generate concepts from the data with preconceived concepts that may not fit or be relevant.

14. In theoretical sampling the process of data collection is controlled by the emerging theory.

15. The grounded theorist simultaneously collects, codes, and analyzes data.

16. Theoretical sampling is continued until the categories are saturated.

17. Criteria for judging grounded theory include fit, work, relevance, and modifiability.

LEARNING ACTIVITIES

Bracketing Exercise

Bracketing helps the researcher become self-aware. This exercise demonstrates to student researchers why bracketing is a necessary first step in a phenomenological study.

1. Identify a lived experience for phenomenological study, such as What is it like to be wheelchair-bound? What is it like to be a pregnant teenager?

2. List anonymously your assumptions and beliefs about the experience and give them to your instructor.

3. The instructor collates the assumptions and beliefs into a master list and distributes it to the class.

4. The instructor leads the class discussion of how varying preconceptions would influence:
   a. The research question.
   b. The openness of the researcher to different experiences.
   c. What data to collect.
   d. How to collect data.
   e. How to interpret data.

Interview Role-Play Exercise

Role-playing in-depth interview techniques helps student researchers develop interviewing skills. Special attention is given to the potential of researcher bias in student questions and interactions with study participants and to listening to problems, such as inattention to detail.

1. Students pair off and interview each other on a common experience, such as What is it like to be a student? What was it like on your first day of clinical nursing?

2. Students record and transcribe their interviews.

3. After listening to the recording and reading the transcript, students identify:
   a. Content areas that could have been more fully explored.
   b. How the interviewer may actually lead the participant away from sharing valuable data.
   c. How to better elicit data.

4. Students share portions of the transcript and their analysis with the class.

5. The instructor leads the discussion and further critiques the students' interview technique.

Review of Literature Exercise

1. Identify a couple of articles from these research-oriented journals within the last 5 years that describes an ethnographic study: *Applied Nursing Research, Nursing Research, Research in Nursing and Health,* and *Western Journal of Nursing Research.*
   a. Did the article follow the definition of ethnographic research as defined by this chapter? Why or why not?
   b. Describe how the researcher was immersed in the subject's way of life.

2. Identify an area of study that would be amenable to the ethnographic approach. Discuss:
   a. The purpose of the study.
   b. The setting for data collection.
   c. The timeline associated with data collection.
   d. How the researcher might function to obtain data.

3. Identify a couple of research studies that use grounded theory methodology, and answer the following questions:
   a. How was the social situation being studied identified by the researcher?
   b. What were the data-gathering techniques used by the researcher?
   c. How long was data collection period?

d. How were subjects and sites determined?

e. How did the researcher attempt to develop a theory about the social situation that was based on observation/interviewing and literature review?

f. How were the researcher's opinions and thoughts about the topic addressed?

REFERENCES

1. Wagner, H: Phenomenology of Consciousness and Sociology of the Life World: An Introductory Study. University of Alberta Press, Edmonton, Canada, 1983.

2. Gaut, D: Philosophical analysis as research method. In Leininger, M (ed): Qualitative Research Methods in Nursing. Grune and Stratton, New York, 1985, pp 73–80.

3. Mariano, C: Qualitative research: Instructional strategies and curricular considerations. Nurs Health Care 11:354, 1990.

4. Munhall, P: Theoretical considerations in qualitative research. In Munhall, P, and Boyd, C (eds): Nursing Research: A Qualitative Perspective, ed. 2. National League for Nursing, New York, 1993, pp 424–453.

5. Guba, E, and Lincoln, Y: Effective Evaluation. Jossey-Bass, San Francisco, 1981.

6. Van Manen, M: Researching the Lived Experience. State University of New York Press, Buffalo, NY, 1990.

7. Emerson, RM: Contemporary Field Research: A Collection of Readings. Little, Brown, Boston, 1983.

8. Denzin, NK, and Lincoln, YS: Handbook of a Qualitative Research. Sage Publications, Thousand Oaks, CA, 1994.

9. Oftand, J: Analytic ethnography: Features, failings and futures. J Contemp Ethnography 24:30, 1995.

10. Honigmann, JJ: The Development of Anthropological Ideas. The Dorsey Press, Homewood, IL, 1976.

11. Mead, M: Blackberry Winter: My Earlier Years. Pocket Books, New York, 1972.

12. Leininger, M: Nursing and Anthropology: Two Worlds to Blend. John Wiley and Sons, New York, 1970.

13. Ragucci, AT: The ethnographic approach and nursing research. Nurs Res 21:485, 1972.

14. Aamodt, AM: The child view of health and healing. Communicating Nurs Res 5:38, 1972.

15. Glaser, B: Basics of Grounded Theory Analysis. Sociology Press, Mill Valley, CA, 1992.

16. Blumer, H: Symbolic Interactionism: Perspectives and Method. Prentice Hall, Englewood Cliffs, NJ, 1969.

17. Glaser, B: Theoretical Sensitivity. Sociology Press, Mill Valley, CA, 1978.

18. Glaser, B, and Strauss, A: The Discovery of Grounded Theory: Strategies for Qualitative Research. Aldine de Gruyter, New York, 1967, p 45.

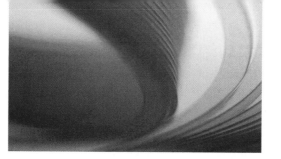

PART 3

Utilization of Nursing Research

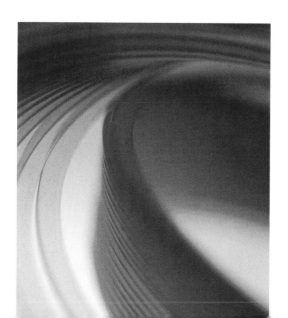

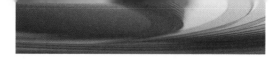

13

INTERPRETING AND REPORTING RESEARCH FINDINGS

JAMES A. FAIN, PHD, RN, BC-ADM, FAAN

LEARNING OBJECTIVES

By the end of this chapter, you will be able to:
1. Explain how to interpret results and discuss findings of a study.
2. Distinguish between statistical and clinical significance.
3. Describe a logical sequence for writing a research report.
4. Identify methods of disseminating research findings.

GLOSSARY OF KEY TERMS

Abstract. A brief summary of a research study; usually includes the purpose, methods, and findings of a study.

Clinical significance. Findings that have meaning for patient care in the absence or presence of statistical significance.

Generalizability. Extent to which research findings can be generalized beyond the given research situation to other settings and subjects; also called external validity.

Limitations. Aspects of a study that are potentially confounding to the main study variables.

Query letter. Letter written to an editor to determine the level of interest in publishing a research report.

Refereed journal. A journal that uses expert peers in specified fields to review and determine whether a particular manuscript will be published.

Research report. A document that summarizes the key aspects of a research study; usually includes the purpose, methods, and findings of a study.

Statistical significance. The extent to which the results of an analysis are unlikely to be the effect of chance.

Writing the interpretation of research findings is important and challenging for researchers. In this final stage of the research process, results are to be conveyed clearly, with accurate interpretations. Research findings are interpreted and discussed based on research question(s) and/or hypotheses cited in a study. In addition, results are discussed in relation to the broader significance, or lack thereof, for nursing practice. This chapter reviews important factors to be considered when evaluating conclusions and interpreting findings from a research study. In addition, it discusses aspects of preparing a research report and how to disseminate findings.

Interpreting Research Findings

Once research data have been collected and analyzed, the researcher proceeds to interpret the results. Interpreted results become findings for others to evaluate. Interpreting research findings involves organizing and explaining the meaning of data. Interpretation of findings is usually found toward the end of a research report, under the heading of results, conclusions, or discussion.

The results section of a research report contains only a report of results. In conducting a study, a researcher gains considerable amounts of information. Unless this information specifically relates to the research question(s) and/or hypotheses, such information is not included in the results. Interpreting the research results includes examining the meaning of results, considering the significance of the findings, generalizing the findings, drawing conclusions, and suggesting implications for practice and/or further study.[1,2]

Examining the Meaning of Results

In quantitative studies, outcomes of statistical tests are included to show or support the statement of results. Although the inclusion of calculated values, degrees of freedom, and the significance level is important, the narrative portion of the results section should emphasize the variables of interest rather than just statistics. The researcher should provide meaning when reporting the results. For example, in a study about whether there is a difference between upper arm and forearm blood pressure measurements (BPMs) among adults, it was reported that forearm mean BPM was higher for most (systolic n = 68, 64%; diastolic n = 74, 70%) but not for all. In Excerpt 13.1, authors discuss the type of statistical analysis (paired t-tests and correlations) performed. Readers are also referred to several tables in which descriptive statistics associated with the paired t-test (e.g., means and standard deviations) are displayed. Information provided in the text and tables is not redundant, but complementary.

Research findings are to be reported as objectively as possible. Quite often, the researcher extrapolates more meaning than is present. Some call this tendency "going beyond the data."[1] For example, a researcher conducts a study to investigate the efficacy of a hydrocolloid dressing in healing a stage 2 pressure sore (dermis is exposed). Results indicate that

EXCERPT 13.1

Describing Meaningful Results of a Study in the Text of an Article

Results

The upper arm systolic and diastolic mean BPMs were lower than the forearm mean BPMs for the sample. . . . Results of the paired t-test showed that the differences between the means were statistically significant at the 0.05 level ($t = 3.22$, $df = 105$, $p = 0.002$, systolic; $t = 2.78$, $df = 105$, $p = 0.006$, diastolic). Pearson r correlation coefficients for the mean BPM differences at the upper arm and forearm sites were statistically significant with correlations of 0.72 for systolic and 0.76 for diastolic. For individual participants, the forearm mean BPM was higher for most (systolic n = 68, 64%; diastolic n = 74, 70%) but not for all. For others (systolic n = 38, 36%; diastolic n = 32, 30%), the upper arms provided the higher BPM.

Source: Domiano, KL, Hinck, SM, Savinske, DL, and Hope, KL: Comparison of upper arm and forearm blood pressure. Clin Nurs Res 17:241, 2008.

the use of hydrocolloid dressings healed a stage 2 pressure sore by 50 percent in 2 days versus 5 days for 4 × 4 gauze dressings ($p < 0.0001$). The researcher interprets the result to mean that hydrocolloid dressings can be used to heal all stages of pressure sores by 50 percent within 2 days. Is this interpretation correct? The finding that hydrocolloid dressings healed stage 2 pressure sores by 50 percent within 2 days is correct. However, the data indicate that only stage 2 pressure sores were studied. Additionally, because the researcher did not include other stages of pressure sores, taking only 2 days to heal 50 percent of the pressure sores is probably unrealistic. This is an example of the researcher going beyond the data. Situations like this are not always this obvious. Researchers should take a more conservative approach when interpreting and discussing research findings.

Considering the Significance of Findings

Another important factor to consider when interpreting research findings is clinical significance. Research findings that have meaning for patient care in the absence or presence of statistical significance are called clinically significant. Achieving statistical significance, however, does not automatically mean that the study has value for the discipline of nursing. **Statistical significance** indicates that the findings from an analysis are unlikely to be the result of chance. Interpretation of findings must make logical sense. For example, results of a study indicate a significant difference between the ages of men and women (M = 57.5 and F = 51.5, respectively). Can you reasonably conclude that this represents clinical significance? Statistical significance can be achieved if there is an adequate sample size. However, is it a clinically significant difference? The word "significant" should be used when reporting statistical results and clarified when describing clinical results. Likewise, a study that is clinically significant does not need to be statistically significant. **Clinical significance** refers to findings that have meaning for patient care in the absence or presence of statistical significance. The reader of research must not only base evaluation of a study on its rigor, but also on its clinical significance.

Generalizing the Findings

An essential feature of results of a study is **generalizability**, the extent to which research findings can be generalized beyond the given research situation to other settings and subjects. This is also termed "external validity." When interpreting the findings of a study, the researcher examines risks to validity that may have been introduced at various stages of the research process, one of which involves selecting the sample. The intent of random sampling is to produce a representative sample. The focus is on the extent to which the sample represents the target population (see Chapter 7), so the results can be applied to the entire target population. If the sample is not representative, researchers can describe only what was found in the sample.

In conducting a study, the researcher needs to consider whether the sample size is too small to allow generalization of findings. For example, 10 subjects were recruited into a study to test the efficacy of a nursing intervention to promote somnolence within 30 minutes. Results indicated that 2 subjects became somnolent after 10 minutes, 3 subjects after 25 minutes, and the remaining 5 subjects after 40 minutes. The researcher could interpret the data by averaging the mean time until somnolence for all 10 subjects to support the effectiveness of the protocol. However, if the sample size had been 100 and the results indicated two subjects became somnolent after 10 minutes, 3 subjects after 25 minutes, with the remaining 95 subjects becoming somnolent after 40 minutes, the protocol would not be considered effective.

Drawing Conclusions

Conclusions are derived from research findings. In order to draw conclusions, the researcher must interpret the results within the context of the study (e.g., organizing framework, literature review, research design). Phrases such as "results of the study indicate" and "study findings demonstrate" link the summary of results and the meaning of those results. In forming conclusions, it is important to remember that research never proves anything, but instead offers support for a position.[1]

Limitations

Limitations are aspects of a study that are potentially confounding to the main study variables. For example, a limitation is created if the time of day a treatment is administered can influence the level of subjects' responses. Additional study limitations include sample deficiencies, design problems, weakness in data collection procedures, and use of unreliable measures. Limitations are generally reported in the discussion section of an article so that the interpretation of results is made with knowledge of the potential impact on the limiting factors.

Research Report

Preparing a research report is an essential component of the research process. A **research report** summarizes key aspects of a study and includes the following elements: title, abstract, introduction (purpose of study and review of literature), methods (sample, setting, data collection), results, discussion, and conclusions. Most research reports consist of 15 to 20 pages. However, theses (required for some master's degree programs) or dissertations (required for most doctoral degrees) are significantly longer (50 to 200 pages). The difference in length is due to the amount of detail given to specific sections of the research report.

Title

The title of a study captures its essence. It is written to attract readers and inform them of the purpose of the study. Most titles tend to be no longer than 15 words and identify key words from the study. Key words are often used by indexing services to categorize the study's contents. A title such as "Diabetes Mellitus" is somewhat vague. A reader is likely to say, "what about diabetes?" Expanded, this title could be "Diabetes Mellitus and School-Aged Children." This is better, but does not suggest a possible research focus. With a few more words, the following title captures the essence of the study: "Coping Strategies of School-Aged Children with Diabetes Mellitus." The title is usually followed by the author name(s), credentials, and academic and/or clinical affiliations.

Abstract

The **abstract** is a brief, succinct summary of a research study. Although abstracts usually consist of only 100 to 300 words, readers are able to decide whether the study meets their needs or interests. A well-written comprehensive abstract provides the reader with an overview of the remaining sections of the report. Excerpt 13.2 gives an example of an abstract in which the authors highlight the purposes of the study and a brief summary of important findings.

Introduction

The introduction section of a research report includes the purpose of the study and literature review. After reading the first one or two paragraphs

EXCERPT 13.2

Example of an Abstract

The purpose of this study was to evaluate the effect of a nurse-directed smoking cessation intervention for adults hospitalized in a small community hospital using a quasi-experimental, prospective, longitudinal design with biochemical validation of self-reported tobacco abstinence. Sixty-eight inpatients were assigned to either a control (n = 30) or an intervention group (n = 38). The control group received smoking cessation literature. The intervention group received smoking cessation literature and a nursing intervention. Each member of the intervention group was randomly assigned to a one- or four-telephone-call subgroup for postdischarge nurse follow-up at 3 months. Fifty-five participants completed the study. Smokers receiving the nurse-directed intervention were significantly more likely to be tobacco abstinent at 3 months (n = 17, 55%) than smokers in the control group (n = 5, 21%). Within the intervention group, tobacco abstinence at 3 months was not significantly different between the one- and four-telephone-call groups. For the total sample, smoking relapse was significantly higher for participants who lived with another smoker.

Source: Gies, CE, Robinson, J, and Smolen, D: Effects of an inpatient nurse-directed smoking cessation program. West J Nurs Res 30:6, 2007.

of the introduction, the reader should have an understanding of the problem being studied and why the problem is important. Information on the incidence and/or prevalence associated with the problem is usually presented here. The purpose of the study is usually included at the beginning or at the end of the introduction section. Some researchers believe that by placing the purpose at the beginning of the introduction section, it quickly draws the attention of the reader. Other researchers end the introduction with a statement of purpose, identifying variables to be investigated. Regardless of where the researcher places the purpose statement, the statement must be clear and understandable. As seen in many journal articles, the statement of purpose is not always identified under a separate heading, nor is it always found under the general heading "Introduction." In Excerpt 13.3 the purpose statement is the last sentence in the introduction.

Literature Review

The literature review identifies what is currently known about the subject under study and reflects relevant background information necessary to support justification for the study. An updated literature review is extremely important to validate the need for a study. Limitations in regarding the problem may be identified in this section. The literature review section usually gives the reader background information on a theoretical/conceptual framework, which helps guide the study. An example of a literature review within the context of a theoretical framework (e.g., health belief model) is displayed in Excerpt 13.4.

EXCERPT 13.3

Placement of Statement of Purpose in Opening Paragraph of Research Report

Hispanics are the fastest growing minority population in the United States (U.S.). In 2000, there were approximately 35 million Hispanics in the U.S., representing 12.5% of the U.S. population. By the year 2025, Hispanics will constitute 21% of the U.S. population.

Diabetes self-management has become associated with glycemic control as a result of findings associated with the Diabetes Control and Complications Trial (DCCT) and the United Kingdom Prospective Diabetes Study (UKPDS). Diabetes self-management refers to a range of activities in which individuals must engage on a regular basis to manage their diabetes. Hispanics differ in their diabetes self-management practices because culture shapes how diabetes is perceived based on beliefs, values, and habits. Understanding cultural beliefs, attitudes, and perceptions is vital to providing diabetes education and identifying barriers among Hispanics that affect self-management.

Clearly, there is a need for measures of diabetes self-management that are comprehensive along with being culturally sensitive, reliable, and valid. Psychometric assessments of existing instruments that measure diabetes self-management are limited and frequently not available for minority populations or individuals that speak a language other than English. There is a need for more measures of diabetes self-management that have been designed or used in minority populations. The purpose of this study is to evaluate the psychometric properties of a Spanish-language version of the Diabetes Self-management Report Tool (D-SMART) for Hispanics with type 2 diabetes.

Source: Fain, JA: Psychometric properties of the Spanish version of the diabetes self-management assessment report tool. Diabetes Educ 33:827, 2007.

Methods

The methods section of the research report is written to inform the reader about the research design, sample, setting, data collection procedures and instruments, and outcome measures. The researcher may also include information on the reliability and validity of instruments. The researcher should outline procedures used in data collection and address any modifications to the original plan. The methods section ends with a discussion of how data will be analyzed, including specific statistical techniques. Depending on the intended audience for the research report, the methods section may vary in length. Research-based nursing journals (e.g., *Applied Nursing Research, Journal of Nursing Scholarship, Nursing Research, Research in Nursing and Health, Western Journal of Nursing Research*) tend to have much lengthier methodology sections than do clinical journals (e.g., *Journal of Gerontological Nursing; Journal of Wound, Ostomy and Continence Nursing; Public Health Nursing; The Diabetes Educator*).

EXCERPT 13.4

Example of Theoretical Framework and Related Literature Section of a Research Report

Theoretical Framework

This study was guided by the health belief model (HBM). There are five core concepts: perceived threat, perceived benefits, perceived barriers, cues to action, and self-efficacy (Rosenstock, Strecher, and Becker, 2004; Strecher and Rosenstock, 1999). The HBM has been previously used to explain and predict health behaviors and health issues by focusing on the knowledge, attitudes, and beliefs of individuals. As suggested by theories based on the HBM, the likelihood that individuals will take action to prevent illness depends on the perception that they are personally vulnerable to the condition, the consequences of the condition would be serious, the precautionary behavior effectively prevents the condition, and the benefits of reducing the threat of the condition exceed the costs of taking action. Clinicians need to appreciate and understand their patients' health beliefs, especially in women age 40 and older who have not been the targets of marketing information about HPV, cervical cancer, and the new vaccine.

Source: Montgomery, K, Bloch, JR, Bhattacharya, A, and Montgomery, O: Human papillomavirus and cervical cancer knowledge, health beliefs, and preventative practices in older women. J Obstet Gynecol Neonat Nurs 39:238, 2010.

Excerpt 13.5 displays the methods section of a descriptive cross-sectional research report describing knowledge of human papillomavirus (HPV) and cervical cancer, health beliefs, and preventative practices in women 40 to 70 years of age. Enough information was provided to enable others to replicate the study. The researchers described the type of study design, setting, sample of subjects participating in the study, data collection procedures, type of data collected, and analysis of data.

Results

The results section of a research report focuses on pertinent findings and answers the research question(s) or tests hypotheses. Data are presented objectively, with little discussion. Tables, graphs, and/or figures are usually presented. The advantage of using tables and graphs is the ability to simplify large amounts of research findings succinctly and logically. Information provided in tables or graphs should not duplicate what is in the text. For example, if the researcher reports means in a table, there is no need to repeat them in the text. Instead, tables, graphs, and figures are used to enhance the text.

Excerpt 13.6 provides an illustration of a results section of a research report. To provide a more complete understanding of the results, the

Example of Methods Section of a Research Report

Methods

Design

This study was a cross-sectional descriptive design. Anonymous data were collected over a 2-month period in 2008 using a self-administered pen and pencil questionnaire.

Setting and Sample

A convenience sample of women age 40 to 70 years was recruited from the waiting room of three ambulatory obstetrics and gynecology offices of a large metropolitan university hospital in the mid-Atlantic section of the United States. All three offices were used in an attempt to get a racially heterogeneous sample in this urban area, which has a rate of cervical cancer 1.7 times higher than the national rate. The inclusion criteria were women age 40 to 70, presenting to their health-care provider for an annual check-up, and who did not have a past or present history of HPV or cervical cancer.

The sample size required for this study was guided by a power analysis using the software program G Power (Version 3.0.10). The power analysis was based on the correlation analysis between the subscales knowledge, susceptibility, and seriousness. Small to medium effect size (Pearson's $r = 0.23$) was postulated in keeping with Cohen's (1992) recommendation for Pearson correlation. Power was set to 0.80, meaning there would be an 80% probability of reaching statistical significance if the subscales correlated in the study. Significance levels were set at 0.05 (two-tail), with an effect size of 0.23 to achieve a power of 0.80. A total of 145 participants were required.

Procedure

Following approval by the university Institutional Review Board (IRB), the study began by training a research assistant (RA) at each of three offices. The training entailed using data on the practice management program to identify potential eligible participants when women are checked in for their visits, inviting potential participants, and keeping all data anonymous by sealing all envelopes and placing them in a research bin in a secured drawer or cabinet based on the specific office. At each of the three sites, there were flyers posted on the walls, and a trained RA invited participants if they met eligibility. If the patient met the two requirements of age and reason for the visit (well-woman check-up), she was given a sheet to read to further determine eligibility (exclusion criteria include a history of HPV or cervical cancer). After she read the sheet, the RA asked if she was eligible. If she said yes, she was given the survey packet with a cover letter. Completion of the survey acted as informed consent for participation. Once the survey was completed, it was placed in a sealed envelope to be returned to the researcher such that no identity was disclosed.

Outcome Measures

Sociodemographic variables collected included age, race, education, health insurance status, religious affiliation, marital status, and income level.

(Continued)

EXCERPT 13.5

Example of Methods Section of a Research Report—cont'd

HPV and Cervical Cancer Knowledge, Health Beliefs, and Preventative Practices

With permission from the authors, the Awareness of HPV and Cervical Cancer Questionnaire was used to measure knowledge and beliefs, as well as preventative measures in regards to HPV and cervical cancer. Ingledue et al developed this self-administered 36-item questionnaire based on the HBM to investigate HPV/cervical cancer knowledge, health beliefs and perceptions, and preventative measures in college-age women. The tool was used in this study because it was specifically designed for HPV and cervical cancer awareness and was congruent with the HBM that guided the study. Although the questionnaire was originally used on college-age women, a panel of experts (obstetricians/gynecologists, physicians, and nurse practitioners) reviewed the questions, concluding they were generalizable to women of all age groups as demonstrated by subsequent studies that used the questionnaire on women from other age groups. Using the same tool allowed comparison of results from this study to other published studies.

Data Analysis

To further understand knowledge, health beliefs (perceived susceptibility and perceived seriousness), and preventative practices in women age 40 to 70, these women were divided into age groups by decade: 40 to 50, 51 to 60, 61 to 70 years. Following testing for assumptions, a one-way analysis of variance (ANOVA) was conducted to compare knowledge and health beliefs among the three subgroups. If the ANOVAs were significant, post hoc analyses were conducted using a Bonferroni adjustment. Preventative practices were compared among the three subgroups using the chi-square analysis. A Fisher's exact test was used when assumptions of chi-square were not met. Levels of significance for all tests were set at an alpha of 0.05.

Source: Montgomery, K, Bloch, JR, Bhattacharya, A, and Montgomery, O: Human papillomavirus and cervical cancer knowledge, health beliefs, and preventative practices in older women. J Obstet Gyn Neo Nurs 39:238, 2010.

---

researchers presented the results in the text and summarized the results in a table. Three research questions were asked:

1. Do hospitalized adult smokers who receive a nurse-directed, smoking cessation intervention reduce or eliminate tobacco use 3 months after hospital discharge?
2. Are adult smokers who receive the nurse intervention and four structured telephone calls after discharge from the hospital during a 3-month period more likely to be tobacco abstinent than those adult smokers who received the nurse intervention and one structured telephone call after discharge from the hospital during a 3-month period?
3. Are there differences between the tobacco-abstinent group and the group who resumed smoking 3 months after hospital discharge?

Example of Results Section of a Research Report

Results

The total sample included 31 (46.5%) males and 37 (54.4%) females who were predominantly white (97.1%) and middle-aged. Thirty-six (52.9%) were married or living with a partner, had at least a high school education, and were employed. Most participants were admitted to the hospital with heart and/or respiratory problems. The sample, on average, had a 34 pack year history (packs per day times smoking years), had tried to quit smoking more than three times, and had a baseline carbon monoxide level of a non-smoker during hospitalization (six parts per million or less). The majority did not live with other smokers, had some confidence in their ability to quit smoking, had tried nicotine patches, and had failed at previous attempts to remain tobacco abstinent because of stress or life changes.

Within the intervention group, differences between the one and four follow-up telephone call subgroups were examined for age, pack years, initial carbon monoxide level, Smoking Abstinence Self-Efficacy Scale (SASE) scores, and Fagerstrom score. The subgroups were significantly different only in mean scores on the positive affect social subscale of the SASE, $t(34)$ = -3.07, $p= 0.00$. The four-telephone-call group (M = 11.72, SD = 2.58) was significantly more tempted to smoke in social situations than the one-telephone-call group (M = 8.88, SD = 2.94).

The first research question asked if a nurse-directed tobacco cessation intervention for hospitalized adult smokers is effective in reducing or eliminating tobacco use. In the total sample, 22 participants (40%) were tobacco abstinent, and 33 (60%) continued to smoke. In the control group, only 5 (21%) participants reported tobacco abstinence at 3 months. Tobacco abstinence was confirmed by CO analysis for 4 of the 5 self-reports (80%). In the nurse intervention group, 17 (55%) reported abstinence at 3 months. Tobacco abstinence was confirmed by CO analysis for 15 of the 17 self-reports (88%).

The second research question asked if hospitalized adult tobacco users who received the nurse-directed intervention and four structured follow-up telephone calls after hospital discharge were more likely to be tobacco abstinent than adult tobacco users who received the nurse-directed intervention and only one follow-up telephone call 3 months after hospital discharge.

At 3 months after discharge, tobacco abstinence was reported by 11 of the 18 participants (61%) in the one-telephone-call subgroup and 6 of the 13 (46%) in the four-telephone-call subgroup.

The difference in reported tobacco abstinence between the two intervention subgroups was not statistically significant, χ^2 (1, N = 31) = 0.68, p = 0.41, which suggests that the number of follow-up telephone calls did not influence tobacco abstinence. A sample size of 31 achieved 13% power to detect the effect size in this study of 0.15 using one degree of freedom chi-square tests with an alpha of 0.05.

(Continued)

EXCERPT 13.6

Example of Results Section of a Research Report—cont'd

To answer the third research question, chi-square and independent *t*-tests were conducted to evaluate differences between the group of study participants who reported tobacco abstinence 3 months after hospital discharge and the group of study participants who were not tobacco abstinent 3 months after hospital discharge, regardless of intervention. There were no statistically significant differences between the tobacco abstinent and the non-tobacco abstinent groups on gender, age, marital status, employment, education, or initial carbon monoxide levels. The study participants who did not maintain tobacco abstinence were more likely to live with other smokers in the home, χ^2 (1, N = 55) = 3.99, p =0 .05.

Source: Gies, CE, Robinson, J, and Smolen, D: Effects of an inpatient nurse-directed smoking cessation program. West J Nurs Res 30:6, 2007.

Discussion

The discussion section focuses on a nontechnical interpretation of the results. Researchers use the discussion section to explain what the results mean in relation to the purpose of the study. In addition to telling the reader what the results mean, many authors use this section to explain why they think the results turned out as they did. Although such a discussion is occasionally found in articles where the data support the researcher's hunches, authors are much more inclined to point out possible reasons for the obtained results when those results are inconsistent with their expectations.[3] Limitations of a study are also addressed. "Conclusion" is sometimes used interchangeably with "Discussion." Excerpt 13.7 displays a discussion section of a research report that includes limitations of the study. Excerpt 13.8 illustrates a research report that includes both a discussion and conclusion sections.

References

The reference list is very important to the research report. This section provides the reader with additional literature related to the particular topic. Information in the reference list also provides the reader with a clearer understanding as to why and how the researcher conducted the particular study. When possible, primary data sources should be used instead of secondary data sources (see Chapter 4). References for the study should be current. However, sometimes older references, or "classics," may be used if they form the foundation for the problem under study.

Disseminating Research Findings

Communicating research findings is the final stage in the research process. By presenting and publishing research findings, researchers

EXCERPT 13.7

Example of a Discussion Section of a Research Report

Discussion

The results of this study conducted in a small community hospital were consistent with published research that found nurse-directed tobacco cessation interventions to be more effective than usual care in reducing or eliminating tobacco use in adult patients after discharge from larger inpatient settings. Two meta-analyses reported similar findings. Carbon monoxide analysis confirmed self-reported tobacco abstinence for 19 of 22 participants (86%) in this study and was noninvasive and cost effective.

Telephone follow-up results in this study differed from the Miller et al study in that the four-telephone-call group was not significantly more successful with tobacco abstinence than the one-telephone-call group. These results should be interpreted with caution given the limited statistical power (13%) in this analysis. To achieve 80% power with the observed effect size, 358 participants would have been required for the intervention group. In spite of randomly assigning participants to the intervention subgroup, the four-telephone-call subgroup had significantly higher temptation to smoke than the one-telephone-call subgroup.

The major limitations identified for this study in addition to small sample size included the use of convenience sampling in a single setting and the lack of ethnic diversity. Participants were not randomly assigned to the intervention and control group. Hospital policy requiring a physician order for the nurse-directed intervention may have biased the results even though the groups appeared similar on major demographic and tobacco use variables. Collecting data during a 3-month period postdischarge presented challenges. Participant attrition may have affected the results of this study, even though attrition was essentially equal in the intervention and control groups.

Source: Gies, CE, Robinson, J, and Smolen, D: Effects of an inpatient nurse-directed smoking cessation program. West J Nurs Res 30:6, 2007.

EXCERPT 13.8

Example of a Research Report That Includes a Discussion and Conclusion Section

Discussion

Findings confirm prior research that has indicated that upper arm BPMs tend to be lower than forearm BPMs and extend present knowledge by identifying for whom upper arm and forearm BP readings have the greatest difference. The largest difference in upper and forearm BPMs was for men and for adults who were middle-aged or obese. Most other investigators have found individual variability in participants but have not reported the personal characteristics associated with the higher readings. Only Palantini and associates (2004) assessed the difference between upper arm and forearm mean BPMs in men and women and found a greater difference for men in the diastolic mean BPM.

(Continued)

EXCERPT 13.8

Example of a Research Report That Includes a Discussion and Conclusion Section—cont'd

There is no consensus in the literature about what numerical value of difference between upper arm and forearm BPMs should be considered clinically significant. Tachovsky (1985) suggested that clinical significance varied among individuals and that differences of 10 to 40 mm Hg may be clinically acceptable when they are caused by anxiety states, exercise, or other environmental factors. Singer et al (1999) recommended that most BPM differences of less than 20 mm Hg indicate that forearm BPMs can be substituted for upper arm measures.

Conclusion

For most individuals, BPMs taken at the upper arm are lower than those taken at the forearm. The difference between the two sites is largest for men, obese adults, and middle-aged adults. These findings alert clinicians to which populations may have the greatest differences between upper arm and forearm BPMs and aid in interpreting clinical data and making decisions about the diagnosis and treatment of hypertension.

Source: Domiano, KL, Hinck, SM, Savinske, DL, and Hope, KL: Comparison of upper arm and forearm blood pressure. Clin Nurs Res 17:241, 2008.

advance the body of knowledge unique to the discipline of nursing. Communicating research findings also promotes the critique and replication of studies, identification of additional research problems, and use of findings in practice. Nursing research is of little value if the results are never presented to other nurses.

Publication

One method of communicating research findings is through publication. Publishing a research report has the advantage of reaching a larger audience, based on the circulation of a particular journal. The disadvantage of publishing a research report is the delay in receiving feedback and potential delay in the actual publication of the report. It is not uncommon to have a research report published 6 months to 1 year after it is originally submitted.

There are currently more than 100 nursing journals in the United States. However, nurse researchers are not limited to publishing nursing research strictly in nursing journals. Nursing research can be found in several medical, health, and lay journals. The decision whether to publish in a research or clinically based journal is left to the researcher. There are, however, similarities in writing the research report for publication.

The preparation of a research report or manuscript for publication differs little among journals. However, depending on the focus of the journal, a researcher may expand a specific section of the research report. For example, a researcher might spend more time (pages) in discussing findings in relation to nursing practice in clinical journals. On the other hand, if journals are research based, the researcher might spend more time (pages) developing the methodology section of the manuscript.

Query Letter

A **query letter** is written to an editor to determine the level of interest the editor has regarding publishing a research report. Although all journals do not require query letters, these letters can save the researcher a lot of time. A query letter should include the title and purpose of the study, name(s) and credentials of investigator(s), and a contact person to whom the editor may respond. In addition, the study should be described or an abstract submitted. If an editor is interested in the manuscript, he or she will ask the researcher to submit the entire manuscript. A response usually occurs within several weeks.

Manuscript Guidelines

Journals provide information for authors, giving instructions on manuscript preparation. In some journals, the information is in every issue; other journals may publish the information only twice a year. Information for authors provides the following: the journal's mission statement, type of articles the journal accepts, readership, and manuscript format (e.g., type of referencing, page limitation, specific instructions on preparing tables and figures, copyright). It is imperative that the researcher follow these directions.

Review Process

Once the researcher submits the manuscript, the review process begins. A peer reviewed, or **refereed journal**, is one that has expert peers in specified fields who review and determine whether a particular manuscript will be published. Most peer-reviewed journals assign two to four reviewers to critique the manuscript. In most instances, the author is blinded to the reviewers of the manuscript. The review process may last from a month to a year. Along with the reviewers, the editorial staff may also critique the manuscript based on its originality, timeliness of the problem, objectivity, honesty, completeness, readability, and rigor of the study.

Oral Presentations

Presentations are another method of communicating a research report. Presentations can be done formally at local, regional, or national levels, as well as informally among peers. Oral presentations have several advantages over publishing. One is the ability to disseminate findings much more quickly. Another advantage is the ability to get feedback from participants either during or after the presentation. This direct feedback can be an invaluable experience and help the researcher rethink the research findings. The disadvantage of using presentation format to communicate research results is that a limited number of people will get the information. Many nursing journals or organizations will send out a "call for papers" to present at a conference. Often they identify a theme or specialty focus for the conference and request abstracts related to the topic.

The format for presenting a research report is very similar to that for presenting a published report. Most presentations are done in a specified amount of time. Conferences allow from 20 minutes to an hour for the researcher to present the report. Thus, the challenge for the researcher is to limit the report to only the essential points of the study. Extraneous explanations of insignificant findings are often avoided. Nurse researchers often use slides, overheads, or handouts to further communicate their findings at presentations.

Poster Presentation

Poster presentations are another method for communicating a research report. Most conferences have poster sessions concurrently with oral presentations. Poster presentations have become increasingly popular in the past 10 years. The advantage of this method derives from the ability of the researcher to engage in an active dialogue with other researchers. The disadvantage is that only a limited number of people will read the poster and only a limited amount of information can be presented.

The goal of the poster presentation is to present the research report visually. Thus, the poster must be presented in a manner that is succinct and easily understood. Often, several people might be reading the poster at the same time. The research report format is also followed for the poster presentation; however, only significant information is provided on the poster. Graphs and photographs are often used to enhance the results. Most researchers supplement the poster presentation with written handouts.

The organization sponsoring the conference gives the nurse researcher guidelines in regard to the size of the poster display. Most often, conferences require that a poster be 4 feet × 6 feet for a mounting board and 3 feet × 6 feet for an easel. There are no standard methods for arranging a poster. Figure 13.1 illustrates a suggested layout for a poster presentation.

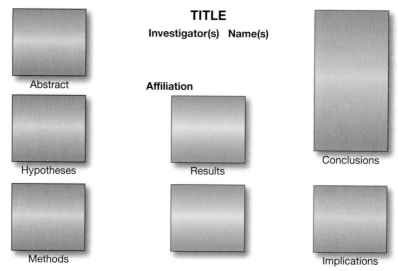

TITLE
Investigator(s)   Name(s)

Abstract

Affiliation

Hypotheses

Results

Conclusions

Methods

Implications

Fig 13•1 Suggested Layout for Poster Presentations.

CRITIQUING THE INTERPRETATION OF RESEARCH FINDINGS

Identify a research study to critique. Read the study to see if you recognize any key terms discussed in this chapter. Remember that all studies may not contain all key terms. The following questions serve as a guide in critiquing interpretation of research results:

1. *Have the results of the study been interpreted appropriately?* Begin by reviewing the methods and results section to judge the validity of the study and to have the necessary information to answer the research questions or test the hypotheses. Look to see if there is a clear statement of the author's major conclusions based on his or her interpretation of the results.

2. *Has the author identified limitations to the study?* Limitations of the study should be identified and explained. Some of these factors may have been identified before the study began, and others will become evident during the course of data collection. Consider the importance of limitations with respect to the interpretation of study results.

3. *Were the results clinically significant?* Findings may or may not have statistical significance; however, they may still have significance for nursing practice. For example, use of a certain sedative in combination with an analgesic consistently reduces the perception of pain in a variety of postoperative conditions. Although differences between groups may not be statistically significant, the trend

consistently favors the use of the sedative in combination with the analgesic; therefore, the results do have clinical significance.[4]

4. *Did the author discuss how the results of the study apply to practice, education, theory, and research?* Were suggestions for further study presented? Read over the discussion section. The importance of the study should be highlighted in terms of the potential contributions to practice, education, theory, and research, as appropriate. This is particularly true if the results are to be used to inform practice or identify new and challenging research questions.

SUMMARY OF KEY IDEAS

1. Research findings are discussed in relation to the purpose, research question(s), and hypotheses of the study.

2. The discussion section of a research report explains the results of a study.

3. Discussion of research findings should not go beyond the data presented.

4. Discussion of research findings should identify any threats to internal or external validity and reliability that might explain the findings.

5. Studies should be clinically significant even though statistical significance has not been achieved.

6. A research report summarizes a research study.

7. Publication, oral presentation, and poster presentation are effective methods of communicating research reports.

LEARNING ACTIVITY

1. Select a nursing research study and identify whether all hypotheses and/or research question(s) have been addressed in the results and discussion sections.

2. In the same nursing research study, identify the strengths and limitations of the authors' results and discussion sections. Do the research findings relate to nursing practice, education, and/or policy?

3. Lyder et al[5] completed a study to evaluate the effect of condom catheters in controlling incontinence odor. The entire nursing staff in a Veterans Administration unit (n = 16) independently rated environmental odor in four rooms before and 1 week after condom catheter removal. Odor was rated on a 4-point scale, from no smell (1) to extreme smell (4). The results indicated that there were statistically significant differences for the factors of room ($p = 0.03$) and time ($p = 0.001$). Mean odor ratings were 2.10 (little smell) before and 3.07 (extreme smell) after condom catheter removal.

The interpretation and discussion section concluded that although the nurse raters were aware of the intervention, removal of condom catheters from urofecal incontinent men resulted in increased unpleasant odor. Additionally, the increased smell was offensive to residents, families, and nursing staff. The study also suggested that the use of condom catheters for separation of incontinent urinary and fecal streams may have protective effects on the skin. Based on the purpose of the study, does the interpretation and discussion section correspond with the purpose of the study? Do the authors go beyond the data? Explain your answer. Based on the interpretation and discussion presented, rewrite this section.

4. Select a conference and attend both an oral and a poster presentation. Identify the components of the research process and delineate the advantages and disadvantages of both presentations. Were the presentations clinically significant?

5. Select a nursing research study from a research-based nursing journal and construct a poster.

REFERENCES

1. Burns, N, and Grove, SK: The Practice of Nursing Research: Conduct, Critique, and Utilization, ed. 4. WB Saunders, Philadelphia, 2001, pp 623–633.
2. Polit, DF, and Beck, CT: Essentials of Nursing Research: Methods, Appraisal, and Utilization, ed. 6. Lippincott Williams & Wilkins, Philadelphia, 2006, p 60.
3. Huck, SW, and Cormier, WH: Reading Statistics and Research, ed. 2.

HarperCollins, New York, 2000, pp 13–14.
4. Gillis, A, and Jackson, W: Research for Nurses: Methods and Interpretation. FA Davis, Philadelphia, 2002, p 590.
5. Lyder, C, McCray, G, and Kutty-Singh, M: Efficacy of condom catheters in controlling incontinence odor. Appl Nurs Res 5:188, 1992.

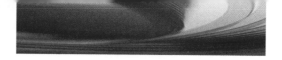

14

CRITIQUING RESEARCH REPORTS

James A. Fain, PhD, RN, BC-ADM, FAAN

LEARNING OBJECTIVES

By the end of this chapter, you will be able to:

1. Distinguish between a research critique and research review.

2. Apply principles that make a critique constructive rather than destructive.

3. Apply a set of guidelines in the critique of research reports.

GLOSSARY OF KEY TERMS

Research critique. Critical evaluation of a piece of reported research.

Research review. Identification and summary of major findings and characteristics of a study.

Nurses are expected to participate in research activities by evaluating and interpreting research reports for applicability to nursing practice. Nurses must decide the appropriateness and adequacy of research findings for use in practice. Publication of research reports in no way guarantees quality, value, or relative worth. Deciding the overall usefulness of a research report requires systematic review and critical appraisal. Failing to critique a research report adequately may adversely affect the outcomes of entire populations of patients. This chapter focuses on conducting a comprehensive evaluation of a research report. Specific attention is directed to providing general critique guidelines. Included are evaluation components for both quantitative and qualitative research.

Research Critiques Vs. Research Reviews

A **research critique** is a critical appraisal of the strengths and weaknesses of a research report.[1,2] Critiquing a research report involves evaluating aspects of the research process. All research studies have strengths and weaknesses; by weighing them, the overall applicability of findings is determined.

Research reports are evaluated based on how well the research process was executed. Using specific criteria and guidelines, the evaluator makes precise and objective judgments about the research study, weighing its strengths and weaknesses. Critiquing research reports does not mean correcting grammar and writing style. However, clarity in writing is essential. A good research critique is two or three pages long and evaluates major aspects of the research process. Outlining the critical components of the research process helps in writing the report in a knowledgeable and professional manner. Inadequate organization is perhaps the most common presentation flaw in research reports. The written evaluation of a study emerges as a research critique.

A distinction is made between research critiques and research reviews. In a **research review**, the study is described by focusing on major aspects of the study and summarizing the most important points.[1,2] One such example is the publication by the American Association of Critical-Care Nurses, *Nursing Scan in Critical Care*. In this publication, a reviewer gives a synopsis of a recently published research study, pointing out major characteristics of the study. A commentary follows, highlighting important features, usually followed by implications for practice.

Research critiques are often difficult to complete because of feelings of insecurity as a beginning researcher. How then do you develop a feeling of competence? Individuals believe that they either can or cannot make scholarly comments, but it is unrealistic to expect to be an expert at any skill without practice. Constructive criticism is a skill and requires practice.

Use of certain words or phrases in a research critique can be important features of sensitive criticism. Use positive terms whenever possible, and begin by commenting on a study's overall strengths. Avoid such terms as "good," "nice," or "bad," as they do not communicate specific information. For example, the statement "the study contained a good review of literature" does not convey any meaning. Instead, the following brief statement contains more information and meaning: "The cited review of literature identified the major published studies related to diabetes education and empowerment." Wilson[3] provides several "dos and don'ts" in critiquing research reports, which are summarized in Table 14.1.

Guidelines for a Critique of a Research Report

Critique guidelines are key components to consider when evaluating research reports. Table 14.2 lists critical components of the research

TABLE 14.1	Dos and Don'ts for Sensitive Research Critiques

Do

1. Try to convey a sincere interest in the study you are critiquing.
2. Be sure to emphasize the points of excellence that you discover.
3. Choose clear, concise statements to communicate your observations rather than ambiguous ones.
4. When pointing out a study's weakness, provide explanations that justify your comments.
5. Include supportive and encouraging comments when they are warranted.
6. Be aware of your own negative attitude toward a particular approach to science or any personal hostilities that could distort your ability to judge a study on its own merits.
7. Offer practical suggestions that are not overly esoteric or unrealistic.
8. Remember that empathy for the researcher is often crucial to being an effective critic.

Don't

1. Nitpick or find fault on trivial details.
2. Ridicule or demean an investigator personally.
3. Try to include flattery that is designed merely to boost a researcher's self-esteem.
4. Base your summary and include recommendations about the study on some loose and perhaps biased attitude toward the state of all science in a particular discipline or on a particular topic.
5. Write your critique in condescending, patronizing, or condemning language.
6. Forget that your purpose is to advise the researcher and to improve the work and nursing science at large.

process to be evaluated. Although each component is equally important in determining a study's worth, researchers need to consider overall strengths and weaknesses as the ultimate determinants. Detailed guidelines and questions associated with critiquing research reports can be found in many nursing research textbooks.[1,2] A simple list of suggested questions is listed here:

A. Title of the Research Report
  1. Does the title accurately describe the type of study? Major variables? Population to which the study applies?
B. Problem Statement
  1. Is the problem clearly stated with pertinent background information?
  2. Is there justification for the study?

TABLE 14.2	Critical Components of the Research Process to Be Evaluated

A. Problem Statement
   Clarity of problem
   Significance of problem for nursing
   Purpose of study
   Conceptual/theoretical framework
   Literature review
   Hypotheses/research questions
B. Research Methodology
   Research design
   Sample/setting
   Data collection procedures
   Data collection instruments
   Data analysis
C. Results, Conclusions, and Interpretations
   Results of data analysis
   Discussion of findings
D. Recommendations/implications for further study in practice, education, research

   3. Is the problem significant to nursing?
   4. Is the problem researchable (can data be collected and analyzed)?
  C. Conceptual/Theoretical Framework
   1. Is there a conceptual model or framework identified?
   2. If not specifically identified, is a model or framework implied?
   3. Is the conceptual model/framework clearly developed?
   4. Is the conceptual model/framework applicable to the research?
  D. Review of Literature
   1. Is the literature cited reviewed critically?
   2. Are classic as well as current citations used?
   3. Does the researcher cite supporting, as well as opposing, studies?
   4. Is the literature review organized logically? Are there appropriate subheadings?
   5. Are most primary sources included?
   6. Does the literature review conclude with a brief summary?
  E. Purpose of the Study
   1. Is there a purpose statement?
   2. Is the purpose statement appropriate for the study (declarative statement, research question, hypothesis)?
  F. Research Questions/Hypotheses
   1. Are the research questions/hypotheses clearly stated?

G. Operational Definitions
  1. Are relevant variables defined operationally?
H. Research Design
  1. Is the type of research design identified?
  2. Does the research design fit appropriately according to the variables studied and purpose of the study?
 I. Sample
  1. Are the target and accessible populations described clearly?
  2. Was the method of choosing the sample (probability vs. non-probability) appropriate?
  3. Were inclusion and exclusion criteria used to select subjects for the study?
  4. Based on the sampling procedures, were there any threats to external validity (generalizability of findings)? If so, does the author acknowledge these threats?
J. Data Collection Procedures
  1. Are the steps in collecting data described clearly and concisely?
K. Data Collection Instruments
  1. Are the instruments/scales used to collect data appropriate for the problem and method?
  2. Are these instruments/scales reliable? Valid?
  3. Are the means of establishing reliability/validity discussed?
  4. Is each instrument described as to how it was scored? Range of possible scores? What does a high/low score mean?
L. Human Subjects
  1. Is evidence of human subject review and approval discussed?
  2. Are issues of subject anonymity or confidentiality addressed?
M. Data Analysis
  1. Is the choice of statistical procedures appropriate for the methodology proposed?
N. Results
  1. Are the characteristics of the sample described?
  2. Are the research questions/hypotheses answered separately?
  3. Do the results limited to data reflect the research questions/hypotheses?
  4. Are generalizations made that are not warranted on the basis of the sample used?
  5. Are tables, charts, and/or graphs used to present data? If so, are they labeled clearly and discussed in the text?
O. Discussion
  1. Are limitations of the study described?
  2. Does the researcher relate findings to the problem and purpose of the study?

3. Does the researcher state whether study results support or refute previous studies?

4. Are there any unexpected (serendipitous) findings?

P. Implications and Recommendations

   1. Are generalizations made beyond the sample identified in the study?

   2. Are suggestions/recommendations made by the researcher for nursing practice, education, and/or further research?

   3. Are these suggestions/recommendations based on the findings of this study?

Research Appraisal Checklist

Duffy[4] proposes a research appraisal checklist for evaluating research reports. The purpose of the checklist is to facilitate students' evaluation of aspects of research reports. The checklist does not provide criteria with which to judge a research report. However, the statements associated with each category represent commonly accepted statements used by researchers when critically appraising strengths and limitations of a research report.

The research appraisal checklist consists of 50 statements that are important to consider. Statements are grouped into eight categories, which are title, abstract, problem, review of literature, methodology, data analysis, discussion, and form and style. Statements are anchored by a rating scale that ranges from 1, "Not Met," to 4, "Completely Met." A rating of NA is used when a statement is not applicable. Comments summarizing reasons why a statement is rated low can be particularly helpful. Use of the research appraisal checklist may be helpful as a way of introducing and identifying steps of the research process that are essential to critique. The checklist provides a set of statements in an easy-to-use format that allows students an opportunity to appraise research reports efficiently and compare their results with others (Table 14.3).

Scoring the Research Appraisal Checklist

A weighted scoring method, also known as "weighting and scoring," is a type of analysis that quantifies the relative importance of certain attributes and characteristics of a research report by assigning a weighted value. The Research Appraisal Checklist is a set of 50 statements grouped in eight categories. The allocation of weights reflects the relative importance of each category along with an allocation of scores.

To derive a total weighted score for the Research Appraisal Checklist, complete the following.

Step 1. Score each statement based on the degree to which the characteristic in the research report being critiqued is present

TABLE 14.3	Research Appraisal Checklist

Criteria	Appraisal Rating
	1 = *Not Met* to
	4 = *Completely Met*

Title

1. The title is readily understood.	1 2 3 4 NA
2. The title is clear.	1 2 3 4 NA
3. The title is clearly related to content.	1 2 3 4 NA
Category Score:	

Abstract

4. The abstract states problem and, where appropriate, hypotheses clearly and concisely.	1 2 3 4 NA
5. Methodology is identified and described briefly.	1 2 3 4 NA
6. Results are summarized.	1 2 3 4 NA
7. Findings and/or conclusions are stated.	1 2 3 4 NA
Category Score:	

Problem Statement

8. The general problem of the study is introduced early in the report.	1 2 3 4 NA
9. Questions to be answered are stated precisely.	1 2 3 4 NA
10. Problem statement is clear.	1 2 3 4 NA
11. Hypotheses to be tested are stated precisely in a form that permits them to be tested.	1 2 3 4 NA
12. Limitations of the study can be identified.	1 2 3 4 NA
13. Assumptions of the study can be identified.	1 2 3 4 NA
14. Pertinent terms are/can be operationally defined.	1 2 3 4 NA
15. Significance of the problem is discussed.	1 2 3 4 NA
16. Research is justified.	1 2 3 4 NA
Category Score:	

Review of the Literature

17. Cited literature is pertinent to research problems.	1 2 3 4 NA
18. Cited literature provides rationale for the research.	1 2 3 4 NA
19. Studies are critically examined.	1 2 3 4 NA
20. Relationship of problem to previous research is made clear.	1 2 3 4 NA
21. A conceptual framework/theoretical rationale is clearly stated.	1 2 3 4 NA
22. Review concludes with a brief summary of relevant literature and its implications to the research problem under study.	1 2 3 4 NA
Category Score:	

(Continued)

TABLE 14.3	Research Appraisal Checklist—cont'd

Criteria	Appraisal Rating
	1 = *Not Met* to
	4 = *Completely Met*

Methodology

Part A: Subjects

23. Subject population (sampling frame) is described.	1 2 3 4 NA
24. Sampling method is described.	1 2 3 4 NA
25. Sampling method is justified (especially for non-probability sampling).	1 2 3 4 NA
26. Sample size is sufficient to reduce type 2 error.	1 2 3 4 NA
27. Standards for protection of subjects are discussed.	1 2 3 4 NA

Category Score:

Part B: Instruments

28. Relevant reliability data from previous research are presented.	1 2 3 4 NA
29. Reliability data pertinent to the present study are reported.	1 2 3 4 NA
30. Relevant previous validity data from previous research are presented.	1 2 3 4 NA
31. Validity data pertinent to present study are reported.	1 2 3 4 NA
32. Methods of data collection are sufficiently described to permit judgment of their appropriateness to the present study.	1 2 3 4 NA

Category Score:

Part C: Design

33. Design is appropriate to study questions and/or hypotheses.	1 2 3 4 NA
34. Proper controls are included where appropriate.	1 2 3 4 NA
35. Confounding/moderating variables are/can be identified.	1 2 3 4 NA
36. Description of design is explicit enough to permit replication.	1 2 3 4 NA

Category Score:

Data Analysis

37. Information presented is sufficient to answer research questions.	1 2 3 4 NA
38. Statistical tests are identified and obtained values are reported.	1 2 3 4 NA
39. Reported statistics are appropriate for hypothesis/ research questions.	1 2 3 4 NA
40. Tables and figures are presented in an easy-to-understand, informative way.	1 2 3 4 NA

Category Score:

TABLE 14.3	Research Appraisal Checklist—cont'd

Criteria	Appraisal Rating
	1 = *Not Met* to
	4 = *Completely Met*

Discussion

41. Conclusions are clearly stated.	1 2 3 4 NA
42. Conclusions are substantiated by the evidence presented.	1 2 3 4 NA
43. Methodological problems in the study are identified and discussed.	1 2 3 4 NA
44. Findings of the study are specifically related to conceptual/theoretical basis of the study.	1 2 3 4 NA
45. Implications of the findings are discussed.	1 2 3 4 NA
46. Results are generalized only to population on which study is based.	1 2 3 4 NA
47. Recommendations are made for further research.	1 2 3 4 NA

Category Score:

Form and Style

48. The report is clearly written.	1 2 3 4 NA
49. The report is logically organized.	1 2 3 4 NA
50. The tone of the report displays an unbiased, impartial, scientific attitude.	1 2 3 4 NA

Category Score:

Grand Score:

using a rating scale of 1 to 4. Number 1 indicates the characteristic is "Not at All" present in the research report; 2 indicates "Very Little" of the characteristic is present in the research report; 3 indicates the characteristic is "Somewhat" present in the research report; and 4 indicates the characteristic is present in the research report "To a Great Extent." For example, under the category Problem Statement, was the general problem of the study introduced early in the research report? Were the research questions in the research report stated precisely? Was the problem statement clearly written?

Step 2. Assign weights to each of the eight categories. Weight the categories to reflect their relative importance. The weighting of categories reflects a group consensus about the relative importance of each category. Thus, each research class may come up with different weights. It is important to express weights in percentage terms so that their sum is 100.

Step 3. Calculate the weighted score. Weighted scores are calculated by tallying the total score associated with each category and multiplying that score by the weighted value assigned to the category.

The assignment of weighted values is essentially a judgmental process; therefore, no set of weighted values can be applied universally. One can identify weighted values to his or her own liking. Some may identify the Problem Statement part of a research report to be highly important; others will be more concerned with the Methodology section of a research report. Thus, weighted values assigned will be arbitrary based on some judgment or rationale. Table 14.4 provides an example of a perfectly scored Research Appraisal Checklist with specified weighted values and a total weighted score. Table 14.5 is an example of a scored Research Appraisal Checklist with specific weighted values associated with the eight categories.

Research Critique of a Quantitative Study

The following is an example of an author's research critique of several sections of a quantitative research report.

Title

Patient Empowerment Program for People with Diabetes

TABLE 14.4	Example of Research Appraisal Checklist Worksheet		
Category	Total Possible Score	Weight	Weighted Score
Title	12/12	5%	5
Abstract	16/16	5%	5
Problem Statement	36/36	10%	10
Review of Literature	24/24	10%	10
Methodology			
Part A	20/20	15%	15
Part B	20/20	15%	15
Part C	16/20	15%	15
Data Analysis	16/20	10%	10
Discussion	28/28	10%	10
Form and Style	12/12	5%	5
TOTALS	200	100%	100

TABLE 14.5	Example of Research Appraisal Checklist Worksheet After Critiquing a Research Report		
Category	Total Possible Score	Weight	Weighted Score
Title	9/12	5%	3.75
Abstract	10/16	5%	3.13
Problem Statement	29/36	10%	8.05
Review of Literature	20/24	10%	8.3
Methodology			
Part A	12/20	15%	9
Part B	14/20	15%	10.5
Part C	12/16	15%	11.25
Data Analysis	8/16	10%	5
Discussion	24/28	10%	8.57
Form and Style	9/12	5%	3.75
TOTALS	200	100%	71.3

CRITIQUE The title is brief but conveys to the reader one of the major variables under study. The sample is implied by the phrase, "people with diabetes." However, the reader cannot ascertain whether the sample being studied refers to those with type 1 or type 2 diabetes.

Problem Statement

Diabetes patient education has long been viewed as a process designed to provide patients with the knowledge, skills, and motivation to manage their diabetes. A compliance/adherence approach regarding the philosophy and practice of diabetes patient education has prevailed for the past two decades. Within this model of care, behavioral strategies were used to increase compliance with recommended treatments. To more adequately understand and improve diabetes self-management, different models of care are needed that improve upon previous research. Recently, patient empowerment has been offered as an alternative to the compliance/adherence approach to diabetes management and patient education. The purpose of this proposed clinical study is to test the feasibility of a patient empowerment program. The program was designed by Feste (1991) and does not focus on the provision of information. Instead, the program helps individuals with diabetes develop skills and self-awareness in the areas of goal-setting, problem-solving, stress management, coping, social support, and motivation.

CRITIQUE The statement of the problem is clearly stated and constitutes an effort to improve patients' diabetes management. This is a very important issue, particularly in the current health-care management cost-containment environment. The problem is researchable and provides direction for specifying the research design and methodology. The purpose statement is clear in stating what the study hopes to accomplish.

Review of the Literature

Type 2 diabetes is the most common form of diabetes and accounts for 90 percent of all diabetes in the United States. However, many cases go undiagnosed. In the United States, the prevalence of type 2 diabetes is lowest in Caucasians (non-Hispanic whites) and elevated in African American, Hispanic American, and Native American populations. Regardless of its prevalence in different populations, type 2 diabetes is a serious disease that warrants the same comprehensive treatment as that given to individuals with type 1 diabetes. There is scientific evidence that early detection, treatment, and rigorous attention to self-care, facilitated by quality diabetes education, can significantly reduce the incidence and progression of diabetes (DCCT Research Group, 1993). Results of the Diabetes Control and Complications Trial (DCCT) led to reevaluation of the team concept and definition of team members' roles. The burden of diabetes can have a negative effect on the life satisfaction of individuals and their families. Individuals with type 2 diabetes need to take personal responsibility for their own disease management.

Patient empowerment has been offered as an alternative to the knowledge model approach to diabetes management and patient education (Anderson, Funnell, Barr, Dedrick, and Davis, 1991; Funnell, Anderson, Arnold, Barr, Donnelly, Johnson, Taylor-Moon, and White, 1992). Whereas it had been common to speak of noncompliance, behavior modification, and glucose control, the empowerment model refers to self-awareness, personal responsibility, informed choices, and quality of life (Feste, 1992). The notion of empowerment is appealing because of its association with such concepts as coping, social support, personal efficacy, and self-esteem (Kieffer, 1984). Rubin and Peyrot (1992) argue that new models of care need to be explored that incorporate psychosocial education as a routine and significant component of diabetes care and education.

CRITIQUE The literature review focuses on the compliance/adherence approach to diabetes education and an empowerment approach to diabetes management. As noted by the researcher, the incidence of diabetes and the severity of complications warrant special attention of efforts to improve health and quality of life. However, references in support of expectations that DCCT results apply to type 2 diabetes patients should be provided.

The effectiveness (or lack) of the compliance/adherence approach used for the past two decades is not clearly described. If this approach has been shown to have an impact on the proposed dependent variables, it would make sense to compare the empowerment approach to the compliance/adherence approach to establish whether the empowerment approach has an effect over and above that of "usual care." Likewise, the researcher does not review studies that have used other diabetes management approaches tailored to individual patients. Primary sources are used, with references complete and integrated into the development of the study.

Hypotheses

Diabetes education that focuses on self-management, self-efficacy, and empowerment issues significantly:

- Increases positive attitudes and self-efficacy as measured by selective subscales of these testing instruments: Diabetes Attitude Scale, Self-Efficacy, and Diabetes Care Profile.
- Decreases negative attitudes as measured by appropriate DCP subscales.
- Improves glycemic control, as measured by a decrease in glycosylated hemoglobin (HbA_{1c}).

CRITIQUE The researcher clearly identifies the study hypotheses with appropriate operational definitions of how variables will be measured.

Methodology: Research Design

The proposed study is an experimental design. Patients will be randomly assigned to either an intervention or a control group. The intervention will be organized as six 2-hour group sessions held weekly. Each session will be presented by the diabetes nurse educator and dietitian to promote consistency of the intervention. At the end of 6 weeks, all subjects (intervention and control) will complete the set of questionnaires a second time. The second set of questionnaires will serve as a post-program test for the intervention group. The control group will then complete the six-session program. At the end of 12 weeks, all subjects will complete the questionnaires for a third time and provide another blood sample. This data will serve as the post-program data for the control group and as 6-week follow-up for the intervention group. The control group will return for its follow-up 6 weeks later, completing the questionnaires another time, along with a blood sample.

CRITIQUE A strength of the proposed study is the experimental design. Criteria for study inclusion and exclusion were described appropriately. The research design describes a 6-week waiting period for control subjects, after which they receive the empowerment program. This design does not offer an uncontaminated control group for the baseline to 12 weeks pre- to post-comparison of major outcome variables. This is a flaw in the design that could be removed by not offering the empowerment program to the control group. If the protocol is followed as written, the experimental group would have a lag of 12 weeks between baseline and follow-up measures of outcome variables, and the control group would have 18 weeks. The times should be equal.

Methodology: Sample

Criteria for inclusion in the clinical study are as follows. All subjects who are diagnosed with type 2 diabetes followed by the Diabetes Clinic will be asked to participate in the study. Type 2 is very different from type 1 diabetes. Type 2 develops classically in an older population and may or may not require use of therapeutic insulin. Individuals are usually controlled by diet, exercise, and an oral hypoglycemic agent. A small percentage of individuals will be on combination therapy (use of insulin and oral hypoglycemic). Criteria for enrollment includes English- or Spanish-speaking adults; diagnosis of diabetes for a minimum of 1 year; and no major complications associated with diabetes. The existence of serious illness or major complication, such as visual impairment, end-stage renal disease, or lower extremity amputation, will be reason for study exclusion.

> CRITIQUE The study sample is not adequately defined. For example, there is no information regarding age, gender, or educational levels and how these will be controlled. Likewise, although subjects must have been diagnosed with diabetes for a minimum of 1 year, there is no stated restriction for length of time since first diagnosed. How will this variable be treated? Although both English- and Spanish-speaking patients will be recruited, there is no indication in the study that the intervention group leaders need to speak Spanish. It is also not clear whether separate Spanish-speaking groups will be formed. The researcher does not specify if the target population is truly representative of the entire diabetic population. Are all subjects at the institution referred to and seen at the Diabetes Clinic? If not, how are referred subjects different from subjects not referred?

Methodology: Data Collection Procedures

The diabetes clinical nurse specialist employed by the institution will help identify eligible subjects from those who attend the Diabetes Clinic. All patients will receive a letter from the principal investigator inviting them to participate in the study. Interested patients will be asked to attend an orientation session, where a discussion about empowerment along with a sample worksheet will be discussed. All patients who choose to participate will sign an informed consent form, complete a set of questionnaires, and have a blood sample drawn for glycosylated hemoglobin (HbA_{1c}). Patients will be randomly assigned to either the intervention or control group.

> CRITIQUE The researcher proposes to invite subjects to an orientation session where issues of empowerment will be discussed. The purpose of this discussion

with all patients is not clear (motivational?). One wonders what the impact of such a session will be on those who are later randomized to the control group. If this session had a positive/motivational impact on control subjects, then the effect of the intervention would be more difficult to detect.

Methodology: Data Collection Instruments
Diabetes Attitude Scale (DAS)
Diabetes patients' attitudes will be measured with selected subscales of the DAS and selected subscales of the Diabetes Care Profile (DCP). The DAS subscale measures (1) patients' attitudes toward compliance, (2) impact of diabetes on their quality of life, and (3) views about patient autonomy. The two DCP subscales measure (1) overall positive and (2) overall negative attitudes about living with diabetes. Both the DAS and DCP are self-administered paper-and-pencil questionnaires composed of several subscales. Patients are asked to read each statement and place a checkmark next to the word or phrase that is closest to their opinion about each statement. Items are scored by assigning five points to "strongly agree," four points to "agree," three points to "neutral," two to "disagree," and one point to "strongly disagree." Internal consistency for each subscale has been determined through the use of Cronbach's alpha coefficients for each subscale and ranges from 0.69 to 0.86 (Anderson, Donnelly and Dedrick, 1990). Self-efficacy measures were developed for the specific content areas of the patient empowerment program. The self-efficacy subscales measured the subject's perceived ability to identify areas of satisfaction related to living with diabetes, identify and achieve personally meaningful goals, cope with emotional aspects of living with diabetes, manage stress, attain appropriate social support, be self-motivated, and make cost/benefit decisions about making behavior changes related to living with diabetes. Glycosylated hemoglobin is a biological marker for diabetes control. It is a routine measure of the average blood glucose control for a previous 3-month period. Subjects in good control will have an $HgbA_{1c}$ value of <8%.

CRITIQUE The outcome measures selected are well described and related to the hypotheses under study. There is, however, no validity information for selected subscales. Only some of the DAS and DCP subscales will be used without explanation as to whether it is appropriate to do so. Why were these subscales selected? What do the scores mean? The description of the self-efficacy measures was equally lacking sufficient psychometric properties. Likewise, the blood glucose control measure needs more discussion. Who, for example, will draw the blood? Who will analyze it? Who will pay for it?

Methodology: Data Analysis
The sample will be described using descriptive statistics. Sociodemographic variables will be described using frequency distributions and

appropriate measures of central tendency and variability. Hypotheses 1 and 2 will be analyzed by Student's *t*-tests. The *t*-test will be used to determine if there are differences between mean scores of attitudes and self-efficacy pre-program and post-program (6 weeks).

> *CRITIQUE* The plan of analysis is appropriate but needs to be clearer in terms of detail. Although not described, the *t*-tests are presumed to compare mean pre-test to post-test change scores for the two groups. In addition, does this mean all self-efficacy subscales will be combined with the subscales from the DAS and DCP for analysis or that separate analysis will be performed for each subscale?

Results and Findings

Demographic characteristics of the sample are displayed. The majority of subjects were older-aged, men, and overweight. All three hypotheses were supported. Those individuals in the intervention group had significantly higher scores on the following self-efficacy subscales: setting goals, managing stress, obtaining support, and making decisions when compared with those subjects in the control group. Likewise, subjects in the intervention group had a more positive attitude toward diabetes and improvement in glycosylated hemoglobin levels. Findings were consistent with Anderson's (1995) study.

> *CRITIQUE* Findings were clearly stated and substantiated by the data presented. The researcher failed to discuss study limitations.

> *OVERALL STRENGTHS* With only about one-half of all patients with chronic diseases actually staying on their treatment regimens, new approaches to diabetes education must be tested. Patient empowerment is one approach that seems relevant to diabetes self-management. The cited literature identified major published studies related to empowerment and diabetes education. The background and experience of the researcher and consultants are strong.

> *OVERALL WEAKNESSES* The overall lack of detail, unfortunately, makes it difficult to evaluate the likelihood that this study will yield new and useful data. The question of how the proposed empowerment program is different from other educational programs designed for people with diabetes has not been adequately addressed nor has the question of whether the program actually "empowers" people to change.

Research Critique of a Qualitative Study

The following is an example of a research critique of several sections of a qualitative research report.[5]

Purpose

The diagnosis of diabetes brings with it a regimen that has a major impact on an individual's daily practices and lifestyle. The purpose of this grounded theory study was to investigate the experience of living with insulin-dependent diabetes mellitus.

CRITIQUE The purpose of this qualitative grounded theory study is clearly articulated.

Identified Problem for Study

At the beginning of this study, I was deeply committed to the value of diabetes education programs, the need for knowledge for clients with diabetes, and the importance of diabetes control for positive health outcomes. However, I had an aversion to the word "compliance" and had begun to doubt the value of compliance/adherence relationships between diabetes clients and their educators. A review of the literature convinced me that the compliance/adherence educational framework typical of current diabetes education programs does not accurately describe, account for, or explain the experience of living with diabetes. Despite extensive research in diabetes education and social learning interventions, neither adherence nor glycemic control has been achieved. Also, a causal relationship link has not been established between these educational approaches and the desired metabolic outcomes. Consequently, a strong rationale exists for taking a new look at diabetes from the perspective of the client rather than from that of the health professional.

CRITIQUE In grounded theory, the research problem is as much discovered as the process that resolves it. The researcher moved into an area of interest with no specific problem in mind as evidenced by the type of question asked, "What is the experience of living with insulin-dependent diabetes mellitus (type 1 diabetes)?"

Sample

Study subjects were recruited through two endocrinologists who had been informed of the study methodology and asked to refer only adults with type 1 diabetes who were in good control. Two females and two males agreed to participate in the study.

CRITIQUE There is insufficient detail about the sampling procedure and study participants. In grounded theory, a predetermined sample size is not calculated. Theoretical sampling is continued until the categories are saturated.

Methodology

Grounded theory was selected as a research methodology. Each participant was seen several times. The purpose of the first meeting was to establish rapport, explain the study, allow opportunity for questions, and obtain written consent. At the next session, an interview was conducted using open-ended questions; this interview was audio-taped and transcribed verbatim. At the end of the interview, instructions were given for writing a personal paper about diabetes and completing a 3- to 5-day journal.

> CRITIQUE The qualitative method is clearly stated. Additional information regarding assumptions associated with grounded theory would be helpful to the reader.

Data Collection Procedures

A comprehensive and accurate picture of the diabetes experience for the participants was obtained by triangulation from three data sources: interviews and two written tasks. The written tasks included preparing a paper about their personal diabetes stories and keeping a three- to five-page journal to document thoughts related to diabetes. Each participant was seen several times, twice for formal interviews and one or more times for more informal meetings.

> CRITIQUE A more detailed discussion of data collection procedures is warranted. Overall, how long was data collection for the entire study? How long were the individual interviews? Were they all audio-taped?

Data Analysis: Organizing/Categorizing/Summarizing

Transcripts of interviews, diabetes papers, and journals were examined and coded line by line to identify underlying processes. Coded data that seemed related were grouped into categories. Throughout the coding, data collected through interviews, diabetes papers, and journals were constantly compared for similarities and differences. As data collection and analysis continued, categories were collapsed into more general categories until the underlying theory of "becoming diabetic" emerged, a theory of integration.

> CRITIQUE The researcher speaks about coding data after the interviews. How many original categories were identified? Very little information is provided on how the data were summarized for ease in theme identification. Reference is made to the underlying theory of "becoming diabetic." However, there is no literature review, which would have facilitated the reader's understanding of how the categories were recognized and accepted. In a grounded theory study, the review of literature does not take place until after problem identification. The grounded theorist begins by collecting data in the field and generating a theory. As the theory becomes sufficiently grounded and developed, the literature in the field is reviewed and related to the developing theory.

Scientific Integrity: Credibility/Transferability/Dependability/Confirmability

> CRITIQUE The researcher does not mention how scientific integrity was addressed in this study. As a qualitative study, several factors are important in

establishing worthiness of findings: triangulation of data, participant observation, and prolonged engagement with participants. The researcher speaks to triangulation of three data sources with little discussion of how he/she became involved with participants in order to understand the problem. A more detailed description of the sample would have made it easier to determine credibility and transferability (external validity) of findings.

Results of the Study

The following themes emerged: a new view of empathy, the diabetes education focuses, and the client-educator relationship. Study participants had a different view of the educator's ability to understand and empathize with them. Laura expressed her opinion about the diabetes educator who does not have diabetes. During the research process I came to a new understanding of empathy as a way of knowing, not merely a way of being. Empathy is a way of knowing of the individual, not of a group, because diabetes cannot be considered a collective experience. In other words, one person's perspective on diabetes cannot be assumed or generalized from others who also have diabetes.

Early in the education of individuals with diabetes, educators promote the notion of the "normalcy" of living with diabetes. Focusing on normalcy may only prolong the integration or becoming process or may make clients feel guilty because they do not feel guilty. Diabetes educators need to view their practice objectively, to become informed by clients' experiences, and to critique their actions. Living with diabetes cannot be defined rigidly within a generalized science of diabetes. Laura succinctly summarized this point, "You can't live the textbook." Laura, Matthew, Mike, and Sandra helped me to understand the inaccuracies of my own assumptions.

CRITIQUE The process of obtaining results was clear and appropriate to a grounded theory approach. The researcher was likewise aware of his/her own knowledge and assumptions regarding the research problem so as to minimize unnecessary bias.

Discussion of Findings

The findings of this grounded theory study provide insight into the experience of living with diabetes, the focus of diabetes education, and the client/education relationships. The recommendations derived from this study represent a significant move away from conventional diabetes education practice. Early in the study I recognized a difference in perspective about diabetes between myself as diabetes educator and the participants. A memo I wrote exemplifies my recognition of these differences: "I am struck by the difference in the way in which Matthew looks at diabetes and the way in which I as a diabetes educator perceive it. I have always seen the diabetes regimen—diet, exercise, insulin, and stress reduction—as

the central focus and presumed that these must somehow be accommo-
dated into a diabetic's lifestyle. Matthew does not talk about these aspects,
but although he is involved with these, I get the feeling that he does not
approach them with the same preoccupation that I do. Matthew's focus
is on his body, paying attention to its needs and demands, whereas we
[diabetes educators] focus on the 'regimen.' "

CRITIQUE Discussion of research findings was consistent with a grounded theory approach. This shows an appropriate use of memoing, where the researcher
recorded his/her ideas while coding and analyzing the data.

SUMMARY OF KEY IDEAS

1. A research critique is a critical appraisal of the strengths and weaknesses of a research report.

2. The writing of a research critique should be clear, concise, well
organized, and grammatically correct.

3. A research review provides a description of the most important
features of a research study.

LEARNING ACTIVITIES

1. Select a quantitative and qualitative research report to critique.

a. Examine the title of the article.

b. Critique the problem and purpose statements.

c. Critique the conceptual/theoretical model and literature review.

d. Evaluate the research questions/hypotheses.

e. Critically evaluate aspects of the research methodology (i.e., design, sample, setting, data collection procedures and instruments,
data analysis).

f. Critique results.

g. Examine study discussion/conclusions.

REFERENCES

1. Polit, DF, and Beck, CT: Essentials of
Nursing Research: Methods, Appraisal,
and Utilization, ed. 6. Lippincott
Williams & Wilkins, Philadelphia,
2006, pp 429–456.
2. Burns, N, and Groves, SK: The Practice
of Nursing Research: Conduct, Critique,
and Utilization, ed. 4. WB Saunders,
Philadelphia, 2001, pp 663–681.

3. Wilson, HS: Introduction to Research
in Nursing, ed. 2. Addison-Wesley
Nursing, Philadelphia, 1993.
4. Duffy, ME: A research appraisal
checklist for evaluating nursing
research reports. In Waltz, CF, and
Jenkins, LS (eds): Measurement of
Nursing Outcomes, Vol 1: Measuring
Nursing Performance in Practice,

Education, and Research, ed. 2. Springer Publishing Company, New York, 2001, pp 313–323.
5. Hernandez, CA: The experience of living with insulin-dependent diabetes: Lessons for the diabetes educator. Diabetes Educ 21:33, 1995.

SUGGESTED READINGS FOR CRITIQUES

Anderson, RM, et al: Learning to empower patients: Results of professional education program for diabetes education. Diabetes Care 14:584, 1991.

Anderson, RM, et al: Patient empowerment: Results of a randomized controlled trial. Diabetes Care 18:943, 1995.

Anderson, RM, Donnelly, MB, and Dedrick, RF: Measuring the attitudes of patients toward diabetes and its treatment. Patient Educ Counseling 16:231, 1990.

Diabetes Control and Complications Trial (DCCT) Research Group: The effect of intensive treatment of diabetes on the development and progression of long-term complications in insulin dependent diabetes mellitus (IDDM). N Engl J Med 329:977, 1993.

Feste, CC: A practical look at patient empowerment. Diabetes Care 15:922, 1992.

Feste, CC: Empowerment: Facilitating a path to personal self-care. Miles Incorporated Diagnostics Division, Elkhart, IN, 1991.

Funnell, MM, et al: Empowerment: An idea whose time has come in diabetes education. Diab Educ 17:37, 1991.

Kieffer, C: Citizen empowerment: A developmental perspective. Prev Human Serv 3:9, 1984.

Rubin, RR, and Peyrot, M: Psychosocial problems and interventions in diabetes. Diabetes Care 15:1640, 1992.

Index

Page numbers followed by "t" denote tables; page numbers followed by "e" denote excerpts